Editors
Jasmine Zain · Larry W Kwak

Management of Lymphomas: A Case-Based Approach

Editors

Jasmine Zain · Larry W Kwak

City of Hope National Medical Center
Duarte, California
USA

Management of Lymphomas: A Case-Based Approach

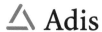

Editors

Jasmine Zain, MD
City of Hope National Medical Center
Duarte, California
USA

Larry W Kwak, MD
City of Hope National Medical Center
Duarte, California
USA

Contributors

Michelle Afkhami, MD
Joseph Alvarnas, MD
Elizabeth Budde, MD
Wing C Chan, MD
Robert Chen, MD
Belen Rubio Gonzalez, MD
Alex F Herrera, MD
Larry W Kwak, MD
Matthew Mei, MD
Auayporn Nademanee, MD
Raju K Pillai, MD
Christiane Querfeld, MD, PhD
Steven T Rosen, MD
Tanya Siddiqi, MD
Joo Y Song, MD
Dennis D Weisenburger, MD
Jasmine Zain, MD

ISBN 978-3-319-26825-5   ISBN 978-3-319-26827-9 (eBook)
DOI 10.1007/978-3-319-26827-9

Printed on acid-free paper

This Adis imprint is published by Springer Nature
The registered company is Springer International Publishing AG
The registered company address is: Gewerbestrasse 11, 6330 Cham, Switzerland

Project editor: Laura Hajba

Contents

Case Study Section Two: Aggressive B-Cell Lymphomas

Case Study Section Three: T-Cell Lymphomas

10 Cutaneous T-cell lymphoma   157

Belen Rubio Gonzalez, Steven T Rosen, and Christiane Querfeld

11 Systemic T-cell lymphoma   173

Jasmine Zain

Case Study Section Four: Hodgkin Lymphoma

12 Hodgkin lymphoma   205
Robert Chen

Case Study Section Five: Lymphomas in Special Clinical Situations

13 Acquired immunodeficiency syndrome-related lymphoma   225
Joseph Alvarnas

14 Central nervous system lymphoma   241

Matthew Mei

15 Conclusion   249

Jasmine Zain and Larry W Kwak

Editor biographies

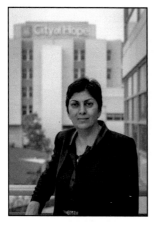

Jasmine Zain MD, is an associate clinical professor in the Department of Hematology & Hematopoietic Cell Transplantation. Additionally, she is the Tim Nesvig Lymphoma Research Fellow, as well as Director of the T cell Lymphoma Program at the Toni Stephenson Lymphoma Center at City of Hope. Dr Zain obtained her medical degree from Fatima Jinnah Medical College for Women in Lahore, Pakistan. She went on to complete an internship and residency at North Shore Hospital of Forest Hills in Forest Hills, NY, followed by a hematology/oncology fellowship at New York University Medical Center. She then took a position at The Brooklyn Hospital as an attending physician, followed by an appointment as assistant professor in the Department of Medicine at the University of Connecticut.

Dr Zain first joined City of Hope where she specialized in the treatment of patients with cutaneous T-cell lymphoma, allogeneic stem cell transplantation, and early phase clinical trials in hematologic malignancies. She left City of Hope to assume a leadership position as Director of the bone marrow transplant program at New York University Langone Medical Center, before joining the faculty at Columbia University in 2012.

Triple-board certified in hematology, oncology and internal medicine, Dr Zain is an active member of several professional associations, and has published more than 78 peer-reviewed publications, abstracts, and book chapters. She served as an Associate Editor for two journals in her field – *Clinical Lymphoma and Myeloma*, and *Clinical Cancer Research* – and has been invited to speak both nationally and internationally.

Dr Zain is a superb clinician, a productive and creative clinical researcher, and an outstanding and experienced teacher.

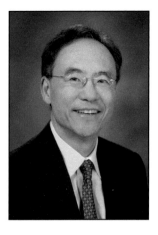

Larry W Kwak MD, PhD, joined City of Hope as inaugural Cancer Center Associate Director, Translational Research & Developmental Therapeutics in April 2015. Dr Kwak graduated from the 6-year combined BS-MD Honors Program in Medical Education from Northwestern University Medical School in 1982 and earned his PhD in tumor cell biology there in 1984. He then completed a residency in internal medicine and a fellowship in medical oncology at Stanford University Medical Center in California. Thereafter, he served as Head of the Vaccine Biology Section, Experimental Transplantation and Immunology Branch, at the National Cancer Institute (NCI) for 12 years. His NCI laboratory is credited with the pioneering bench-to-clinic development of a therapeutic cancer vaccine for B-cell malignancies, which was recently reported as positive in a landmark national Phase III clinical trial. This was one of three recently positive Phase III clinical trials of cancer vaccine immunotherapy.

From 2004–14 Dr Kwak served as Chairman of the Department of Lymphoma and Myeloma and Co-Director of the Center for Cancer Immunology Research at the University of Texas, MD Anderson Cancer Center in Houston, Texas, where he also held the Justin Distinguished Chair in Leukemia Research. As Chair, his department successfully captured extensive research support, including large team science grants, such as two SPORE grants in Lymphoma and Multiple Myeloma, respectively, from the NCI and a SCOR program project grant awarded by the Leukemia and Lymphoma Society. He also led the expansion of the department's laboratory research space and launched biospecimens banks to support translational research.

A committed physician, scientist, and mentor, his vision is to assemble and lead research teams to integrate basic discoveries from academic laboratories with translational clinical development to first-in-human clinical trials of novel 'homegrown' therapeutics, such as next generation cancer immunotherapies. He plays a key role in the future direction of

City of Hope's translational and precision medicine and 'teamwork science' initiatives. He is an expert in the clinical management of patients with low grade lymphomas.

In 2010 Dr Kwak was named to the TIME 100, one of the world's 100 most influential people by TIME magazine, for his 20 year commitment to the science of cancer immunotherapy. In 2016, he was awarded the Ho-Am Prize in Medicine for his pioneering research in cancer immunotherapy.

Abbreviations

2HG	2-hydroxyglutarate
2KG	2 ketoglutarate
A2aR	Adenosine A2a receptor
ABC-DLBCL	Activated B-cell type of DLBCL
ABVD	Adriamycin, bleomycin, vinblastine, and dacarbazine
AEs	Adverse events
AID	Activation-induced cytidine deaminase enzyme
AILD	Angioimmunoblastic lymphadenopathy with dysproteinemia
AITL	Angioimmunoblastic T-cell lymphoma
AKT1	v-akt murine thymoma viral oncogene homolog 1
ALC	Absolute lymphocyte count
ALCL	Anaplastic large cell lymphoma
alloHCT	Allogeneic hematopoietic cell transplantation
AMC	AIDS Malignancy Consortium
APC	Antigen-presenting cell
ARA-C	Cytarabine
ARID1A	*AT-rich interactive domain 1A gene*
ASCT	Autologous stem cell transplantatio
AspMet Dex	Asparginase, dexamethsone, and methotrexate
ATLL	Adult T-cell leukemia/lymphoma
AZT	Zidovudine
B-PLL	B-cell prolymphocytic leukemia
BCCA	The British Columbia Cancer registry
BCL10	B-cell lymphoma/leukemia 10
BCNU	Thiotepa and carmustine
BCR	B-cell receptor
BEACOPP	Etoposide, doxorubicin, cyclophosphamide, vincristine, procarbazine, and prednisone
BIRC3	Baculoviral IAP repeat containing 3
BL	Burkitt lymphoma
BM	Bone marrow

BR	Bendamustine and rituximab
BRAF	B-Raf proto-oncogene, serine/threonine kinase
BSA	Body surface area
BTK	Bruton's kinase receptor
BTLA	B- and T-lymphocyte-associated
CAR-T	Chimeric antigen receptor T cells
CARD11	Caspase recruitment domain family, member 11
CAP	Cyclophosphamide, adriamycin, and cisplatin
CBC	Complete blood count
CBM	CARD11-BCL10-MALT1 multi-protein complex
CBV	Cyclophosphamide, carmustine, and etoposide
CHOEP	Cyclophosphamide, doxorubicin, vincristine, prednisone, and etoposide
CHOP	Cyclophosphamide, doxorubicin, vincristine, and prednisolone
CIRS	Cumulative Illness Rating Scale
CLL	Chronic lymphocytic leukemia
CMP	Comprehensive metabolic panel
CMT	Combined modality therapy
CNS	Central nervous system
CNV	Copy number variations
CODOX-M	Cyclophosphamide, vincristine doxorubicin, and methotrexate
CR	Complete remission
CRS	Cytokine release syndrome
CSF	Cerebral spinal fluid
CT	Computed tomography
CTCL	Cutaneous T-cell lymphoma
CTLA-4	Cytotoxic T-lymphocyte-associated protein 4
CVP	Cyclophosphamide, vincristine, and prednisone
DA/SC-EPOCH-R	Dose-adjusted/short course etoposide, doxorubicin, cyclophosphamide, vincristine, prednisone, and rituximab
DeVic	Dexamethasone, etoposide, ifosfamide, and carboplatin

DFS	Disease-free survival
DHAP	Cisplatin, cytarabine, and dexamethasone
DLBCL	Diffuse large B-cell lymphoma
DNMT1	DNA methyl transferase 1
EATL	Enteropathy-associated T-cell lymphoma
EBV	Epstein-Barr virus
ECOG	Eastern Cooperative Oncology Group
ECP	Extracorporeal photopheresis
EFRT	Extended field radiotherapy
EFS	Event-free survival
EKG	Electrocardiogram
EORTC	European Organisation for Research and Treatment of Cancer
ERK	Extracellular signal-regulated kinase
ESHAP	Etoposide, methylprednisolone, cisplatin, and cytarabine
ESR	Erythrocyte sedimentation rate
FC	Fludarabine and cyclophosphamide
FCM	Fludarabine, cyclophosphamide, and mitoxantrone
FCR	Fludarabine, cyclophosphamide, and rituximab
FDA	Food and Drug Administration
FDG	Fluorodeoxyglucose
FFS	Failure-free survival
FISH	Fluorescence in situ hybridization
FL	Follicular lymphoma
FLIPI	Follicular Lymphoma International Prognostic Index
FNA	Fine needle aspiration
Gal-9	Lectin, galactoside-binding, soluble 9
GCLLSG	German CLL study Group
GELA	Groupe d'Etude des Lymphomes, de l'Adulte
GELF	Groupe d'Etude des Lymphomes Folliculares
GELOX	Gemcitabine, asparaginase, and oxaliplatin
GFR	Glomerular filtration rate
GHSG	German Hodgkin Study Group
GIT	Gastrointestinal tract

GMALL	The German Multicenter Study Group for Adult ALL
GVHD	Graft versus host disease
GVL	Graft versus lymphoma
GWAS	Genome-wide association data
HAART	Highly active retroviral therapy
HCL	Hairy cell leukemia
HCT	Hematopoietic stem cell transplantation
HCV	Hepatitis C virus
HD	Hodgkin disease
HDT	High-dose therapy
HGB	Hemoglobin
HIV	Human immunodeficiency virus
HL	Hodgkin lymphoma
HLA	Human leukocyte antigen
HSTCL	Hepatosplenic T cell lymphoma
HTLV1	Human T-lymphotropic virus
ICE	Ifosphamide, carboplatin, and etoposide
ICOS	Inducible T-cell co-stimulator
ICOSL	Inducible T-cell co-stimulator ligand
ID3	Inhibitor of DNA binding 3
IFN-α	Interferon-alpha
IFRT	Involved-field radiotherapy
IHC	Immunohistochemistry
IKK	Inhibitor of NF-κB kinase
IL-6	Interleukin 6
IMiDs	Immunomodulatory drugs
IPI	International Prognostic Index
IRAK	Interleukin-1 receptor-associated kinase 1
ISRT	Involved site radiotherapy
ITAM	Immunoreceptor tyrosine-based activation motifs
IVAC	Ifosfamide, cytarabine, and etoposide
IVE	Ifosfamide, epirubacin, and etoposide
iwCLL	International workshop on CLL
JAK	Janus kinase
KSHV	Kaposi sarcoma-associated herpes virus

LCT	Large cell transformation
LDH	Lactate dehydrogenase
LFT	Liver function test
LPL	Lymphoplasmacytic lymphoma
m-BACOD	Methotrexate, bleomycin, doxorubicin, cyclophosphamide, vincristine, and dexamethasone
MAb	Monoclonal antibody
MALT	Mucosa-associated lymphoid tissue
MALT1	Mucosa-associated lymphoid tissue lymphoma translocation protein 1
MAP3K14	Mitogen-activated protein kinase kinase kinase 14
MAPK	Mitogen-activated protein kinase
MBL	Monoclonal B-cell lymphocytosis
MCL	Mantle cell lymphoma
MCHC	Mean corpuscular hemoglobin concentration
MCV	Mean corpuscle volume
MEK	Mitogen-activated protein kinase kinase kinase 1
MF	Mycosis fungoides
MF-LCT	Mycosis fungoides with large cell transformation
MGUS	Monoclonal gammopathy of undetermined significance
MHC	Major histocompatibility locus
MIPI	Mantle Cell Lymphoma International Prognostic Index
MMAE	Monomethyl auristatin E
MOMP	Mitochondrial outer membrane permeabilization
MOPP	Nitrogen mustard, vincristine, procarbazine, and prednisone
MRD	Minimal residual disease
MRI	Magnetic resonance imaging
mSWAT	Modified severity-weighted assessment tool
mTOR	Mechanistic target of rapamycin
MUGA	Multigated acquisition
MYD88	*Myeloid differentiation primary response 88 gene*
NB-UVB	Narrowband-ultraviolet light B

NCI	National Cancer Institute
NCIC	National Cancer Institute of Canada
NCCN	National Comprehensive Cancer Network
NF-kB	Nuclear factor-kappa B
NHEJ	Non-homologous end-joining genes
NHL	Non-Hodgkin lymphoma
NK	Natural killer
NLPLHL	Nodular lymphocyte-predominant HL
NMA	Non-myeloablative conditioning
NOS	Not otherwise specified
NRAS	Neuroblastoma RAS viral (v-ras) oncogene homolog
NSTEMI	Non-ST segment elevation myocardial infarction
ORR	Overall response rate
pcALCL	Primary cutaneous anaplastic large cell lymphoma
PCNSL	Primary central nervous system lymphoma
PCR	Pentostatin, cyclophosphamide, and rituximab
PD	Progressive disease
PD-1	Programmed-death 1
PD-L1/L2	Programmed-death 1 ligand 1/2
PFT	Pulmonary function test
PEST	C-terminal proline, glutamic acid, serine, and threonine-rich
PET	Positron emission tomography
PFS	Progression-free survival
PI3K	Phosphoinositide 3 kinase
PKCβ	Protein kinase C beta
PLCg	Phospholipase C gamma
PMBL	Primary mediastinal B-cell lymphoma
PR	Partial response
PRC2	Polycomb repressive complex 2
PS	Performance status
PTCL	Peripheral T-cell lymphoma
PUVA	UV-A phototherapy
R-CHOP	Rituximab, cyclophosphamide, doxorubicin, vincristine, and prednisolone

R-CODOX-M	Rituximab, cyclophosphamide, vincristine doxorubicin, and methotrexate
R-CVP	Rituximab, cyclophosphamide, vincristine, and prednisone
R-DHAP	Rituximab, dexamethasone, cytarabine, and cisplatin
R-HDMTX	Rituximab plus high-dose methotrexate
R-HyperCVAD	Rituximab, hyperfractionated cyclophosphamide, vincristine, doxorubicin, and dexamethasone
RAG	Recombination activating gene enzymes
REAL	The revised Europe-American Lymphoma Classification
RIC	Reduced intensity conditioning
RT	Radiation therapy
SBLs	Small B-cell lymphomas
SHM	Somatic hypermutation
SHP-1	Src homology region 2 domain-containing phosphatase-1
SLL	Small lymphocytic lymphoma
SMILE	Dexamethasone, methotrexate, ifosfamide, l-asparaginase, and etoposide
SMZL	Splenic marginal zone lymphoma
SNP	Single nuclear polymorphisms
SNV	Single nucleotide variants
SS	Sézary syndrome
STAT	Signal transducer and activator of transcription
STNI	Subtotal nodal irradiation
SUV	Standardized uptake value
SYK	Spleen tyrosine kinase
T-PLL	T-cell prolymphocytic leukemia
TCF3	Transcription factor 3 protein
TET	Tet methylcytosine dioxygenase enzymes
TF	Tissue factor
TFH	Follicular helper T-cell
TGF	Transforming growth factor

TIM-3	T-cell immunoglobulin and mucin domain-containing protein 3
TLR	Toll-like receptor
TLS	Tumor lysis syndrome
TNFR	Tumor necrosis factor receptor
TNFAIP3	TNF alpha-induced protein 3
TRAF	TNF receptor-associated factor
TRM	Transplant-related mortality
TSBA	Total body surface area
TSEBT	Total skin electron beam therapy
TTNT	Time to next treatment
ULN	Upper limit of normal
WBC	White blood cell count
WBRT	Whole-brain radiotherapy
WHO	World Health Organization
WM	Waldenström's macroglobulinemia

Chapter 1

Overview of lymphoma

Jasmine Zain and Larry W Kwak

Diseases characterized by non-infectious enlargement of lymph nodes were recognized as lymphosarcoma and psudoleukemia by Virchow and Cohenheim in 1864 and 1865. Around the same time Thomas Hodgkin described clinical histories and post-mortem findings of seven patients with enlarged lymph nodes and splenomelgaly without inflammation where the disease spread to contiguous lymph nodes and his colleague Samuel Wilks called it Hodgkin disease (HD). Consequently other neoplastic or inflammatory enlargements of lymph nodes came to be known as non-Hodgkin lymphoma (NHL) although the term malignant lymphoma was first used by Bilroth in 1872 [1].

Lymphoma is a cancer of the mature lymphocytes that inhabit the primary lymphoid organs including lymph nodes, bone marrow liver spleen as well as various lymphoid aggregates in other organs such as the intestinal tract, lungs, and skin. Lymphoma can arise in any organ as is reflected in the various subtypes of lymphoma although the most common presentation consists of adenopathy followed by cytopenias. Lymphomas may be accompanied by constitutional symptoms called B symptoms consisting of fevers, weight loss, and night sweats, which generally portend a worse prognosis. Etiology of B symptoms is unknown but is thought to be related to increased levels of interleukin 6 (IL-6) [2] and other inflammatory cytokines. A myriad of paraneoplastic syndromes can also be seen in cases of lymphoma. Neurologic disorders including

© Springer International Publishing AG 2017
J. Zain and L.W. Kwak (eds.), *Management of Lymphomas:
A Case-Based Approach*, DOI 10.1007/978-3-319-26827-9_1

Gulliam Barre syndrome and polyneuropathy [3], skin and soft tissue lesions [4], and nephrotic syndrome [5] are the most notable and respond to primary therapy directed towards the underlying lymphoma.

NHL is the sixth most common cancer diagnosed worldwide. In the US in 2016 the projected annual incidence is of 80,900 cases of NHL and 8500 cases of Hodgkin lymphoma (HL) [6]. This was comparable in the EU in 2012 with 78,768 cases of NHL and 12,271 cases of HL [7,8]. The probability of developing NHL increases with each decade of life and it causes an estimated 3.4% of all cancer deaths [9] in the US each year [10]. Median age at presentation is over 50 years of age except for high grade lymphoblastic lymphoma and Burkitt lymphoma, which are more common in children and young adults. There is a male predominance (age-adjusted incidence was 45% higher in men than women between 2007 and 2011). The incidence of lymphoma doubled between 1970s and 1990 but has stabilized since then. Partly, this increase may have been related to improved diagnostic techniques as well as the increased incidence of human immunodeficiency virus (HIV)-related lymphomas, but additional factors may be responsible [11]. Using statistical methods of analysis, rates of new cases of NHL have not changed much over time in the past 10 years but the death rates have been falling on an average of 2.4% each year from 2004–2013 [6].

Possible etiologic factors for lymphomas include pesticides and herbicides (possibly limited to t(14,18)-positive NHL) [12]. There is an association between lymphomagenesis and immunity. Congenital states of immune deficiency such as ataxia telegenctasia, wiskot aldrich syndrome, and severe combined immunedeficiency are associated with an increased risk of lymphoma. HIV infection is associated with a relative 75–100 times increase in the risk of lymphoma as compared with the general population with a decrease seen with the implementation of highly active retroviral therapy (HAART). Iatrogenic immunosuppression seen after organ or stem cell transplant [13] results in a 1–10% increase in the risk of lymphoma. Secondary cases of NHL can be seen in patients who have received prior chemotherapy or radiation. Certain autoimmune states such as Sjögren's syndrome, rheumatoid arthritis, and systemic lupus erythematosus also increase the risk of NHL [14]. Finally the use of disease-modifying agents in autoimmune diseases such as low dose methotrexate, thiopurines, and tumor necrosis factor antagonist therapy is also associated with an increased risk of NHL [15]. Viruses are known to cause genetic instability, increase in cell proliferation, alteration in DNA repair and evasion of host immunity, and are implicated in the pathogenesis of several types of NHL [16]. Viral particles from Epstein-Barr virus (EBV) are demonstrated in Burkitt lymphoma, post-transplant lymphoproliferative disorder, some cases of diffuse large B-cell lymphoma (DLBCL), natural killer (NK)-T-cell lymphoma, and peripheral T-cell lymphoma [17]. The human T-lymphotropic virus (HTLV1) in adult T-cell leukemia/lymphoma (ATLL) [18], and Kaposi sarcoma-associated herpes virus (KSHV) in primary effusion lymphoma and Castleman's disesase are other examples of viruses driving lymphomagenesis. Hepatitis C virus (HCV) is associated with marginal zone lymphomas (13–15% according to one meta-analysis). HCV may predispose B cells to malignant transformation by enhancing signal transduction on binding to the CD81(TAPA-1) [16]. Chronic antigenic stimulation and inflammation may also lead to lymphomagenesis. In this regard, certain bacterial infections are associated with lymphomas. *Borellia burgdorfi* is detected in 35% of patients with cutaneous B cell lymphomas [19]. *Helicobacter pylori* infection is strongly associated with gastric mucosa-associated lymphoid tissue (MALT) lymphoma [20] and there is a possible association between *Chalmydophilia psittaci* and ocular lymphoma [21]. In some of these cases lymphomas have responded to antibiotic therapy pointing to chronic inflammation as a cause of lymphomagenesis. There is now increasing identification of genetic variations that increase the susceptibility to develop lymphoma. Using genome-wide association data (GWAS), predisposing single nuclear polymorphisms (SNPs) have been identified for various subtypes of NHL. These include genes involved in immune function, inflammation, oxidative stress, and metabolism. Examples include *CXCR5*, *ETS1*, *ACTA2/FAS*, *BCL2*, and others [22].

The complicated and evolving classification of NHL is reflective of the evolution of diagnostic techniques over time ranging from microscopic appearances to immunological diagnostic techniques, cytogenetics, and now molecular techniques. Rappaport first classified lymphomas in 1966 by categorizing them into nodular diffuse and histiocytic based on the architectural organization and cell size of the neoplastic infilterate [23]. The 1974 Lukes and Collins classification combined cell of origin (B versus T cell), site of origin in the node, cell size, and nuclear shape to reflect transformation [24]. The concept of tumor grading was introduced in the Keil classification while adding the category of extranodal and T-cell lymphomas to the classification [25]. The working formulation for clinical use was created in 1978 by a group of experts appointed by the National Institute of Health [26] categorizing lymphomas as low, intermediate, and high grade based on cell size and clinical behavior. The revised Europe-American Lymphoma Classification (REAL) was the foundation of the current World Health Organization (WHO) 2001, 2008, and now 2016 classification that has tapped into clinical features, morphology, immunophenotyping, and molecular information recognizing over 70 different types of NHL [27,28].

Current staging of NHL is based on the subtype of lymphoma. The classic Ann Arbor staging system applies only to nodal lymphomas [29]. Other presentations require individualized staging criteria as will be described in the following chapters. Ever-evolving prognostic systems for various lymphomas such as the International Prognostic Index (IPI), Follicular Lymphoma International Prognostic Index (FLIPI), Mantle Cell Lymphoma International Prognostic Index (MIPI), and others reflect our deepening understanding of the clinical and pathological differences between these diseases that have allowed clinicians to decide therapies that will best benefit certain groups of patients and perhaps prevent overtreatment of others. In the era of genotyping and personalized medicine, it is possible that clinical criteria may lose their importance as treatments are directed more and more by defining genetic mutations and finding targeted treatments as is being illustrated by therapies in chronic lymphocytic leukemia (CLL) and other low grade lymphomas. All of this is the subject of the following chapters.

Treatment strategies for lymphomas have evolved alongside the classification and reflect the evolution of anticancer treatments. Radiotherapy was the first modality used to treat HL as early as 1902 [30] and became more popular in the 1940s onwards with the first cures of HD demonstrated in 1963 using radiotherapy [31]. The first use of a cytotoxic agent used to treat a human cancer was demonstrated against lymphoma. Naval personnel exposed to mustard gas were found to have changes in their blood counts and this observation led to the first use of a compound called nitrogen mustard to treat a case of lymphoma in 1942 at Yale University [32]. Other cytotoxic agents were to follow and in 1965 the concept of combination chemotherapy was initiated based on the principles of combining antibiotics to overcome microbial resistance in treating infections. Multiple cytotoxic agents were combined with a differing mechanism of action and this concept was extended to lymphomas in 1963 when it was demonstrated that nitrogen mustard, vincristine, procarbazine, and prednisone (MOPP) could cure patients with lymphoma [33]. Lymphoma therapy continued to revolve around various combinations of chemotherapy and radiation until the next milestone when a monoclonal antibody rituximab that targets CD20 was approved in 1997 for the treatment of B-cell lymphomas. The landmark randomized trial of rituximab + cyclophosphamide, doxorubicin, vincristine, and prednisolone (CHOP) chemotherapy versus CHOP alone demonstrated an increased complete remission rate, progression free, and overall survival of patients with diffuse large B cell lymphomas [34]. Meanwhile high dose chemotherapy followed by autologous stem cell transplant was shown to have a superior outcome in patients with chemosensitive disease in NHL as compared with salvage therapy alone firmly establishing the role of autologous stem cell transplant in the treatment of relapsed lymphomas [35]. This indication has been extended to several lymphoma subtypes and is a mechanism to deliver high dose chemotherapy in situations where standard dose chemotherapy is not expected to cure patients. The first allogeneic stem cell transplant for lymphoma was performed in 1982 and increasing data regarding the use of this modality appeared in both HL and NHL in the 1990s. Differences in outcome were noted based on various factors including histology and the role of graft versus lymphoma effect was identified as a therapeutic goal at least in some subtypes especially in low grade lymphomas. This has led to the increasing use of reduced intensity conditioning regimens for lymphoma transplants [36].

Besides stem cell transplant, other types of immunotherapy have been explored for the treatment of lymphomas including cancer vaccines [37,38], non-specific immunomodulatory agents including interferon [39], and immunomodulatory drugs (IMiDs) such as lenalidomide [40] with varying success. The first successful use of monoclonal antibodies to target specific proteins on lymphoma cells was established by rituximab. Currently, there are at least two other anti-CD20 antibodies that have been approved as well as two radioisotope conjugates that can target CD20 [41]. Other antibodies to target specific proteins on lymphoma cells such as CD25, CD52, and CXCR4 are also available for clinical and research purposes and are in various stages of development. Further modification of monoclonal antibodies has led to the antibody drug conjugate; the first approved agent for lymphoma being brentuximab vedotin, which combines a monoclonal antibody against CD30 with a cytotoxic agent monomethyl auristatin E (MMAE) thus directly targeting the malignant cell in HL [42]. Its approval in 2013 was a major landmark in the success of the ADC technology and has led to a plethora of similar agents for innumerable targets in other cancers and lymphomas. The latest approach is to engineer T cells to target proteins on malignant B cells (chimeric antigen receptor T cells [CAR-T]) as adoptive immunotherapy to treat lymphomas [43]. Finally, with the approval of nivolumab for the treatment of relapsed refractory HL, immune checkpoint inhibitor therapy has arrived in the realm of anti-lymphoma therapy [44].

Finally, no discussion of anti-lymphoma therapies can be completed without targeted therapies and epigenetic agents. Understanding the dysfunctional pathways in lymphomagenesis has enabled the use of small molecules that can target these pathways leading to meaningful clinical responses in patients. These are great examples of bench to bedside research. Currently, the field is dominated by the orally administered ibrutinib that selectively targets Bruton's tyrosine kinase receptor (BTK) and is approved for mantle cell lymphoma, CLL, marginal zone lymphoma and is active in many other B-cell malignancies. PI3 kinase (PI3K) is another active target with idelalisib being the first approved agent and many others in trials that target different isoforms of the enzymes. Other targeted agents include PI3K/AKT pathway inhibitors, proteosome inhibitors, histone deacetylase inhibitors, and agents targeting the janus kinase (JAK)/signal transducer and activator of transcription (STAT) pathways a [45]. With such a plethora of options the future remains limitless in terms of combinations of various modalities and agents towards curative and safe therapies for all lymphoma patients.

The future of lymphoma therapy holds great promise. Precision medicine allows an accurate delineation of altered genetic pathways in each patient's tumor and microenvironment as well as an understanding of the host immune milieu. This can allow a tailored prescription of a single or combination of targeted agents that can be given to 'fix' the altered genetic pathway, and stimulate an adequate immune response to keep the tumor in check without the toxic regimens of chemotherapy and stem cell transplant that are the current treatment paradigms.

The following chapters present a concise discussion of the various lymphomas and challenges in clinical management. Case presentations and continuing commentary on the case will be included in italics throughout the book. We hope that the reader will find this a useful compendium to their daily clinical work.

References

1   Lakhtakia R, Burney I. A Historical Tale of Two Lymphomas: Part II: Non-Hodgkin lymphoma. *Sultan Qaboos University Medical J.* 2015;15:e317-321.
2   Kurzrock R, Redman J, Cabanillas F, Jones D, Rothberg J, Talpaz M. Serum interleukin 6 levels are elevated in lymphoma patients and correlate with survival in advanced Hodgkin's disease and with B symptoms. *Cancer Res.* 1 1993;53:2118-2122.
3   Kelly JJ, Karcher DS. Lymphoma and peripheral neuropathy: a clinical review. *Muscle Nerve.* 2005;31:301-313.
4   Thomas I, Schwartz RA. Cutaneous paraneoplastic syndromes: uncommon presentations. *Clin Dermatol.* 2005;23:593-600.
5   Gagliano RG, Costanzi JJ, Beathard GA, Sarles HE, Bell JD. The nephrotic syndrome associated with neoplasia: an unusual paraneoplastic syndrome. Report of a case and review of the literature. *Am J Med.* 1976;60:1026-1031.
6   National Cancer Institute. Surveillance, Epidemiology, and End Results Program. SEER Stat Fact Sheets: Hodgkin Lymphoma. https://seer.cancer.gov/statfacts/html/hodg.html. Accessed March 7, 2017.
7   International Agency for Research on Cancer, World Health Organization. Non-Hodgkin lymphoma. http://eco.iarc.fr/eucan/Cancer.aspx?Cancer=38. Accessed March 7, 2017.
8   International Agency for Research on Cancer, World Health Organization. Hodgkin lymphoma. http://eco.iarc.fr/eucan/Cancer.aspx?Cancer=37. Accessed March 7, 2017.
9   Adzersen KH, Friedrich S, Becker N. Are epidemiological data on lymphoma incidence comparable? Results from an application of the coding recommendations of WHO, InterLymph, ENCR and SEER to a cancer registry dataset. *J Cancer Res Clin Oncol.* 2016;142:167-175.
10 Siegel RL, Miller KD, Jemal A. Cancer statistics, 2015. *CA Cancer J Clin.* 2015;65:5-29.

11 Evens AM, Winter JS, Gordon LI, et al. Non-Hodgkin Lymphoma. http://www.cancernetwork. com/cancer-management/non-hodgkin-lymphoma. Accessed March 7, 2017.

12 Roulland S, Kelly RS, Morgado E, et al. t(14;18) Translocation: A predictive blood biomarker for follicular lymphoma. *J Clin Oncol*. 2014;32:1347-1355.

13 Dierickx D, Tousseyn T, Gheysens O. How I treat posttransplant lymphoproliferative disorders. *Blood*. 2015;126:2274-2283.

14 Askling J, Fored CM, Baecklund E, et al. Haematopoietic malignancies in rheumatoid arthritis: lymphoma risk and characteristics after exposure to tumour necrosis factor antagonists. *Ann Rheum Dis*. 2005;64:1414-1420.

15 Lakatos PL, Miheller P. Is there an increased risk of lymphoma and malignancies under anti-TNF therapy in IBD? *Curr Drug Targets*. 2010;11:179-186.

16 Morales-Sanchez A, Fuentes-Panana EM. Human viruses and cancer. *Viruses*. 2014;6:4047-4079.

17 Ali AS, Al-Shraim M, Al-Hakami AM, Jones IM. Epstein-Barr virus: clinical and epidemiological revisits and genetic basis of oncogenesis. *Open Virol J*. 2015;9:7-28.

18 Panfil AR, Martinez MP, Ratner L, Green PL. Human T-cell leukemia virus-associated malignancy. *Curr Opin Virol*. 2016;20:40-46.

19 Schollkopf C, Melbye M, Munksgaard L, et al. Borrelia infection and risk of non-Hodgkin lymphoma. *Blood*. 2008;111:5524-5529.

20 Morgner A, Bayerdorffer E, Neubauer A, Stolte M. Helicobacter pylori associated gastric B cell MALT lymphoma: predictive factors for regression. *Gut*. 2001;48:290-292.

21 Collina F, De Chiara A, De Renzo A, De Rosa G, Botti G, Franco R. Chlamydia psittaci in ocular adnexa MALT lymphoma: a possible role in lymphomagenesis and a different geographical distribution. *Infect Agent Cancer*. 2012;7:8.

22 Cerhan JR, Berndt SI, Vijai J, et al. Genome-wide association study identifies multiple susceptibility loci for diffuse large B cell lymphoma. *Nat Genet*. 2014;46:1233-1238.

23 Rappaport H. Tumors of the Heamtopoeitic System. Atlas of Tumor Pathology. *Ann Intern Med*. 1967;67(3_Part_1):686-687.

24 Lukes RJ, Collins RD. Immunologic characterization of human malignant lymphomas. *Cancer*. 1974;34:1488-1503.

25 Stansfeld AG, Diebold J, Noel H, et al. Updated Kiel classification for lymphomas. *Lancet*. 1988;1:292-293.

26 [no authors listed]. National Cancer Institute sponsored study of classifications of non-Hodgkin's lymphomas: summary and description of a working formulation for clinical usage. The Non-Hodgkin's Lymphoma Pathologic Classification Project. *Cancer*. 1982;49:2112-2135.

27 Harris NL, Jaffe ES, Stein H, et al. A revised European-American classification of lymphoid neoplasms: a proposal from the International Lymphoma Study Group. *Blood*. 1994;84:1361-1392.

28 Swerdlow SH, Campo E, Harris NL, et al (Eds). *WHO Classification of Tumors of Hematopoeitic and Lymphoid Tissues*. 4th edn. World Health Organization, France: IARC Press 2008.

29 Juliusson G, Abrahamsen AF, Cavallin-Stahl E, et al. Management of non-Hodgkin lymphoma in adults in Scandinavia, United Kingdom, and The Netherlands. Report from the European School of Oncology intercity meeting at Huddinge Hospital, 3rd June, 1988. *Acta Oncologica*. 1989;28:135-140.

30 Pusey WA. Cases of sarcoma and of Hodgkin's disease treated by exposures to x-rays-a preliminary report. *JAMA*. 1902;38:166-169 .

31 Easson EC, Russell MH. Cure of Hodgkin's disease. *Br Med J*. 1963;1:1704-1707.

32 Gilman A. The initial clinical trial of nitrogen mustard. *Am J Surg*. 1963;105:574-578.

33 DeVita VT, Jr., Chu E. A history of cancer chemotherapy. *Cancer Res*. 2008;68:8643-8653.

34 Coiffier B, Lepage E, Briere J, et al. CHOP chemotherapy plus rituximab compared with CHOP alone in elderly patients with diffuse large-B-cell lymphoma. *N Engl J Med*. 2002;346:235-242.

35 Philip T, Guglielmi C, Hagenbeek A, et al. Autologous bone marrow transplantation as compared with salvage chemotherapy in relapses of chemotherapy-sensitive non-Hodgkin's lymphoma. *N Engl J Med*. 1995;333:1540-1545.

36 Chakraverty R, Mackinnon S. Allogeneic transplantation for lymphoma. *J Clin Oncol.* 2011;29:1855-1863.

37 Schuster SJ, Neelapu SS, Santos CF, Popa-McKiver MA, McCord AM, Kwak LW. Idiotype vaccination as consolidation therapy: time for integration into standard of care for follicular lymphoma? *J Clin Oncol.* 2011;29:4845-4846.

38 Schuster SJ, Neelapu SS, Gause BL, et al. Vaccination with patient-specific tumor-derived antigen in first remission improves disease-free survival in follicular lymphoma. *J Clin Oncol.* 2011;29:2787-2794.

39 Armitage JO, Coiffier B. Activity of interferon-alpha in relapsed patients with diffuse large B-cell and peripheral T-cell non-Hodgkin's lymphoma. *Ann Oncol.* 2000;11:359-361.

40 Nowakowski GS, LaPlant B, Macon WR, et al. Lenalidomide combined with R-CHOP overcomes negative prognostic impact of non-germinal center B-cell phenotype in newly diagnosed diffuse large B-Cell lymphoma: a phase II study. *J Clin Oncol.* 2015;33:251-257.

41 Wiseman GA, White CA, Sparks RB, et al. Biodistribution and dosimetry results from a phase III prospectively randomized controlled trial of Zevalin radioimmunotherapy for low-grade, follicular, or transformed B-cell non-Hodgkin's lymphoma. *Crit Rev Oncol Hematol.* 2001;39:181-194.

42 Younes A, Bartlett NL, Leonard JP, et al. Brentuximab vedotin (SGN-35) for relapsed CD30-positive lymphomas. *N Engl J Med.* 2010;363:1812-1821.

43 Kochenderfer JN, Dudley ME, Feldman SA, et al. B-cell depletion and remissions of malignancy along with cytokine-associated toxicity in a clinical trial of anti-CD19 chimeric-antigen-receptor-transduced T cells. *Blood.* 2012;119:2709-2720.

44 Younes A, Santoro A, Shipp M, et al. Nivolumab for classical Hodgkin's lymphoma after failure of both autologous stem-cell transplantation and brentuximab vedotin: a multicentre, multicohort, single-arm phase 2 trial. *Lancet Oncology.* 2016;17:1283-1294.

45 Younes A. Beyond chemotherapy: new agents for targeted treatment of lymphoma. *Nat Rev Clin Oncol.* 2011;8:85-96.

Chapter 2

Pathogenesis of lymphomas
Raju K Pillai and Wing C Chan

Genetic alterations lead to development of lymphomas

Cancer is, in essence, a genetic disease in which an accumulation of mutations leads to activation of oncogenic pathways and impairment of normal controls in growth and survival. Recent developments in high throughput sequencing technologies have produced an increasingly detailed record of the genomic alterations present in malignant lymphomas. Acquired (somatic) genetic alterations seen in malignancies include single nucleotide variants (SNV), small insertions and deletions (indels), copy number variations (CNV), and other large structural variations. Epigenetic alterations are heritable changes in gene expression that are due to mechanisms other than changes in the DNA sequence and include DNA methylation, histone modifications, and altered expression of non-coding RNA. Every tumor has acquired genetic and epigenetic alterations that lead to its pathogenesis and dictate most of its behavior including metastases, response to therapy, and resistance. A study of these genomic alterations has led to novel approaches in the treatment of cancers including lymphomas.

Most of these changes are 'passenger' mutations that occur incidentally. A very small fraction of these alterations are 'driver' mutations that are defined in a broad sense as cell-autonomous or non-cell-autonomous alterations that contribute to tumor evolution at any stage – including

© Springer International Publishing AG 2017
J. Zain and L.W. Kwak (eds.), *Management of Lymphomas:
A Case-Based Approach*, DOI 10.1007/978-3-319-26827-9_2

initiation, progression, metastasis, and resistance to therapy – by promoting a variety of functions including proliferation, survival, invasion, or immune evasion [1]. Only about 1–2% of human genes have been shown to act as drivers [2]. Alterations in these driver genes affect a limited number of pathways that control cell proliferation, differentiation, and apoptosis.

The frequency of genetic alterations varies widely among lymphoid malignancies. Hairy cell leukemia (HCL) and Waldenström's macroglobulinemia (WM) are characterized by low mutation load but are highly specific; *BRAF V600E* and *MYD88* L265P are seen in most cases of HCL and WM, respectively. Burkitt lymphoma (BL) and splenic marginal zone lymphoma (SMZL) have approximately 25–30 non-silent mutations per case [3,4] whereas 'high mutators' such as diffuse large B-cell lymphoma (DLBCL) have increased mutational load (approximately 50–100 non-silent mutations per case) [5–7].

It has been proposed that the accumulation of genetic alterations occurs in three phases [2]. In the breakthrough phase, a cell acquires a driver gene mutation and begins to expand and survive abnormally, undergoing many rounds of cell division, typically over many years. In the second expansion phase, secondary driver gene mutations enable the cells to expand in the local environment even under adverse conditions. In the invasive phase, additional mutations enable cells to invade normal tissue leading to distorted architecture and widespread dissemination, which are, by definition, features of a malignancy. An analogous situation has been described in the pathogenesis of malignant lymphomas. In follicular lymphoma (FL), the initial driver mutation, which is the t(14; 18) (*IGH;BCL2*) translocation occurs in the bone marrow during early B-cell development. Increased *BCL2* expression enables the precursor cell to survive multiple rounds of cell division in the germinal center – these t(14;18)-positive cells now circulate in the peripheral blood and are seen in up to 50% of the normal adult population [8]. Colonization of lymph nodes leads to in-situ FL and accumulation of further mutations results in development of FL. Similarly, in-situ mantle cell lymphoma (MCL) and monoclonal B-cell lymphocytosis have been described as precursors of MCL and chronic lymphocytic leukemia (CLL), respectively. Malignant lymphoma, therefore, represents the clinically detectable late stages in a continuum of increasing genetic complexity, which also raises the question of when it would be most appropriate to therapeutically intervene in the oncogenic process.

Mechanisms of genetic alterations in B-cell lymphomas

The B-cell receptor in the pre-B cell is assembled from various combinations of variable (V), diversity (D), and joining (J) gene segments. Two additional processes, somatic hypermutation (SHM) and class switching (CS), which occur in the germinal centers of secondary lymphoid organs, generate additional structural and functional diversity. The generation of a large antibody repertoire necessary for immunity involves DNA strand breaks and nucleotide alterations, which increase the risk for oncogenic alterations. These are described in the following section.

The variable region of the heavy chain (Vh) is assembled from approximately 40 variable, 23 diversity, and 6 joining gene segments and the variable region of the light chains is assembled from approximately 30–35 variable and 5 joining gene segments. These segments are rearranged by a process of double-stranded DNA breaks followed by recombination mediated by the recombination activating gene (RAG) enzymes. Aberrant recombination leads to chromosomal translocations, as exemplified by the RAG-mediated t(14;18) translocation in FL and t(11;14) translocation in MCL. In most cases, the coding region of the oncogene is not altered but the tightly regulated expression pattern is altered by association with the partner gene. Further development of the B cell occurs in the germinal center where the affinity of the B-cell receptor is further improved by selection of cells that have undergone SHM of the IgV region genes mediated by the activation-induced cytidine deaminase (AID) enzyme. Heavy chain class switching alters the functional properties of the antibody molecule. Both of these processes also create double-stranded breaks and aberrant chromosomal translocations. Somatic mutations mediated by AID may also affect non-immunoglobulin genes in germinal center B cells. Up to 10% of actively transcribed genes may be affected by aberrant somatic hypermutation.

The various B-cell development stages described above have been histogenetically correlated with various B-cell lymphomas as shown in Figure 2.1.

Signaling pathways involved in development of B-cell lymphomas

In this section, the major physiologic signaling pathways in B cells and examples of their alteration in lymphomas are described. An understanding of these pathways in lymphomas will enable rational therapeutic intervention.

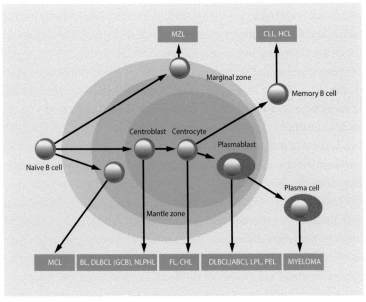

Figure 2.1 B-cell differentiation and relationship to major B-cell neoplasms. Lymphoblasts undergo VDJ recombination in the bone marrow. After maturation, naive B cells traverse to the germinal center of secondary lymphoid organs where two additional processes, somatic hypermutation and class switching, occur and generate additional structural and functional diversity. The vast majority of B-cell neoplasms arise form germinal center B cells with the remaining arising from mantle zone cells, marginal zone cells, or memory B cells. ABC, activated B cell; BL, Burkitt lymphoma; CLL, chronic lymphocytic leukemia; DLBCL, diffuse large B-cell lymphoma; GCB, germinal center B cell; HCL, Hairy cell leukemia; LPL, lymphoplasmacytic lymphoma; MCL, mantle cell lymphoma; MZL, marginal zone lymphoma; NLPHL, nodular lymphocyte-predominant Hodgkin lymphoma; PEL, primary effusion lymphoma; VDJ, variable, diversity, and joining gene segments.

B-cell receptor pathway

The B-cell receptor complex consists of the immunoglobulin molecule linked to a signaling subunit, which is a heterodimer of Ig-alpha (CD79A) and Ig-beta (CD79B) proteins. Antigen binding to the Ig molecule leads to phosphorylation of immunoreceptor tyrosine-based activation motifs (ITAM) in CD79A and CD79B by src family kinases such as LYN followed by activation of spleen tyrosine kinase (SYK), Bruton's tyrosine kinase (BTK), phospholipase C gamma (PLCg), and protein kinase C beta (PKCb) (Figure 2.2).

Activation of PKCb leads to caspase recruitment domain family, member 11 (CARD11) phosphorylation, recruitment of mucosa-associated lymphoid tissue lymphoma translocation protein 1 (MALT1) and B-cell lymphoma/leukemia 10 (BCL10) into the CARD11-BCL10-MALT1 (CBM) multi-protein complex and nuclear factor-kappa B (NF-kB) pathway activation. Mature B cells require 'tonic' signaling from the BCR complex for survival throughout their lifespan [9]. BCR signaling is also critical for survival and proliferation of B-cell lymphomas. A prominent feature of the activated B-cell type of DLBCL (ABC-DLBCL) is the constitutive activation of NF-kB signaling pathway and a 'chronic active' form of BCR signaling reminiscent of antigen-stimulated B cells that signal through the CBM complex to activate NF-kB. More than 20% of ABC-DLBCL patients harbor somatic mutations in *CD79B* and to a lesser extent in *CD79A* [10], and approximately 9% have oncogenic mutations in the *CARD11* gene [11]. Interruption of the BCR signaling pathway is specifically toxic to ABC-DLBCL cells in vitro [10]. In FL, it has been shown that the 'protective' allele that encodes the expressed B-cell receptor is not involved in the translocation with the *BCL2* gene and maintains BCR signaling [12].

The transcription factor 3 protein (TCF3) modulates germinal center gene expression and regulates survival and proliferation of lymphoid cells through the BCR and PI3K signaling pathway and by modulating cell cycle regulators such as CCND3. TCF3 also induces its own inhibitor, called inhibitor of DNA binding 3 (ID3), creating an autoregulatory loop that inactivates TCF3 in the resting state (Figure 2.2). Release of TCF3 from the ID3–TCF3 complex promotes BCR signaling by upregulating the expression of immunoglobulin heavy and light chain genes and repression of the BCR signaling inhibitor src homology region 2 domain-containing phosphatase 1 (SHP1). Most patients with BL (70%) harbor *ID3* and *TCF3* mutations leading to the activation of the TCF3 pathway, which ultimately results in intensification of 'tonic' BCR signaling [13].

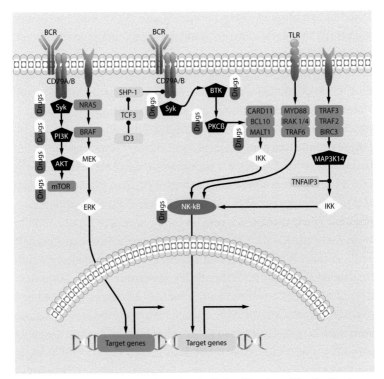

Figure 2.2 Intracellular signaling pathways involved in B-cell lymphoproliferative disorders and therapeutic targets: see text for details. AKT1, v-akt murine thymoma viral oncogene homolog 1; BCL10, B-cell CLL/lymphoma 10; BCR, B-cell receptor; BIRC3, baculoviral IAP repeat containing 3; BRAF, B-Raf proto-oncogene, serine/threonine kinase; BTK, Bruton's tyrosine kinase; CARD11, caspase recruitment domain-containing protein 11; ERK/MAPK, extracellular signal-regulated kinase/mitogen-activated protein kinase; ID3, inhibitor of DNA binding 3; IKK, inhibitor of NF-κB kinase; IRAK, interleukin-1 receptor-associated kinase 1; MALT1, mucosa-associated lymphoid tissue lymphoma translocation protein 1; MAP3K14, mitogen-activated protein kinase kinase kinase 14; MEK, mitogen-activated protein kinase kinase kinase 1; mTOR, mechanistic target of rapamycin; MYD88, myeloid differentiation primary response 88; NF-κB, nuclear factor of kappa light polypeptide gene enhancer in B cells; NRAS, neuroblastoma RAS viral (v-ras) oncogene homolog; PI3K, phosphoinositide 3-kinase; PKCβ, protein kinase C β; SHP-1, Src homology region 2 domain-containing phosphatase-1; SYK, spleen tyrosine kinase; TCF3, transcription factor 3; TLR, toll-like receptor; TNFAIP3, TNF alpha-induced protein 3; TRAF, TNF receptor-associated factor.

Toll-like receptor pathway

Toll-like receptors (TLRs) recognize a variety of pathogen-associated molecular patterns derived from bacteria, viruses, and fungi in a BCR-independent manner. Ligand binding causes aggregation of TLRs and activation of cytoplasmic adapters such as *myeloid differentiation primary response gene 88* (*MYD88*) and triggering NF-kB pathway activation (Figure 2.2). The MYD88 pathway can also be activated by cytokines such as interleukin 1 (IL-1). *MYD88* mutations are seen in approximately 90% of all WM, approximately 30% of ABC-DLBCL, and 10% of SMZL [4,7,14,15].

Notch signaling

Notch receptor proteins are transmembrane receptors that function as ligand-activated transcription factors. Ligand binding causes proteolytic cleavage of the Notch intracellular domain, which then translocates to the nucleus and induces transcription of target genes including MYC and NF-kB pathway components. Notch signaling plays an important role in a number of cellular functions including cell fate specification, proliferation and apoptosis, and the physiological development of the splenic marginal zone. The C-terminal proline, glutamic acid, serine, and threonine-rich (PEST) domain of the Notch protein is recognized by ubiquitin ligase leading to proteolytic degradation. Most mutations in lymphoma target the PEST domain resulting in truncation with impaired degradation and dysregulated Notch signaling. Notch pathway mutations have been identified in SMZL, CLL, and MCL. *Notch 1* mutations are seen in 5–10% of patients with CLL and this number increases with relapse and transformation. F-box and WD repeat domain-containing 7 (FBXW7) is an F-Box protein that forms one of the subunits of the ubiquitin ligase complex and promotes proteolytic degradation of Notch protein; loss of function mutations are seen in ~2% of patients with CLL [16,17].

Nuclear factor-kappa B pathway

NF-kB is a homo or heterodimer of Rel-like domain-containing proteins including RELA/p65, RELB, c-Rel, NF- kB1, and NF-kB2 that function downstream of the BCR, TLR, and Notch signaling pathways. NF-kB proteins are bound in a complex with an inhibitor protein, IkB alpha, which keeps them in the cytoplasm. Activation of IkB kinase (IKK) by external stimuli leads to phosphorylation of IkB alpha and its subsequent ubiquitination and proteasomal degradation lead to the release of NF-kB transcription factors that translocate to the nucleus and regulate gene transcription (Figure 2.2).

The role of the NF-kB pathway in ABC-DLBCL and SMZL has been discussed earlier. Negative regulators of NF-kB signaling are inactivated by mutations/deletions in many B-cell lymphomas as described below. TNFAIP3 is homozygously inactivated or deleted in 30% of patients with ABC-DLBCL [18]. BIRC3, TRAF2, and TRAF3 are negative regulatory proteins that form an inhibitory complex with the enzyme MAP3K14 (Figure 2.2) in association with the CD40 and BAFF receptors that mediate the non-canonical NF-kB signaling pathway. Activation of these receptors leads to disruption of the complex and release and stabilization of MAP3K14, which in turn activates IKKa. Loss of function mutations in *TRAF3* and *BIRC3* are detected in SMZL leading to activation of MAP3K14 and NF-kB signaling [19]. The *BIRC3* gene is inactivated in CLL by mutations and *BIRC3* mutations correlate with the clinical course and chemo refractoriness in CLL [20]. Activator mutations such as *CARD11* mutations are present in ABC-DLBCL and have been described above.

G-protein coupled receptors

G-protein coupled receptors (GPCR) are the largest family of cell surface receptors involved in signal transduction with over 800 members. In conjunction with their cognate heterotrimeric G proteins, GPCRs activate multiple downstream targets that regulate cells survival, proliferation, and differentiation. Sequencing studies have revealed mutations or copy number alterations in members of the *S1PR2-GNA13* (encodes the Gα13 G-protein)-*RHOA* pathway in DLBCL as well as in BL [5,13]. Impairment of this pathway affects B-cell localization and migration and leads to simultaneous activation of the AKT pathway [21]. GNA13 knockout mice develop DLBCL supporting the importance of this pathway in lymphomagenesis [22].

Mitogen-activated protein kinase signaling pathway

The mitogen-activated protein kinase pathway (MAPK) consists of receptor tyrosine kinases transmitting a variety of signals from the external environment to the nucleus. MAPK signaling in B cells is initiated at the BCR and propagated through RAS and RAF proteins. The *BRAF* V600E mutation is the pathognomonic genetic event for HCL. *BRAF* is also frequently mutated in Langerhans cell histiocytosis [23].

PI3k-AKT1-MTOR signaling pathway

The PI3K-AKT1-MTOR (phosphatidylinositol 3'-kinase/v-akt murine thymoma viral oncogene homolog 1/mechanistic target of rapamycin) pathway is a key component of tonic BCR signaling, a process that is required for B-cell survival. Conditional inactivation of the B-cell receptor leads to profound reduction of peripheral B cells, which can be rescued by transgenic expression of PI3K [24]. B-cell receptor signaling in BL activates the PI3K pathway, as demonstrated by phosphorylation of AKT1 and p70S6 kinase [25]. Activating mutations in *TCF3* as well as deleterious mutations in the *TCF3* inhibitor *ID3* potentiates B-cell receptor signaling by repression of SHP1 and enhancement of Ig production (Figure 2.2). 70% of BL cases have mutations in TCF3 or ID3 proteins, as described previously. Activation of the PI3K pathway due to loss of PTEN expression has been described in 37% of the DLBCL and 19% of MCL [26,27]. Activating mutations in exons 9 and 20 of *PI3K* have also been reported [26].

Role of MYC In lymphomagenesis

The MYC family includes C-MYC, N-MYC, L-MYC and S-MYC, which are involved in the control of cell growth, differentiation, and apoptosis. MYC-MAX heterodimers bind DNA sequences called E-box motifs to activate transcription of a large number of targets, estimated at 10–15% of all human genes. Enhanced *MYC* expression is seen in up to 70% of human malignancies and usually requires co-operation with other genetic lesions for oncogenic transformation.

MYC plays a crucial role in the initial stages of formation of the germinal center, where it is rapidly suppressed by *BCL6* expression in centroblasts. In the light zone, *MYC* is again expressed in a subset of centrocytes, accompanied by *BCL6* downregulation, NF-κB activation, and *IRF4* expression. These cells later re-enter the dark zone for further antigen receptor maturation. MYC-negative centrocytes in the light zone will exit the germinal cell to differentiate into memory B cells or long-lived plasma cells [28].

BL is characterized by a translocation that places the *MYC* gene under the control of the immunoglobulin enhancer. *MYC* deregulation is frequent in DLBCL; *MYC* translocations are seen in 5–14% of DLBCL, and *MYC* gain and amplification in 21–38% of DLBCL. Concurrent translocations of *BCL2* or *BCL6* gene with *MYC*, which are designated 'double-hit lymphomas' impart a significantly worse clinical prognosis. High *MYC* expression without *MYC* gene abnormalities, presumably induced by other mechanisms, is observed in 28–41% of DLBCL cases. In addition, the BCL2 protein is overexpressed concurrently in 60% of *MYC*-positive DLBCL cases, independent of the presence of gene rearrangement. These cases described as 'double expressor lymphoma' behave more aggressively than cases with single protein overexpression. *MYC* alterations are also seen in plasmablastic lymphoma (PBL), and anaplastic lymphoma kinase (ALK)-positive large B-cell lymphoma.

Role of p53 and DNA repair pathways

p53 is induced and activated by a number of stress signals, including DNA damage, oxidative stress, telomere shortening, hypoxia, and activated oncogenes leading to cell cycle arrest, cellular senescence, or apoptosis. Inactivation of p53 is seen in a variety of lymphomas such as BL, DLBCL, including those derived from transformation of FL, MCL, CLL, peripheral T-cell lymphoma (PTCL), and natural killer cell lymphoma/leukemia (NKCL). HDM2, the negative regulator of TP53, is often amplified in lymphoma.

DNA repair pathways preserve genomic integrity – there are at least six major DNA repair mechanisms in human cells. Somatic and germline mutations have been identified in various DNA repair pathways, mainly in DLBCLs [29]. Mutations in mismatch repair genes (*EXO1*, *MSH2*, and *MSH6*) were associated with microsatellite instability, increased number of somatic insertions/deletions, and altered mutation signatures in tumors. Somatic mutations in non-homologous end-joining (NHEJ) genes (*DCLRE1C/ARTEMIS*, *PRKDC/DNA-PKcs*, *XRCC5/KU80*, and *XRCC6/KU70*) were almost exclusively associated with translocations involving the immunoglobulin-heavy chain locus [29]. *ATM* abnormalities are often seen and are particularly common in patients with MCL and CLL.

Regulation of apoptosis

Apoptosis is a genetically controlled mechanism of cell death involved in the regulation of tissue homeostasis controlled by enzymes called caspases. Caspases are cysteine proteases that cleave proteins at the Aspartate residues – at least 17 caspases have been described in mammals. Caspases include 'executioner caspases' (caspases 3, 6, and 7), which are activated by 'initiator caspases'. There are two major pathways of apoptosis: the extrinsic pathway initiated by Fas and the other tumor necrosis factor receptor (TNFR) superfamily members leading to caspase-3 activation, and the intrinsic mitochondria-associated pathway, which is activated by apoptotic stimuli that induce mitochondrial outer membrane permeabilization (MOMP) followed by the release of molecules that facilitate the cell death program such as, cytochrome c, SMAC, and Omi. Cytochrome c interacts with Apaf-1 and caspase-9 to activate caspase-3. As a common final pathway, caspase-3 activation leads to the degradation of cellular proteins necessary for cell survival and maintenance of cellular integrity.

The BCL2 family of proteins, which include pro-apoptotic (BAX, BAK, BIM, and BID) and anti-apoptotic (BCL-2, BCL-XL, BCL-w, MCL-1, and BFL-1) members, regulate apoptosis by controlling MOMP. Translocations affecting the *BCL2* gene represent the genetic hallmark of FL and are seen in 80–90% cases, it is also detected in about 30% of GCB-DLCBL. Ectopic *BCL2* expression prevents apoptosis of germinal center B cells leading to accumulation of other genetic abnormalities. High expression of anti-apoptotic proteins such as MCL1 and inactivation of BIM and other pro-apoptotic proteins have also been reported.

Impairment of differentiation to plasma cells

BCL6 is the master regulator of the germinal center reaction. As a transcriptional repressor, BCL6 negatively regulates multiple target genes involved in BCR and CD40 signaling, T-cell mediated B-cell activation and induction of apoptosis in response to DNA damage. BCL6 therefore maintains the proliferative status of centroblasts and prevents terminal differentiation to plasma cells via suppression of PRDM1/BLIMP1, the master regulator of plasma cell differentiation. The *PRDM1/BLIMP1* gene on 6q21 is bi-allelically inactivated in ~25% of ABC-DLBCL cases [30] and represents another mechanism of impairing differentiation with the tumor cells arrested at the plasmablastic stage.

Epigenetic alterations

The epigenome is composed primarily of cytosine modifications, histone modifications, and expression of non-coding RNA molecules, which are particularly important in the germinal center reaction [31,32]. In a normal somatic cell, approximately 70–80% of cytosines that occur as a CpG dinucleotide are methylated whereas CpG islands are largely unmethylated [33] and this methylation status is mediated by DNA methylases and demethylases. Hemi-methylated DNA is the target of DNA methyl transferase 1 (DNMT1) and is needed to maintain methylation patterns during DNA replication. DNA methyl transferases 3A and 3B (DNMT3A and DNMT3B) target primarily unmethylated CpG's. A deeper understanding of the epigenetic modifications would enable rational use of epigenetic therapies.

Histone octamers composed of H2A, H2B, H3, and H4 proteins form the scaffold upon which DNA is wound to form nucleosomes. Histones can be chemically modified by acetylation, methylation, phosphorylation, sumoylation, or ubiquitinylation. Trimethylation of H3 lysine 27 (H3K27me3) by the polycomb repressive complex 2 (PRC2), which includes EZH2, SUZ12, and EED is associated with transcriptional repression. EZH2 is upregulated in centroblasts and mediates H3K27 methylation and epigenetic silencing of genes required for memory and plasma cell differentiation. *EZH2* gain of function mutations have been observed in >20% of patients with FL and 23% of those with GCB-DLBCL but are rare in ABC-DLBCL [5]. EZH2 inhibition in GCB-DLBCL alters the gene expression profile and induces proliferation arrest and plasma cell differentiation. In contrast to H3K27me3, trimethylation of H3 lysine 4 (H3K4me3) by the MLL family of histone methyltransferases is associated with active chromatin and gene expression. Loss of function mutations in *MLL* and *MLL2* are frequent in FL but seen less often in DLBCL patients. The outcome of epigenetic modifications is related to the 'geography' and 'topology' of the genome [34]. For example, cytosine methylation of transcription factor binding sites can result in either transcriptional activation or repression. Epigenetic modifications have different degrees of plasticity and may be reprogrammed based on environmental signals. In addition, epigenetic marks are combinatorial [35]. For example, the combination of H3K27me3, which is a repressive mark and an activation mark H3K4me3 in gene promoters leads to a bivalent chromatin domain that is transcriptionally poised but transiently repressed. Subsequent loss of an H3K27me or H3K4me3 mark leads to more durable activation or repression, respectively. Such bivalent chromatin marks are common in genes associated with differentiation.

EP300 and *CREBBP* are histone acetyltransferases, which are commonly mutated in FL and DLBCL [32] and may alter the enhancer profile of the tumor. Such loss of function mutations also lead to defective acetylation of other proteins including BCL6 and TP53 that may promote germinal center B-cell lymphomagenesis [36]. Additional chromatin modifiers that are often mutated in lymphoma include components of the SNF/SWI complex, *ARID1A* and *B*, and *SMARC* family proteins.

Host/tumor interaction

Lymphomas typically arise in secondary lymphoid tissues, extranodal sites or uncommonly in the bone marrow. The microenvironment in lymphomas is composed of a mixture of stromal cells (follicular dendritic cells, fibroblastic reticular cells, and mesenchymal cells), immune cells (antigen-presenting cells, macrophages, T- and B-lymphoid cells, plasma cells, and mast cells), and extracellular matrix proteins as well as blood vessels [37]. Interactions between the neoplastic cells and the microenvironment promote tumor cell survival and malignant cells constantly evolve to evade anti-tumor immunity. Mutations or loss of molecules important in immune response are common in tumor cells; these include *B2M*, *CD58*, *CIITA*, and *HLA* components. There may also be increased immunosuppressive cells or cytokines in the stroma, which could be orchestrated by STAT3 activation among others.

Recent advances in understanding the interactions between the host immune system and tumors has enabled therapeutic interventions designed to enhance the anti-tumor response. The adaptive immune response, mediated primarily by T cells, requires three kinds of signals for activation and differentiation. The primary signal is provided by engagement of the T-cell receptor with the peptide-major histocompatibility locus (MHC) complex and the second signal is provided by various costimulatory molecules, the most well-characterized of which are members of the B7 family (Figure 2.3) expressed on antigen-presenting cells. Signal 3 is delivered mostly by cytokines such as IL-6, IL-12, IL-4,

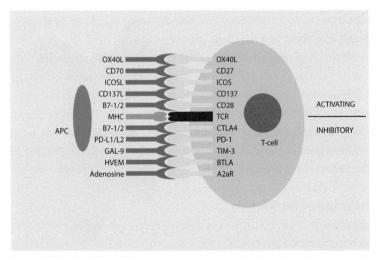

Figure 2.3 The role of PD-1, CTLA-4, and other immune checkpoint pathways is represented.
A2aR, adenosine A2a receptor; APC, antigen-presenting cell; BTLA, B- and T-lymphocyte-associated; CTLA-4, cytotoxic T-lymphocyte-associated protein 4; Gal-9, lectin, galactoside-binding, soluble 9; HVEM, tumor necrosis factor receptor superfamily, member 14; ICOS, inducible T-cell co-stimulator; ICOSL, inducible T-cell co-stimulator ligand; MHC, major histocompatibility locus; OX40, tumor necrosis factor receptor superfamily, member 4; PD-1, programmed-death 1; PD-L1/L2, programmed-death 1 ligand 1/2; TCR, T-cell receptor; TIM-3, T-cell immunoglobulin and mucin domain-containing protein 3. Adapted from © The American Society of Hematology, 2015. All rights reserved. Armand [38].

and transforming growth factor (TGF)-beta and promotes T-cell differentiation into effector subsets. Activation of CD28 receptors on T cells by B7 molecules induces expression of IL-2 and the high affinity IL-2 receptor. T-cell co-stimulation is also modified by inhibitory molecules such as cytotoxic T-lymphocyte associated protein 4 (CTLA-4), which binds B7 molecules with 20 times more avidity than CD28. Signaling through the programmed-death 1 (PD-1) protein leads to decreased T-cell proliferation, cytotoxicity, and cytokine production, and increased susceptibility to apoptosis. Other inhibitory signals are mediated by T-cell immunoglobulin and mucin-domain containing-3 (TIM-3), B- and T-lymphocyte-associated (BTLA), and adenosine A2a receptor (A2aR) molecules on the T cells (Figure 2.3).

Tumors can selectively block anti-tumor immune responses through expression of the checkpoint receptor ligands such as CTLA4 and programmed death-1 ligand-1/2 (PD-L1/PD-L2). Immune checkpoint blockade using anti-CTLA-4, anti-PD1, and anti-PDL1 antibodies and their combinations have been shown to be effective in stimulating a cellular immune response in many hematological malignancies including classical Hodgkin lymphoma (cHL), FL, and DLBCL [38].

Pathogenesis of T-cell and natural killer cell lymphomas

PTCL represents about 10% of all non-Hodgkin lymphomas (NHLs), with angioimmunoblastic T-cell lymphoma (AITL) and anaplastic large cell lymphoma (ALCL) being the two most common entities. A large group of T-cell lymphomas cannot be classified further by current criteria and are designated as PTCL-not otherwise specified (PTCL-NOS). In comparison to B-cell lymphomas, much less is known about the pathogenetic mechanisms in T-cell lymphomas.

Next generation sequencing studies in AITL have shown frequent mutations of *TET2*, *DNMT3A*, *IDH2*, and *RHOA* with *IDH2* mutations exclusively involving R172 [39]. In contrast to the situation in AML, *IDH2* and *TET2* mutations are not exclusive and frequently occur together. Tet methylcytosine dioxygenase (TET) enzymes are alpha-ketoglutarate-dependent dioxygenases that catalyze demethylation of 5-methylcytosine. *IDH2* gain of function mutations increase 2-hydroxyglutarate (2HG) levels leading to competitive inhibition of 2 ketoglutarate (2KG) dependent enzymes including TET enzymes and histone demethylases thus leading to aberrant histone lysine and DNA cytosine methylation and alteration in gene expression [40]. Other mutations are far less common and some mutations such as *CD28* are unique to PTCL. *CD28* mutations appear to enhance its signaling either through increased binding affinity to its ligand CD80/86 on antigen-presenting cells or its interaction with cytoplasmic adaptor molecules such as GRB2 eventually resulting in increased activation of the NF-kB pathway [41]. Uncommon fusions involving the extracellular domain of *CTLA4* and the cytoplasmic domain of *CD28* are expected to markedly increase the affinity of binding to CD80/86 and thus CD28 signaling [41].

The genetic hallmark of ALK-positive ALCL is a chromosomal translocation involving the *ALK* gene. Translocations involving *DUSP2* and *TP63* have been described in some cases of ALK-negative ALCL with good and poor prognosis, respectively [42]. Additional translocations often involving a kinase and a tissue factor (TF) have recently been described [43].

Many cytokines signal through the Janus-associated kinase (JAK)-signal transducer and activator of transcription (STAT) pathway, which includes four cytoplasmic JAK kinases and seven STAT proteins. Cytokine/receptor binding leads to activation of the associated JAK kinase, docking and phosphorylation of the cognate STAT protein, and translocation of the dimer to the nucleus where it functions as a transcription factor. A systematic genomic analysis in ALK-ALCLs identified activating mutations of *JAK1* and/or *STAT3* genes in 18% of ALK-ALCLs and 5% of cutaneous ALCLs. Of the positive cases, co-occurrence of *JAK1* and *STAT3* mutations were seen in 38% of systemic ALK-ALCLs but not in cutaneous ALCLs [43]. Recurrent chimeras combining a transcription factor (*NFkB2* or *NCOR2*) with a tyrosine kinase (*ROS1* or *TYK2*) that lead to the constitutive activation of the *JAK/STAT3* pathway were also observed [43]. *STAT3* is also one of the key downstream targets of activated ALK.

Two major subgroups have been described within the PTCL-NOS category by gene expression profiling. The first group is characterized by the high expression of *GATA3* and some of its target genes and is associated with poor prognosis. The second group demonstrates high expression of *TBX21* and some of its target genes – increased expression of the cytotoxic gene signature in this group also showed poor clinical outcome [44]. The mutational landscape of PTCL-NOS is not well defined but some of the mutations see in AITL and other lymphomas including epigenetic mediators (*MLL*, *TET2*, and *DMNT3A*), signaling pathway proteins (TNFAIP3, APC, and CHD8), and tumor suppressors (*TP53*, *FOXO1*, and *ATM*) have been detected [45,46]. Multiple studies on cutaneous T-cell lymphoma/Sezary syndrome have been reported recently [47–50]. Recurrent SNVs in *CD28*, *RHOA*, *PLCG1*, *TP53*, *DNMT3A*, and *FAS* were reported by Choi et al in cutaneous T-cell lymphomas. However, in this study copy number variations (CNVs) were much more frequent than single-nucleotide variations (SNVs) [50]. A large study detailing the mutations and CNVs in adult T-cell leukemia/lymphoma (ATLL) has also been published [51].

The gene expression profiles of NK cell-derived and γδ T-cell-derived lymphomas have been shown to be alike indicating that lymphoma derived from cells of the innate immune system may be biologically similar [52]. Recent whole-exome sequencing studies of extranodal natural killer/T-cell lymphoma (ENKTCL) found frequent mutations involving the *DDX3X*, *TP53*, *STAT3*, and *STAT5B* genes. In addition, a number of mutations in epigenetic modifiers including *MLL2*, *ARID1A*, *EP300*, and *ASXL3* were also reported [53]. Targeted DNA sequencing from a larger group of cases confirmed the high frequency of *STAT3* and *STAT5B* mutations, especially the *N642H* mutation, in γδ lineage lymphomas including cutaneous, intestinal, and hepatosplenic lymphomas [54,55]. Mutation results in increased binding affinity of the dimers between the SH2 domain and phosphotyrosine leading to increased persistence of the activated dimeric molecule and prolonged occupancy of the STAT binding site on the target genes.

Pathogenesis of Hodgkin lymphoma

Classical HL arises from post-germinal center B cells as evidenced by clonally rearranged and somatically mutated immunoglobulin genes. Surface Ig is not expressed indicating independence from antigen stimulation.

Other important pathogenetic features include loss of expression of many B-cell specific genes, activation of the NF-kB pathway, Epstein-Barr virus infection in a subset of cases, and genetic changes that modulates the tumor environment to favor HL cell survival.

Constitutive activation of the NF-κB pathway occurs through multiple mechanisms in cHL, including *REL* amplification [56], increased expression of the positive NF-κB regulator BCL3, or inactivating mutations in negative regulators such as *NFKBIA* (20% of cases), *NFKBIE* (15%), and *TNFAIP3* (40%) [57]. Interestingly, TNFAIP3 loss and EBV positivity were mutually exclusive. A recent study revealed alterations in genes involved in antigen presentation, chromosome integrity, transcriptional regulation, and ubiquitination [58]. *Beta2-microglobulin* was the most commonly altered gene in Hodgkin and Reed/Stenberg (HRS) cells, with inactivating mutations leading to loss of class I MHC expression. Genomic studies have identified PD-L1 and PD-L2 as key targets of 9p24.1 amplification, which is a recurrent abnormality seen in cHL [59]. PD-L1 transcription is also enhanced by amplification of the Janus kinase 2 (JAK2) locus as part of the 9p24.1 amplification as well as by EBV infection. Recent clinical trials with PD-1 checkpoint blockade have validated the effectiveness of this approach. The novel highly recurrently mutated genes *DUSP2, SGK1,* and *JUNB* were recently described in nodular lymphocyte-predominant HL (NLPLHL) [60].

Conclusions

Most lymphomas arise from a combination of somatic mutations and aberrantly regulated genes that lead to activation of biochemical and signaling pathways promoting tumor growth. Panomic studies have mostly confirmed the validity of traditional histologic classification of lymphomas. Future diagnostic paradigms are expected to incorporate an integrated analysis of the mutations, copy number changes, and transcriptomic and epigenomic alterations in addition to traditional histology and immunophenotyping. These results interpreted in the context of the patient's clinical features and knowledge of available pharmacological interventions will likely enable multipoint targeting of tumor drivers.

References

1 Alizadeh AA, Aranda V, Bardelli A, et al. Toward understanding and exploiting tumor heterogeneity. *Nat Med*. 2015;21:846-853.

2 Vogelstein B, Kinzler KW. The path to cancer–three strikes and you're out. *N Engl J Med*. 2015;373:1895-1898.

3 Richter J, Schlesner M, Hoffman S, et al. Recurrent mutation of the ID3 gene in Burkitt lymphoma identified by integrated genome, exome and transcriptome sequencing. *Nat Genet*. 2012;44:1316-1320.

4 Rossi D, Trifonov V, Fangazio M, et al. The coding genome of splenic marginal zone lymphoma: activation of NOTCH2 and other pathways regulating marginal zone development. *J Exp Med*. 2012;209:1537-1551.

5 Lohr JG, Stojanov P, Lawrence MS, et al. Discovery and prioritization of somatic mutations in diffuse large B-cell lymphoma (DLBCL) by whole-exome sequencing. *Proc Natl Acad Sci USA*. 2012;109:3879-3884.

6 Morin RD, Mendez-Lago M, Mungall AJ, et al. Frequent mutation of histone-modifying genes in non-Hodgkin lymphoma. *Nature*. 2011;476:298-303.

7 Pasqualucci L, Trifonov V, Fabbri G, et al. Analysis of the coding genome of diffuse large B-cell lymphoma. *Nat Genet*. 2011;43:830-837.

8 Limpens J, Stad R, Vos C, et al. Lymphoma-associated translocation t(14;18) in blood B-cells of normal individuals. *Blood*. 1995;85:2528-2536.

9 Gauld SB, Dal Porto JM, Cambier JC. B cell antigen receptor signaling: roles in cell development and disease. *Science*. 2002;296:1641-1642.

10 Davis RE, Ngo VN, Lenz G, et al. Chronic active B-cell-receptor signalling in diffuse large B-cell lymphoma. *Nature*. 2010;463:88-92.

11 Lenz G, Davis RE, Ngo VN, et al. Oncogenic CARD11 mutations in human diffuse large B cell lymphoma. *Science*. 2008;319:1676-1679.

12 Roulland S, Navarro JM, Grenot P, et al. Follicular lymphoma-like B cells in healthy individuals: a novel intermediate step in early lymphomagenesis. *J Exp Med*. 2006;203:2425-2431.

13 Love C, Sun Z, Jima D, et al. The genetic landscape of mutations in Burkitt lymphoma. *Nat Genet*. 2012;44:1321-1325.

14 Ngo NV, Young RM, Schmitz R, et al. Oncogenically active MYD88 mutations in human lymphoma. *Nature*. 2011;470:115-119.

15 Treon SP, Xu L, Yang G, et al. MYD88 L265P somatic mutation in Waldenstrom's macroglobulinemia. *N Engl J Med*. 2012;367:826-833.

16 Fabbri G, Rasi S, Rossi D, et al. Analysis of the chronic lymphocytic leukemia coding genome: role of NOTCH1 mutational activation. *J Exp Med*. 2011;208:1389-1401.

17 Wang L, Lawrence MS, Wan Y, et al. SF3B1 and other novel cancer genes in chronic lymphocytic leukemia. *N Engl J Med*. 2011;365:2497-2506.

18 Compagno M, Lim WK, Grunn A, et al. Mutations of multiple genes cause deregulation of NF-kappaB in diffuse large B-cell lymphoma. *Nature*. 2009;459:717-721.

19 Arcaini L, Rossi D. Nuclear factor-kappaB dysregulation in splenic marginal zone lymphoma: new therapeutic opportunities. *Haematologica*. 2012;97:638-640.

20 Rossi D, Fangazio M, Rasi S, et al. Disruption of BIRC3 associates with fludarabine chemorefractoriness in TP53 wild-type chronic lymphocytic leukemia. *Blood*. 2012;119:2854-2862.

21 O'Hayre M, Inoue A, Kufareva I, et al. Inactivating mutations in GNA13 and RHOA in Burkitt's lymphoma and diffuse large B-cell lymphoma: a tumor suppressor function for the Galpha/RhoA axis in B cells. *Oncogene*. 2015; doi:10.1038/onc.2015.442 [Epub ahead of print].

22 Muppidi JR, Schmitz R, Green JA, et al. Loss of signalling via Galpha13 in germinal centre B-cell-derived lymphoma. *Nature*. 2014;516:254-258.

23 Badalian-Very G, Vergilio JA, Degar BA, et al. Recurrent BRAF mutations in Langerhans cell histiocytosis. *Blood*. 2010;116:1919-1923.

24 Srinivasan L, Sasaki Y, Calado DP, et al. PI3 kinase signals BCR-dependent mature B cell survival. *Cell*. 2009;139:573-586.

25 Schmitz R, Young RM, Ceribelli M, et al. Burkitt lymphoma pathogenesis and therapeutic targets from structural and functional genomics. *Nature*. 2012;490:116-120.

26 Abubaker J, Bavi PP, Al-Harbi S, et al. PIK3CA mutations are mutually exclusive with PTEN loss in diffuse large B-cell lymphoma. *Leukemia*. 2007;21:2368-2370.

27 Rudelius M, Pittaluga S, Nishizuka S, et al. Constitutive activation of Akt contributes to the pathogenesis and survival of mantle cell lymphoma. *Blood*. 2006;108:1668-1676.

28 Ott G, Rosenwald A, Campo E. Understanding MYC-driven aggressive B-cell lymphomas: pathogenesis and classification. *Blood*. 2013;122:3884-3891.

29 de Miranda NF, Peng R, Georgiou K, et al. DNA repair genes are selectively mutated in diffuse large B cell lymphomas. *J Exp Med*. 2013;210:1729-1742.

30 Mandelbaum J, Bhagat G, Tang H, et al. BLIMP1 is a tumor suppressor gene frequently disrupted in activated B cell-like diffuse large B cell lymphoma. *Cancer Cell*. 2010;18:568-579.

31 Chi P, Allis CD, Wang GC. Covalent histone modifications--miswritten, misinterpreted and mis-erased in human cancers. *Nat Rev Cancer*. 2010;10:457-469.

32 Jiang Y, Melnick A. The epigenetic basis of diffuse large B-cell lymphoma. *Semin Hematol*. 2015;52:86-96.

33 Taylor KH, Briley A, Wang Z, Cheng J, Shi H, Caldwell CW. Aberrant epigenetic gene regulation in lymphoid malignancies. *Semin Hematol*. 2013;50:38-47.

34 Shen H, Laird PW. Interplay between the cancer genome and epigenome. *Cell*. 2013;153:38-55.

35 Maze I, Noh KM, Soshnev AA, Allis CD. Every amino acid matters: essential contributions of histone variants to mammalian development and disease. *Nat Rev Genet*. 2014;15:259-271.

36 Pasqualucci L, Dominguez-Sola D, Chiarenza A, et al. Inactivating mutations of acetyltransferase genes in B-cell lymphoma. *Nature*. 2011;471:189-195.

37 Blonska M, Agarwal NK, Vega F. Shaping of the tumor microenvironment: Stromal cells and vessels. *Semin Cancer Biol*. 2015;34:3-13.

38 Armand P. Immune checkpoint blockade in hematologic malignancies. *Blood*. 2015;125:3393-3400.

39 Cairns RA, Iqbal J, Lemonnier F, et al. IDH2 mutations are frequent in angioimmunoblastic T-cell lymphoma. *Blood*. 2012;119:1901-1903.

40 Wang C, McKeithan TW, Gong Q, et al. IDH2R172 mutations define a unique subgroup of patients with angioimmunoblastic T-cell lymphoma. *Blood*. 2015;126:1741-1752.

41 Rohr J, Guo S, Huo J, et al. Recurrent activating mutations of CD28 in peripheral T-cell lymphomas. *Leukemia*. 2016;30:1062-1070.

42 Zeng Y, Feldman AL. Genetics of anaplastic large cell lymphoma. *Leuk Lymphoma*. 2016;57:21-27.

43 Crescenzo R, Abate F, Lasora E, et al. Convergent mutations and kinase fusions lead to oncogenic STAT3 activation in anaplastic large cell lymphoma. *Cancer Cell*. 2015;27:516-532.

44 Iqbal J, Wright G, Wang C, et al. Gene expression signatures delineate biological and prognostic subgroups in peripheral T-cell lymphoma. *Blood*. 2014;123:2915-2923.

45 Palomero T, Couronné L, Khiabanian H, et al. Recurrent mutations in epigenetic regulators, RHOA and FYN kinase in peripheral T cell lymphomas. *Nat Genet*. 2014;46:166-170.

46 Schatz JH, Horwitz SM, Teruya-Feldstein J, et al. Targeted mutational profiling of peripheral T-cell lymphoma not otherwise specified highlights new mechanisms in a heterogeneous pathogenesis. *Leukemia*. 2015;29:237-241.

47 da Silva Almeida AC, Abate F, Khiabanian H, et al. The mutational landscape of cutaneous T cell lymphoma and Sezary syndrome. *Nat Genet*. 2015;47:1465-1470.

48 Wang L, Ni X, Covington KR, et al. Genomic profiling of Sezary syndrome identifies alterations of key T cell signaling and differentiation genes. *Nat Genet*. 2015;47:1426-1434.

49 Vaque JP, Gómez-López G, Monsálvez V, et al. PLCG1 mutations in cutaneous T-cell lymphomas. *Blood*. 2014;123:2034-2043.

50 Choi J, Goh G, Walradt T, et al. Genomic landscape of cutaneous T cell lymphoma. *Nat Genet*. 2015;47:1011-1019.

51 Kataoka K, Nagata Y, Kitanaka A, et al. Integrated molecular analysis of adult T cell leukemia/lymphoma. *Nat Genet.* 2015;47:1304-1315.

52 Iqbal J, Weisenburger DD, Chowdhury A, et al. Natural killer cell lymphoma shares strikingly similar molecular features with a group of non-hepatosplenic gammadelta T-cell lymphoma and is highly sensitive to a novel aurora kinase A inhibitor in vitro. *Leukemia.* 2011;25:348-358.

53 Jiang L, Gu ZH, Yan ZX, et al. Exome sequencing identifies somatic mutations of DDX3X in natural killer/T-cell lymphoma. *Nat Genet.* 2015;47:1061-1066.

54 Küçük C, Jiang B, Hu X, et al. Activating mutations of STAT5B and STAT3 in lymphomas derived from gammadelta-T or NK cells. *Nat Commun.* 2015;6:6025.

55 Nicolae A, Xi L, Pittaluga S, et al. Frequent STAT5B mutations in gammadelta hepatosplenic T-cell lymphomas. *Leukemia.* 2014;28:2244-2248.

56 Martin-Subero JI, Gesk S, Harder L, et al. Recurrent involvement of the REL and BCL11A loci in classical Hodgkin lymphoma. *Blood.* 2002;99:1474-1477.

57 Schmitz R, Stanelle J, Hansmann ML, Küppers R. Pathogenesis of classical and lymphocyte-predominant Hodgkin lymphoma. *Annu Rev Pathol.* 2009;4:151-174.

58 Reichel J, Chadburn A, Rubinstein PG, et al. Flow sorting and exome sequencing reveal the oncogenome of primary Hodgkin and Reed-Sternberg cells. *Blood.* 2015;125:1061-1072.

59 Green MR, Monti S, Rodig SJ, et al. Integrative analysis reveals selective 9p24.1 amplification, increased PD-1 ligand expression, and further induction via JAK2 in nodular sclerosing Hodgkin lymphoma and primary mediastinal large B-cell lymphoma. *Blood.* 2010;116:3268-3277.

60 Hartmann S, Schuhmacher B, Rausch T, et al. Highly recurrent mutations of SGK1, DUSP2 and JUNB in nodular lymphocyte predominant Hodgkin lymphoma. *Leukemia.* 2016;30:844-853.

Chapter 3

Classification of Hodgkin and non-Hodgkin lymphoma

Joo Y Song and Dennis D Weisenburger

Introduction

The World Health Organization (WHO) classification of lymphoid neoplasms [1,2] was built upon earlier classifications such as the Lukes-Collins [3], Kiel [4], and Revised European-American Lymphoma (REAL) [5] classifications. It represents a worldwide consensus on the diagnosis of lymphoid neoplasms, which is updated and refined periodically by incorporating emerging concepts and new data. The anticipated most recent 2016 classification is listed in Tables 3.1 and 3.2 (unpublished data; adapted from [2]).

The foundation of the WHO classification is the cell of origin of the neoplasm, which places different lymphoid neoplasms into B-cell, T-cell, and natural killer (NK)-cell groups defined by morphologic and immunohistochemical features to detect important differences in the expression of cell proteins on the cell surface. It then incorporates clinical features, genetic, and more recently molecular data to further define distinctive disease entities as has been shown by successive changes in the WHO classification for example, in 2001, 2008, and the upcoming 2016 classification. This is complicated by the fact that although many genetic and chromosomal changes may be indicative of a disease process, they are not specific. As an example, recurrent genetic aberrations have been

© Springer International Publishing AG 2017
J. Zain and L.W. Kwak (eds.), *Management of Lymphomas:
A Case-Based Approach*, DOI 10.1007/978-3-319-26827-9_3

Mature B-cell neoplasms
Chronic lymphocytic leukemia/small lymphocytic lymphoma
Monoclonal B-cell lymphocytosis*
B-cell prolymphocytic leukemia
Splenic marginal zone lymphoma
Hairy cell leukemia
Hairy cell leukemia-variant
Splenic B-cell lymphoma/leukemia, unclassifiable
Splenic diffuse red pulp small B-cell lymphoma
Lymphoplasmacytic lymphoma
Plasma cell neoplasms
Monoclonal gammopathy of undetermined significance (MGUS), IgM*
Monoclonal gammopathy of undetermined significance (MGUS), IgG/A
Gamma heavy chain disease
Mu heavy chain disease
Alpha heavy chain disease
Plasma cell myeloma
Solitary plasmacytoma of bone
Extraosseous plasmacytoma
Monoclonal immunoglobulin deposition diseases
Extranodal marginal zone lymphoma of mucosa-associated lymphoid tissue (MALT lymphoma)
Nodal marginal zone lymphoma
Pediatric nodal marginal zone lymphoma
Follicular lymphoma
In situ follicular neoplasia*
Pediatric type follicular lymphoma
Large B-cell lymphoma with IRF4 rearrangement*
Primary cutaneous follicle center lymphoma
Mantle cell lymphoma
In situ mantle cell neoplasia*
Diffuse large B-cell lymphoma (DLBCL), not otherwise specified (NOS)
T-cell/histiocyte-rich large B-cell lymphoma
Primary DLBCL of the central nervous system
Primary cutaneous DLBCL, leg type
Epstein-Barr virus (EBV)-positive DLBCL, not otherwise specified*
EBV-positive mucocutaneous ulcer*
*Potential changes in the 2016 WHO classification

Table 3.1 World Health Organization classification of mature B-cell neoplasms. Adapted from © International Agency for Research on Cancer, 2008. All rights reserved. Swerdlow et al [2].

Mature B-cell neoplasms
T-cell prolymphocytic leukemia
T-cell large granular lymphocytic leukemia
Chronic lymphoproliferative disorder of NK cells
Aggressive NK-cell leukemia
EBV-positive T-cell lymphoproliferative diseases of childhood
Chronic active EBV infection, cutaneous
Chronic active EBV infection, systemic
Hydroa vacciniforme-like lymphoma
Severe mosquito bite hypersensitivity
Systemic EBV-positive T-cell lymphoma of childhood
Adult T-cell leukemia/lymphoma
Extranodal NK/T-cell lymphoma, nasal type
Enteropathy-associated T-cell lymphoma
Monomorphic epitheliotropic intestinal T-cell lymphoma*
Indolent T-cell lymphoproliferative disorder of the gastrointestinal tract*
Hepatosplenic T-cell lymphoma
Subcutaneous panniculitis-like T-cell lymphoma
Mycosis fungoides
Sézary syndrome
Primary cutaneous CD30-positive T-cell lymphoproliferative disorders
Lymphomatoid papulosis
Primary cutaneous anaplastic large cell lymphoma
Primary cutaneous gamma-delta T-cell lymphoma
Primary cutaneous CD8-positive aggressive epidermotropic cytotoxic T-cell lymphoma
Primary cutaneous acral CD8-positive T-cell lymphoma*
Primary cutaneous CD4-positive small/medium T-cell lymphoproliferative disorder*
Peripheral T-cell lymphoma, NOS
Angioimmunoblastic T-cell lymphoma
Follicular T-cell lymphoma*
Anaplastic large cell lymphoma, anaplastic lymphoma kinase (ALK)-positive
Anaplastic large cell lymphoma, ALK-negative
Breast implant-associated anaplastic large cell lymphoma*

Table 3.2 World Health Organization classification of mature T/NK-cell neoplasms and Hodgkin lymphoma (continues overleaf). Adapted from © International Agency for Research on Cancer, 2008. All rights reserved. Swerdlow et al [2].

Hodgkin lymphoma
Nodular lymphocyte predominant Hodgkin lymphoma
Classical Hodgkin lymphoma
Nodular sclerosis classical Hodgkin lymphoma
Lymphocyte-rich classical Hodgkin lymphoma
Mixed cellularity classical Hodgkin lymphoma
Lymphocyte-depleted classical Hodgkin lymphoma
*Potential changes in the 2016 WHO classification

Table 3.2 World Health Organization classification of mature T/NK-cell neoplasms and Hodgkin lymphoma (continued). Adapted from © International Agency for Research on Cancer, 2008. All rights reserved. Swerdlow et al [2].

identified in many lymphomas such as the t(14;18)(q32;q21) in follicular lymphoma and the t(2;5)(p23;q35) in anaplastic large cell lymphoma (ALCL). Although these translocations are considered a genetic hallmark of the disease, they are not always definitive. The *MYC* translocations are known to be important in Burkitt lymphoma but can also be seen in some cases of diffuse large B-cell lymphomas (DLBCL), as well as plasmablastic lymphomas. The *BCL2/IGH* translocation is found in the majority of follicular lymphomas, but is absent in some cases and is also seen in a subset of de novo DLBCL. Hence arriving at an accurate diagnosis requires a multidisciplinary approach with careful attention to clinical features and other aspects of the disease. In the following section, an attempt will be made to give an overview of the new 2016 WHO classification and to highlight some of the changes that will be incorporated in this classification.

Clinical features in lymphoma
Role of clinical features in the classification of lymphoma
The site of involvement at presentation is important in many subtypes of lymphoma and defines the unique clinical and biologic features of that subtype. These include primary mediastinal B-cell lymphoma, primary central nervous system large cell lymphoma as well as marginal zone lymphomas of mucosa-associated lymphoid tissue (MALT), and cutaneous T-cell lymphomas. Epstein-Barr virus (EBV)-positive mucocutaneous ulcer [6] has histologic overlap with classical Hodgkin lymphoma but the

latter typically does not involve the skin, oral cavity, or gastrointestinal tract. As with the immunophenotype and genetic abnormalities, the clinical presentation can be important in defining the subtype of lymphoma.

Age at presentation can be an important diagnostic criteria in some of the newer disease entities. Children can also develop lymphomas similar to their adult counterparts but they are clinically distinct in regard to biology and prognosis. The pediatric variant of follicular lymphoma [7] typically lacks the *BCL2/IGH* translocation and often involves extranodal sites such as the testis, gastrointestinal tract, and Waldeyer's ring. Pediatric follicular lymphoma also differs from adult follicular lymphoma in that, despite the high-grade cytology (typically grade 3), the former is associated with limited stage disease and a good prognosis. Pediatric marginal zone lymphoma [8] also differs from the adult variant in that the former is usually localized and well controlled with conservative management. However, it is important to note that the future WHO classification will eliminate the term 'elderly' from EBV-positive DLBCL as these lesions can also been seen in patients younger than 50 years of age [9,10].

Early lesions

These are now recognized as early lymphoproliferative lesions that may or may not progress to overt lymphoma over time. Two examples are monoclonal B-cell lymphocytosis (MBL) and monoclonal gammopathy of undetermined significance (MGUS). Both of these disorders are considered precursor lesions to overt malignancy but not all cases progress. MBL can have the same genetic aberrations as chronic lymphocytic leukemia (CLL) but most cases never progress to overt leukemia [11]. The same is true of MGUS, which also has overlapping cytogenetic abnormalities with plasma cell myeloma [12]. Both of these examples are distinguished from their malignant counterpart by clinical features such as the absolute lymphocyte count or identification of end-organ involvement (hypercalcemia, renal failure, anemia, or bony lesions). Other precursor lesions have been listed as entities in the most recent WHO classification, such as in situ mantle cell [13] and follicular neoplasia [14]. In situ follicular neoplasia has been seen simultaneously with or prior to the development of overt follicular lymphoma [15]. However, most patients with in situ follicular neoplasia will never develop follicular lymphoma as additional genetic 'hits' are necessary for lymphomagenesis [16]. In situ mantle cell neoplasia also has a low risk of progression to overt mantle cell lymphoma and does not require treatment when found in isolation but should prompt routine follow-up [13].

As mentioned previously, genetic aberrations such as translocations are not disease-defining or necessarily indicative of overt lymphoma. Healthy individuals can have a low level of circulating lymphoid cells with classical translocations, such as *BCL2/IGH* or *NPM/ALK1*, which would be disease-defining as follicular lymphoma [17] or ALCL [18], respectively, in the right clinical context. Therefore, these findings emphasize that additional genetic aberrations are needed for the development of overt lymphoma.

New lymphoproliferative disorders with an indolent behavior

Recently, an atypical lymphoma-like lesion involving the skin and mucosa was described in older patients with various types of immunosuppression. This lesion, named mucocutaneous ulcer [6], has morphologic features of Hodgkin-like cells and can mimic cutaneous or mucosal involvement of classical Hodgkin lymphoma but the lesions are usually localized and regress after a taper of the immunosuppressive therapy.

Although the majority of T- and NK-cell lymphomas have an aggressive clinical course, some cases have been found to have a more indolent clinical pattern [19,20]. A recent study by Perry et al described 10 cases of a T-cell lymphoproliferative disorder that mimics intestinal T-cell lymphoma [20]. These cases had disease localized to the gastrointestinal tract and had an indolent clinical course that did not require treatment.

Another example of a T-cell proliferation with an excellent prognosis is primary cutaneous CD4-positive small/medium T-cell lymphoma ('lymphoproliferation' in the updated 2016 WHO classification). These cases are localized, indolent, spontaneously regress, and may be difficult to distinguish from pseudolymphomas or reactive lymphoid hyperplasia [21]. They may have a clonal T-cell receptor gene rearrangement with increased programmed cell death (PD-1)-positive T-cells [22].

Recently, cases of a CD8-positive T-cell proliferation involving the ear with histology mimicking a high-grade T-cell lymphoma have been reported [23,24]. These cases typically have a cytotoxic phenotype with clonal T-cell gene rearrangements, but are localized to the ear or other acral sites and also have an indolent behavior. These T-cell lymphoproliferative disorders can mimic overt T-cell lymphoma but are usually localized and have an indolent clinical behavior requiring little to no treatment. They are to be incorporated in the upcoming WHO classification to emphasize the importance of identifying such cases so that they do not receive unnecessary or aggressive treatment.

Large B-cell lymphomas

In the 2008 WHO classification [2], a category of 'gray zone' lymphomas was created which includes B-cell lymphomas intermediate between classical Hodgkin lymphoma (CHL) and primary mediastinal B-cell lymphoma (PMBL), and B-cell lymphoma intermediate between Burkitt lymphoma and DLBCL. Recently, studies have found a morphologic and immunophenotypic overlap between CHL and PMBL [25–28]. These cases typically involve the mediastinum, in young adults and have a more aggressive behavior than either CHL or PMBL [29].

Burkitt lymphoma usually has a characteristic *MYC* translocation with an immunoglobulin partner. Recently, however, cases resembling Burkitt lymphoma with a gene expression profile consistent with this type of lymphoma but lacking a *MYC* translocation and having aberrations of chromosome 11q have been described [30]. These cases may be included as a provisional entity of Burkitt-like lymphomas with 11q aberration in the upcoming WHO classification. *MYC* translocations may also be found in cases of typical DLBCL. Therefore, the morphologic, cytogenetic, and immunophenotypic findings need to be taken into consideration when making a diagnosis of Burkitt lymphoma [31,32]. 'Double hit' DLBCL, defined by either translocations of *BCL2* and/or *BCL6* and *MYC*, has been found to have a poor prognosis despite the cell-of-origin in such cases (germinal center versus non-germinal center) [33–35]. Cases with overexpression of *BCL2* and *MYC* also have a worse outcome compared with typical DLBCL [33,36].

Salaverria et al have recently described a germinal center-derived DLBCL that occurs predominately in the pediatric setting and carries an *IG/IRF4* translocation. Such cases are frequently seen concurrently with pediatric follicular lymphoma and were found to have a favorable outcome [37,38]. This form of DLBCL with IRF4 rearrangements may be a distinct entity from other types of DLBCL (Figure 3.1).

Peripheral T-cell lymphomas

Many cases of peripheral T-cell lymphomas (PTCL) cannot be classified as a specific disease entity and are placed in the 'not otherwise specified (NOS)' category, which has been somewhat of a 'wastebasket' category. The other major types of PTCL are ALCL, anaplastic lymphoma kinase (ALK)-positive and ALK-negative subtypes, angioimmunoblastic T-cell lymphoma (AITL), adult T-cell lymphoma/leukemia, and hepatosplenic T-cell lymphoma.

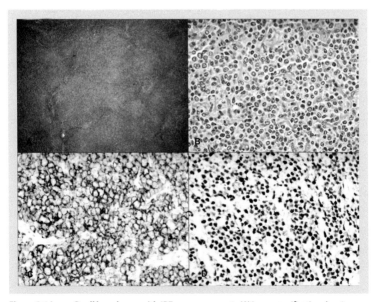

Figure 3.1 Large B cell lymphoma with *IRF* rearrangement. (A) Low magnification showing a vaguely nodular pattern composed of (B) large atypical cells. These cells are positive for (C) CD20 and (D) MUM1, and have an *IRF* rearrangement by FISH analysis (not shown).

Angioimmunoblastic T-cell lymphoma has a follicular helper T-cell (TFH) phenotype, but there are cases that lack some of the classic features of AITL (lack of expanded follicular dendritic meshworks or lack of EBV-positive B-cells). Cases of PTCL that do not have the classical features of AITL and cases of the follicular variant of PTCL, NOS, will likely be incorporated as a new entity of follicular T-cell lymphoma in the updated WHO classification.

Recently, two major molecular subtypes have been identified within PTCL, NOS, which have either high expression of *GATA3* or *TBX21* [39,40]. A high expression of GATA3 was typically associated with a poor clinical outcome. Continued genetic and molecular data will help delineate the category of PTCL, NOS.

Breast implant-associated ALCL was first described in 1997 and the number of cases has grown with the popularity of cosmetic surgery (Figure 3.2) [41]. Most patients with breast implant-associated ALCL achieve a complete remission after capsulectomy and removal of the

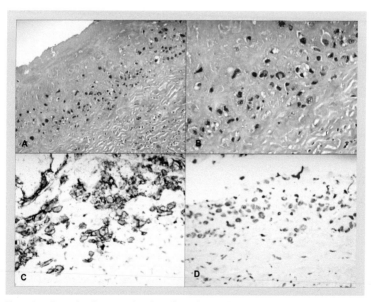

Figure 3.2. Breast implant-associated anaplastic large cell lymphoma. (A) The capsule of the implant shows large atypical cells (B) with some characteristic hallmark cells. (C) The cells are CD30 positive and (D) negative for ALK1 protein.

implant, but patients who present with tumor mass typically have a more aggressive clinical course and these will likely require chemotherapy [42].

Enteropathy-associated T-cell lymphoma (EATL) has two distinct subtypes: type I and type II. Type I is the most common form, typically negative for both CD4 and CD8, frequently shows admixture of eosinophils, and has a strong association with celiac disease. Type II EATL has a monomorphic morphology, predominately CD8- and CD56-positive, and has a weak association with celiac disease [2]. Recently, many cases of EATL type II were found to express the gamma-delta T-cell receptor [43]. Given the differences in clinicopathologic and epidemiologic findings between EATL type I and type II, the latter will likely be separated from this disease entity and designated as 'monomorphic epitheliotropic intestinal T-cell lymphoma'.

Conclusion

The WHO classification is the result of an international collaboration of clinicians, pathologists, and scientists to create a common language of disease entities in lymphoma. The classification of lymphoid neoplasms will continue to evolve as our knowledge in the fields of cellular and molecular biology advances.

References

1 Jaffe ES, Harris NL, Stein H, Vardiman JW (eds). *Pathology and Genetics of Tumours of Haematopoietic and Lymphoid Tissues*. Lyon, France: IARC Press; 2001.

2 Swerdlow SH, Campo E, Harris NL, et al (eds) *WHO Classification of Tumours of Haematopoietic and Lymphoid Tissues, Fourth Edition*. Lyon, France: IARC Press; 2008.

3 Lukes RJ, Collins RD. Immunologic characterization of human malignant lymphomas. *Cancer*. 1974;34:suppl:1488-1503.

4 Stansfeld A, Diebold J, Noel H, et al. Updated Kiel classification for lymphomas. *The Lancet*. 1988;331:292-293.

5 Harris NI , Jaffe ES, Stein H, et al. A revised European-American classification of lymphoid neoplasms: a proposal from the International Lymphoma Study Group. *Blood*. 1994;84:1361-1392.

6 Dojcinov SD, Venkataraman G, Raffeld M, Pitaluga S, Jaffe ES. EBV positive mucocutaneous ulcer–a study of 26 cases associated with various sources of immunosuppression. *Am J Surg Pathol*. 34:405-417.

7 Liu Q, Salaverria I, Pittaluga S, et al. Follicular lymphomas in children and young adults: a comparison of the pediatric variant with usual follicular lymphoma. *Am J Surg Pathol*. 2012;37:333-343.

8 Swerdlow SH. Pediatric follicular lymphomas, marginal zone lymphomas, and marginal zone hyperplasia. *Am J Clin Pathol*. 2004;122 Suppl:S98-S109.

9   Kojima M, Kashimura M, Itoh H, et al. Epstein-Barr virus-related reactive lymphoproliferative disorders in middle-aged or elderly patients presenting with atypical features. A clinicopathological study of six cases. *Pathol Res Pract*. 2007;203:587-591.

10 Asano N, Yamamoto K, Tamaru J, et al. Age-related Epstein-Barr virus (EBV)-associated B-cell lymphoproliferative disorders: comparison with EBV-positive classic Hodgkin lymphoma in elderly patients. *Blood*. 2009;113:2629-2636.

11 Karube K, Scarfò L, Campo E, Ghia P. Monoclonal B cell lymphocytosis and "in situ" lymphoma. *Semin Cancer Biol*. 2014;24:3-14.

12 Avet-Loiseau H, Facon T, Grosbois B, et al. Oncogenesis of multiple myeloma: 14q32 and 13q chromosomal abnormalities are not randomly distributed, but correlate with natural history, immunological features, and clinical presentation. *Blood*. 2002;99:2185-2191.

13 Carvajal-Cuenca A, Sua LF, Silva NM, et al. In situ mantle cell lymphoma: clinical implications of an incidental finding with indolent clinical behavior. *Haematologica*. 2012;97:277-278.

14 Cong P, Raffeld M, Teruya-Feldstein J, Sorbara L, Pittaluga S, Jaffe ES. In situ localization of follicular lymphoma: description and analysis by laser capture microdissection. *Blood*. 2002;99:3376-3382.

15 Jegalian AG, Eberle FC, Pack SD, et al. Follicular lymphoma in situ: clinical implications and comparisons with partial involvement by follicular lymphoma. *Blood*. 2011;118:2976-2984.

16 Mamessier E, Song JY, Eberle FC, et al. Early lesions of follicular lymphoma: a genetic perspective. *Haematologica*. 2014;99:481-488.

17 Roulland S, Navarro JM, Grenot P, et al. Follicular lymphoma-like B cells in healthy individuals: a novel intermediate step in early lymphomagenesis. *J Exp Med*. 2006;203:2425-2431.

18 Trümper L, Pfreundschuh M, Bonin FV, Daus H. Detection of the t(2;5)-associated NPM/ALK fusion cDNA in peripheral blood cells of healthy individuals. *Br J Haematol*. 1998;103:1138-1144.

19 Mansoor A, Pittaluga S, Beck PL, Wilson WH, Ferry JA, Jaffe ES. NK-cell enteropathy: a benign NK-cell lymphoproliferative disease mimicking intestinal lymphoma: clinicopathologic features and follow-up in a unique case series. *Blood*. 2011;117:1447-1452.

20 Perry AM, Warnke RA, Hu Q, et al. Indolent T-cell lymphoproliferative disease of the gastrointestinal tract. *Blood*. 2013;122:3599-3606.

21 Lan TT, Brown NA, Hristov Ac. Controversies and considerations in the diagnosis of primary cutaneous CD4(+) small/medium T-cell lymphoma. *Arch Pathol Lab Med*. 2014;138:1307-1318.

22 Cetinozman F, Jansen PM, Willemze R. Expression of programmed death-1 in primary cutaneous CD4-positive small/medium-sized pleomorphic T-cell lymphoma, cutaneous pseudo-T-cell lymphoma, and other types of cutaneous T-cell lymphoma. *Am J Surg Pathol*. 2012;36:109-116.

23 Petrella T, Maubec C, Conillet-Lefebvre P, et al. Indolent CD8-positive lymphoid proliferation of the ear: a distinct primary cutaneous T-cell lymphoma? *Am J Surg Pathol*. 2007;31:1887-1892.

24 Greenblatt D, Ally M, Child F, et al. Indolent CD8(+) lymphoid proliferation of acral sites: a clinicopathologic study of six patients with some atypical features. *J Cutan Pathol*. 2013;40:248-258.

25 Savage KJ, Monti S, Kutok JI, et al. The molecular signature of mediastinal large B-cell lymphoma differs from that of other diffuse large B-cell lymphomas and shares features with classical Hodgkin lymphoma. *Blood*. 2003;102:3871-3879.

26 Savage KJ, Al-Rajhi N, Voss N, et al. Favorable outcome of primary mediastinal large B-cell lymphoma in a single institution: the British Columbia experience. *Ann Oncol*. 2006;17:123-130.

27 Eberle FC, Salaverria I, Steidl C, et al. Gray zone lymphoma: chromosomal aberrations with immunophenotypic and clinical correlations. *Mod Pathol*. 2011;24:1586-1597.

28 Eberle FC, Rodriguez-Canales J, Wei L, et al. Methylation profiling of mediastinal gray zone lymphoma reveals a distinctive signature with elements shared by classical Hodgkin's lymphoma and primary mediastinal large B-cell lymphoma." *Haematologica*. 2011;96:558-566.

29 Dunleavy K, Grant C, Eberle FC, Pittaluga S, Jaffe ES, Wilson WH. Gray zone lymphoma: better treated like hodgkin lymphoma or mediastinal large B-cell lymphoma? *Curr Hematol Malig Rep*. 2012;7:241-247.

30 Salaverria I, Martin-Guerrero I, Wagener r, et al. A recurrent 11q aberration pattern characterizes a subset of MYC-negative high-grade B-cell lymphomas resembling Burkitt lymphoma. *Blood*. 2014;123:1187-1198.

31 Dave SS, Fu K, Wright GW, et al. Molecular diagnosis of Burkitt's lymphoma. *N Engl J Med*. 2006;354:2431-2442.

32 Horn H, Staiger AM, Vöhringer M, et al. Diffuse large B-cell lymphomas of immunoblastic type are a major reservoir for MYC-IGH translocations. *Am J Surg Pathol*.

33 Johnson NA, Slack GW, Savage KJ, et al. Concurrent expression of MYC and BCL2 in diffuse large B-cell lymphoma treated with rituximab plus cyclophosphamide, doxorubicin, vincristine, and prednisone. *J Clin Oncol*. 2012;30:3452-3459.

34 Pillai RK, Sathanoori M, Van Oss SB, Swerdlow SH. Double-hit lymphomas with BCL6 and MYC translocations are aggressive, frequently extranodal lymphomas distinct from BCL2 double-hit B-cell lymphomas. *Am J Surg Pathol*. 2013;37:323-332.

35 Caponetti GC, Dave BJ, Perry AM, et al. Isolated MYC cytogenetic abnormalities in diffuse large B-cell lymphoma do not predict an adverse clinical outcome. *Leuk Lymphoma*. 2015;56:3082-3089.

36 Horn H, Ziepert M, Becher C, et al. MYC status in concert with BCL2 and BCL6 expression predicts outcome in diffuse large B-cell lymphoma. *Blood*. 2013;121:2253-2263.

37 Salaverria I, Philipp C, Oschlies I, et al. Translocations activating IRF4 identify a subtype of germinal center-derived B-cell lymphoma affecting predominantly children and young adults. *Blood*. 2011;118:139-147.

38 Salaverria I, Martin-Guerrero I, Burkhardt B, et al. High resolution copy number analysis of IRF4 translocation-positive diffuse large B-cell and follicular lymphomas. Genes Chromosomes Iqbal J, Wright G, Wang C, et al. Gene expression signatures delineate biological and prognostic subgroups in peripheral T-cell lymphoma. *Blood*. 2014;123:2915-2923.

39 Wang T, Feldman AL, Wada DA, et al. GATA-3 expression identifies a high-risk subset of PTCL, NOS with distinct molecular and clinical features. *Blood*. 2014;123:3007-3015.

40 Keech JA Jr, Creech BJ. Anaplastic T-cell lymphoma in proximity to a saline-filled breast implant. *Plast Reconstr Surg*. 1997;100:554-555.

41 Miranda RN, Aladily TN, Prince HM, et al. Breast implant-associated anaplastic large-cell lymphoma: long-term follow-up of 60 patients. *J Clin Oncol*. 2014;32:114-120.

42 Chan JK, Chan AC, Cheuk W, et al. Type II enteropathy-associated T-cell lymphoma: a distinct aggressive lymphoma with frequent gammadelta T-cell receptor expression. *Am J Surg Pathol*. 2011;35:1557-1569.

Indolent B-cell lymphomas

Chapter 4

Small B-cell lymphocytic lymphoma and chronic lymphocytic leukemia

Tanya Siddiqi and Steven T Rosen

Case presentation

A 72-year-old man with a history of diabetes mellitus, hypertension, and hypercholesterolemia self-palpated a left submandibular lump in 2012. Complete blood count (CBC) in his internist's office showed solitary leukocytosis (white count 22) with predominant lymphocytes for which he was referred to a hematologist. Peripheral blood flow cytometry on 04/11/12 confirmed chronic lymphocytic leukemia (CLL)/small lymphocytic lymphoma (SLL): abnormal cell population comprising 63% of CD45 positive leukocytes, co-expressing CD5 and CD23 in CD19-positive B cells. CD38 was negative but other prognostic markers were not assessed at that time. The patient was observed regularly for the next 3 years and his white count trend was as follows: 22.8 (4/2012) → 28.5 (07/2012) → 32.2 (12/2012) → 36.5 (02/2013) → 42 (09/2013) → 44.9 (01/2014) → 75.8 (2/2015). His other counts stayed normal until early 2015 when he also developed anemia (hemoglobin [HGB] 10.9) although platelets remained normal at 215. He had been noticing enlargement of his cervical, submandibular, supraclavicular, and axillary lymphadenopathy for several months since 2014 and a positron emission tomography (PET)/computed tomography (CT) scan done in 12/2014 had shown extensive diffuse lymphadenopathy

© Springer International Publishing AG 2017
J. Zain and L.W. Kwak (eds.), *Management of Lymphomas: A Case-Based Approach*, DOI 10.1007/978-3-319-26827-9_4

within the neck, chest, abdomen, and pelvis. Maximum standardized uptake value (SUV max) was similar to low baseline activity within the vasculature of the neck and chest. In the abdomen and pelvis, however, there was mild to moderately hypermetabolic adenopathy measuring up to SUV of 4. The largest right neck nodes measured up to 2.3 x 3 cm and left neck nodes measured up to 2.3 x 1.5 cm. His right axillary lymphadenopathy measured up to 5.5 x 2.6 cm and on the left measured up to 4.8 x 3.4 cm. Lymph nodes on the right abdomen and pelvis measured up to 6.7 cm and seemed to have some mass effect with compression on the urinary bladder without symptoms. He underwent a bone marrow biopsy on 02/03/15, which revealed hypercellular marrow (60%) with involvement by CLL (30%); flow cytometry showed CD38 and ZAP-70 positivity; fluorescence in situ hybridization (FISH) analysis showed 13q deletion/monosomy 13; IgVH was unmutated; karyotype was 46XY.

He came to see us for treatment recommendations in 06/2015 and reported some episodes of non-drenching night sweats and progressing fatigue over the last several months. He denied any unexplained weight loss or frequent/lingering/recurrent infections except for one episode of an upper respiratory tract infection requiring antibiotics this year. Eastern Cooperative Oncology Group (ECOG) performance status was 1. Based on his examination that day and most recent laboratory tests, he was determined to be at Binet stage A (Rai stage 1).

Introduction and epidemiology

According to the World Health Organization (WHO) classification, CLL is a low grade leukemic lymphocytic lymphoma and is distinguishable from SLL by its leukemic presentation [1]. SLL is essentially a nodal form of the same disease. CLL/SLL is a disease of malignant clonal B lymphocytes and is the most common hematologic malignancy of the Western world with an incidence of about 5/100,000 persons per year in the United States [2]. Incidence increases with age significantly and the median age at diagnosis is 72 years although about 10% CLL/SLL patients present at age <55 years. There is a male predominance in an approximately 2:1 pattern. The incidence is higher among Caucasians than other races. About 10% patients with CLL/SLL report a family history of some lymphoproliferative disorder [3] so it is suspected that some genetic predisposition occurs in individuals although the exact etiology of CLL/SLL development is largely unknown.

Work up and diagnosis

At the time of diagnosis, it is important to confirm that the patient has CLL/SLL and not a masquerading lymphoproliferative disorder like hairy cell leukemia or the leukemic phase of mantle cell lymphoma, marginal zone lymphoma, or follicular lymphoma. All patients should undergo a history and physical examination (historical review of prior CBCs may shed some light on how long the patient may have had lymphocytosis for before the actual diagnosis of CLL/SLL) as well as laboratory testing for complete blood counts/differential, peripheral blood smear review, and peripheral blood flow cytometry/immunophenotyping. A bone marrow biopsy is typically not needed to diagnose CLL but should be performed if another lymphoproliferative disorder is suspected as well as for the evaluation of cytopenias, especially prior to starting any therapy. Also, bone marrow biopsy is recommended in patients with persisting cytopenias after treatment in order to uncover disease-related versus therapy-related causes.

The diagnosis of CLL requires peripheral blood lymphocytosis with the presence of ≥ 5000 monoclonal B-cells/uL for at least 3 months duration. The leukemia cells in peripheral blood are typically small, mature lymphocytes with scant cytoplasm, dense chromatin, and lack prominent nucleoli. Admixed with these mature lymphocytes, there may be some larger or atypical lymphocytes, cleaved lymphocytes, or prolymphocytes. Prolymphocytes in excess of 55% of total lymphocyte count would favor a diagnosis of B-cell prolymphocytic leukemia (B-PLL). Cellular debris called smudge cells are often found in the peripheral blood smear of CLL patients as well.

Presence of monoclonal lymphocytosis but with <5000 B-cells/uL in the peripheral blood and no accompanying lymphadenopathy or organo-megaly by physical examination or radiographical imaging, cytopenias, or disease-related symptoms is defined as monoclonal B-lymphocytosis (MBL). The incidence of MBL in the United States is about 3.5% in individuals younger than 40 years and increases with age [4]. In Europe, depending on the sensitivity of the test used, the prevalence ranges from 6.7–12% in individuals older than 40 years of age. Progression of MBL to frank CLL can occur at a rate of 1–2% per year. Presence of lymphadenopathy and/or splenomegaly with or without peripheral blood and some lymphocytosis (if present, must be <5000 B-cells/uL of total lymphocytes) may be pure SLL and should be diagnosed formally with a lymph node biopsy. The presence of any cytopenia caused by bone marrow infiltration by disease is consistent with a diagnosis of CLL regardless of the peripheral blood B-lymphocytosis level or the presence/absence of lymphadenopathy [5]. The entity formerly known as T-cell CLL has been re-classified by the WHO as T-PLL.

Immunophenotyping

Leukemic CLL cells co-express the T-cell antigen CD5 along with the B-cell surface antigens CD19, CD20, and CD23. The clonal leukemic cells express either surface kappa or lambda immunoglobulin (Ig) light chains with variable intensity. Levels of surface Ig, CD20, and CD79b are characteristically of low intensity in CLL cells compared with normal B-cells. In contrast, B-PLL cells do not express CD5 in 50% cases and have brighter CD20 and surface Ig expression. On the other hand, leukemic mantle cell lymphoma cells do not express CD23 even though they do co-express other B-cell surface antigens and CD5.

Additional testing

If indicated, baseline testing should also include direct Coombs test, lactate dehydrogenase (LDH), haptoglobin, reticulocyte, and bilirubin to evaluate for the presence of autoimmune hemolytic anemia. Quantitative immunoglobulin levels should be measured periodically to follow progressive hypogammaglobulinemia and/or any monoclonal gammopathy.

Prognostic markers

- Cytogenetics/FISH : interphase FISH assessment of CLL cells can show cytogenetic abnormalities in more than 80% cases. The most common abnormality is a deletion in the long arm of chromosome

13 (del13q14) (~55%) that harbors the miRNAs miR-15a and 16-1, which may be involved in the pathogenesis of CLL/SLL [6]. In general, isolated del13q is a good prognostic marker characterizing a benign disease course and is often found early in the course of the disease. Other aberrations include:

1. trisomy of chromosome 12 (+12; 10–20%) – prognostic relevance of this is uncertain;

2. deletion in the long arm of chromosome 11 (del11q23; 10–25%) harboring the *ATM* gene – these patients typically have bulky lymphadenopathy, rapid disease progression, and reduced overall survival;

3. deletion in the long arm of chromosome 6 (del6q); and

4. deletion in the short arm of chromosome 17 (del17p13; 5–10%) harboring the tumor suppressor gene *TP53* – del17p is considered the most significant negative prognostic factor in CLL. The TP53 protein normally responds to DNA damage by inducing cell cycle arrest and facilitating DNA repair. It can also induce apoptosis in cells with damaged DNA and in this way mediates the cytotoxicity of many anticancer agents. Resistance to treatment is a particular characteristic of *TP53* deletion and has been observed for agents including purine analogs (del11q can also confer some resistance to standard chemoimmunotherapy regimens, especially those containing purine analogs). Deletion 17p typically occurs upon relapse after therapy or at the time of disease progression (clonal evolution) although it can be an initial cytogenetic abnormality in ~5% patients. A subset of patients may have the very poor prognostic *TP53* gene mutations (4–37%) that can be missed on FISH analysis and, therefore, it is advisable to perform conventional cytogenetics in addition to FISH before any new treatment is undertaken as there could be therapeutic ramifications of *del17p* and *TP53* mutations. *TP53* mutations are associated with higher genomic complexity in CLL.

- Lymphocyte doubling time: a lymphocyte doubling time of <12 months is associated with a poor prognosis.

- IgV_H gene rearrangement status: somatic hypermutation of IgV_H is a normal process in B-cell physiology and is responsible for the diverse immunoglobulin pool. CLL cells that retain this normal process (mutated IgV_H) have a better prognosis than CLL cells that lack this capability (unmutated IgV_H). Prospective clinical trials are needed to validate and standardize the assessment of this parameter and to determine if it should affect the management of patients with CLL.

- ZAP70: this encodes a T-cell receptor-associated protein tyrosine kinase that is involved in intracellular signaling. Expression of ZAP70 confers a poor prognosis as it is thought to be correlated with unmutated IgV_H status in 70% cases. However, this test has poor reproducibility in different laboratories.

- CD38 expression: this is a cyclic ADP ribose hydrolase on cell surfaces and is detectable by flow cytometry. Expression of CD38 is also correlated with unmutated IgV_H status in 70% cases and so also confers a poor prognosis.

- B2 microglobulin: levels >3.5 mg/L are associated with a poorer prognosis.

- *Notch 1* mutation: next generation sequencing has led to the identification of novel somatic mutations that can predict behavior of CLL/SLL in patients [7]. *Notch 1* mutations are the most frequent somatic aberrations in CLL, affecting 5–10% newly diagnosed patients, 15–20% progressing patients in need of frontline therapy, and 30% Richter transformation patients [7]. *SF3B1* is another recurrently mutated gene in CLL/SLL (5–10% newly diagnosed patients, 15% progressing patients in need of frontline therapy, and 20–25% relapsed and fludarabine-refractory patients). In addition to the poor prognostic effects of mutations in DNA-repair genes (*TP53* and *ATM*), *Notch 1*-activating mutations can lead to apoptosis resistance with increased survival of tumor cells. Clinically, *Notch 1*-mutated CLL/SLL patients show features associated with poor prognosis and have a high risk of Richter transformation and poor outcome [7,8]. *Notch 1* mutations are associated with unmutated IgV_H and trisomy 12 while *SF3B1* mutations are more preferentially associated with *del11q* and *ATM* mutations [8]. The precise biological consequence of *SF3B1* mutations in CLL is currently unknown.

- Bone marrow biopsy: typically >30% of nucleated cells in the bone marrow are CLL/SLL cells. Diffuse pattern of marrow infiltration reflects tumor burden and may be prognostic but the above mentioned newer markers have superseded the prognostic value of bone marrow biopsies in general.

Staging

Rai and Binet staging systems are the commonly used staging systems and both divide CLL/SLL patients into low, intermediate, and high risk categories (see Table 4.1 and Table 4.2).

Recommended treatment and discussion:

Treatment of CLL/SLL is indicated for patients who have active disease as defined by guidelines developed by the International workshop on CLL (iwCLL) [5]:

- evidence of progressive marrow failure as manifested by the development of, or worsening of, anemia and/or thrombocytopenia;
- massive (≥6cm below left subcostal margin), progressive, or symptomatic splenomegaly;

Binet stage	Clinical features
A	HGB≥10 g/dl, platelets ≥100/L, <3 areas of lymphadenopathy/ organomegaly*
B	HGB≥10 g/dl, platelets ≥100/L, ≥3 areas of lymphadenopathy/ organomegaly*
C	Anemia (<10g/dl), thrombocytopenia (<100,000/L), or both

Table 4.1 Binet staging system. *nodal areas: cervical [head and neck], axillary, inguinal (including femoral lymph nodes), spleen, liver. HGB, hemoglobin.

Rai stage	Risk category	Clinical features
0	Low	Lymphocytosis alone
1	Intermediate	Lymphadenopathy
2	Intermediate	Hepato/splenomegaly
3	High	Anemia (<11g/dl)
4	High	Thrombocytopenia (<100,000/L)

Table 4.2 Rai staging system.

- massive (≥10cm in longest diameter), progressive, or symptomatic lymphadenopathy;
- progressive lymphocytosis with an increase of >50% over a 2-month period or lymphocyte doubling time (LDT) of <6 months; if absolute lymphocyte count (ALC) is <30,000/L, LDT should not be used as a single parameter to define treatment indication; other factors contributing to lymphocytosis or lymphadenopathy (eg, infections) should be excluded;
- autoimmune hemolytic anemia and/or thrombocytopenia that is poorly responsive to corticosteroids or other standard therapy; and
- constitutional symptoms defined as ≥one of the following:
  - unintentional weight loss of ≥10% within the previous 6 months;
  - significant fatigue (ECOG performance status ≥2; inability to work or perform usual activities);
  - fevers >100.5°F or 38°C for ≥2 weeks without other evidence of infection; and
  - night sweats for >1 month without evidence of infection.

As the goal of therapy is not curative, for patients with no indication for treatment based on the criteria above, observation or a 'watch and wait' strategy should be employed.

This is how our patient in the case presentation at the start of this chapter was managed for the first 3–4 years after diagnosis. However, with time he has developed signs and symptoms indicating need for treatment: worsening lymphocytosis, lymphadenopathy, anemia, and fatigue. There is no standard treatment regimen for CLL patients with indication for treatment. Therapeutic options include radiation (limited to one area of symptomatic disease generally), chemotherapy, immunotherapy, novel targeted agents, immunomodulatory agents, and various combinations of these components. In the current era of rapidly emerging novel therapeutics and novel combinations of treatments, the best treatment is thought to be enrolment of eligible patients into clinical trials if available. This was our recommendation to the patient in the case presented for the frontline management of his active disease.

Treatment components (systemic)
Chemotherapy
Alkylating agents
Chlorambucil

This was the gold standard in CLL treatment for decades previously and can still be used in frail, elderly, unfit patients as it is a convenient and cheap oral agent and has relatively low toxicity [9]. Extended use can lead to prolonged cytopenias, myelodysplastic syndrome (MDS), or acute leukemia. Therefore, its use is generally limited to no more than 12 months duration. Complete remissions (CR) are rare with this agent although the responses are much better if combined with an anti-CD20 monoclonal antibody, especially obinutuzumab (see below).

Bendamustine

In a randomized trial comparing bendamustine with chlorambucil among previously untreated CLL/SLL patients, overall response rate (ORR) and median progression-free survival (PFS) were significantly better on the bendamustine arm (67% and 22 months, respectively) than for those receiving chlorambucil (30% and 8 months, respectively), $p<0.0001$ for both [10].

The combination of bendamustine and rituximab (BR) has been studied in both frontline and relapsed settings [11,12]. In the frontline setting, ORR was 88% (23.1% CR), but only 37.5% in del17p patients. Median event-free survival (EFS) was 33.9 months. Severe infections occurred in 7.7% patients and grade 3/4 cytopenias were seen in up to 22.2% patients. In the relapsed setting, ORR was 59% (9% CR), but only 7.1% among del17p patients. Median EFS was 14.7 months. Severe infections occurred in 12.8% patients and grade 3/4 cytopenias were seen in up to 28% patients. The direct comparison of BR with FCR (CLL10 trial) is discussed below.

Purine analogs
Fludarabine

This is the most studied purine analog in CLL/SLL. Single-agent fludarabine produced better ORRs than some other agents initially, including more CR rates (7–40% compared with cyclophosphamide, doxorubicin, and vincristine [CHOP], cyclophosphamide, adriamycin, and cisplatin [CAP], or chlorambucil), but did not improve survival [13,14]. The combination of fludarabine and cyclophosphamide (FC) improved the CR rate up to 50% [15] as did the addition of mitoxantrone to FC (50% durable CR rate) [16]. Three randomized trials of FC compared with fludarabine alone have shown improved ORR, CR, and PFS [17–19]. A re-analysis of the CLL4 trial by the German CLL study Group (GCLLSG) suggested that the frontline therapy of CLL with FC may improve OS in patients not exhibiting *del17p* or *TP53* mutations [6]. The combination of FC with rituximab yielded even better results and is discussed below (CLL 8 trial).

Pentostatin

In order to reduce myelotoxicity seen in the fludarabine, cyclophosphamide, and rituximab (FCR) regimen, fludarabine was replaced by pentostatin. In a Phase III trial comparing FCR to pentostatin, cyclophosphamide, and rituximab (PCR) in previously untreated/minimally treated CLL/SLL patients, ORR and OS were similar in the two arms [20]. A lower infection rate was not demonstrated on the PCR arm.

Cladribine (2-CdA)

Monotherapy with 2-CdA has produced higher CR rate than chlorambucil+prednisone (47% versus 12%) without improving survival [21]. Combining 2-CdA with cyclophosphamide +/– mitoxantrone improved activity in CLL, but results with FC were better [22,23].

Monoclonal antibodies

Anti-CD20

Rituximab

Single agent rituximab in CLL produced an unimpressive ORR of 12% at doses used in non-Hodgkin lymphoma (NHL) [24]. At higher doses however, the responses have been better, but the best results with this agent are seen when it is combined with other agents.

In the GCLLSG CLL8 trial, 817 physically fit, previously untreated patients were randomized between FC and FCR [25]. The ORR was superior with FCR compared with FC (92.8% versus 85.4%) and CR rate was also higher (44.5% vs 22.9%), $p<0.001$. Also, 2-year PFS was better with FCR (76.6% versus 62.3%, $p<0.01$) and this PFS benefit was seen across all prognostic subgroups except those with the *del17p* mutation. A recent update reported median PFS of 56.8 months (FCR) versus 32.9 months (FC), $p<0.001$ [26]. Median OS has not been reached for the FCR group and is 86 months for the FC group, $p=0.001$. However, there was a significantly higher rate of prolonged neutropenia during the 1st year after treatment in the FCR group compared with the FC group (16.6% versus 8.8%), $p=0.007$. Another Phase III trial proved the benefit of FCR over FC among previously treated CLL patients as well [27]. A dose modified FCR-lite regimen has also been studied for better tolerance in elderly patients with comorbidities and showed a lower neutropenia rate in the 50 previously untreated CLL patients than full-dose FCR had in other studies. It also demonstrated an excellent ORR (100%) and CR rate (77%) [28].

The GCLLSG CLL10 trial directly compared BR with FCR in 564 previously untreated, physically fit CLL patients [29]. The ORR in both arms was 97.8% (40% CR with FCR and 31.5% CR with BR, $p=0.026$). Data on minimal residual disease (MRD) status by four-color flow cytometry was available in 355 patients – of these, in the FCR versus BR arms, 74.1% versus 62.9% patients were MRD-negative on peripheral blood specimens ($p=0.024$) and 58.1% versus 31.6% patients were MRD-negative on bone marrow biopsy samples ($p<0.001$). Median PFS was 53.7 months in the FCR arm and 43.2 months in the BR arm ($p=0.001$) but there was no statistically significant difference in PFS between the two groups among patients ≥ 65 years of age, those with Cumulative Illness Rating Scale (CIRS) 4–6 or with >1 CIRS item. The greatest benefit, therefore, was observed in the physically fit subgroups (<65 years age, CIRS ≤ 3, or 1 CIRS item only). There was no difference in OS between the two treatment arms at 36 months (90.6% for FCR and 92.2% for BR, $p=0.910$). Severe neutropenia and severe infections (latter seen up to 6 months follow-up time point, especially in older patients) occurred significantly more frequently in the FCR arm.

Ofatumumab

A fully humanized anti-CD20 monoclonal antibody (MAb), this antibody has increased binding affinity to its target and increased cell kill compared with rituximab. Single agent ofatumumab in CLL produced an ORR of 51% in patients refractory to both fludarabine and alemtuzumab, and an ORR of 44% in patients with fludarabine-refractory and bulky disease [30]. It received US FDA approval in this setting but more recently has also received approval in combination with chlorambucil when an international trial showed this combination to be better than chlorambucil alone [31]. Randomization was done in 447 patients and ORR was 82% for the combination therapy compared with 69% for chlorambucil alone ($p=0.001$). Also, PFS was significantly prolonged (22.4 months versus 13.1 months, $p<0.001$). The European Commission granted conditional approval for ofatumumab use in CLL in the European Union initially but this was switched to full approval in April 2015.

Obinutuzumab

This is a humanized, glycoengineered MAb that has higher affinity binding to its target and causes more apoptosis than rituximab [6]. In the GAUGUIN monotherapy trial, it has been shown to have an ORR of 62% (Phase I) and 30% (Phase II) [32].

In the GCLLSG CLL11 Phase III trial of 781 previously untreated patients with CIRS >6 or creatinine clearance 30–69 ml/minute, obinutuzumab + chlorambucil (arm 1) was compared directly with rituximab + chlorambucil (arm 2) and with chlorambucil alone (arm 3) [33]. There was significant improvement in ORR and prolongation of PFS on arm 1 compared with arm 3 as well as on arm 2 compared with arm 3. Median PFS was 26.7 months on arm 1 versus 11.1 months on arm 3 ($p<0.001$) and 16.3 months on arm 2 versus 11.1 months on arm 3 ($p<0.001$). Treatment on arm 1 improved OS compared with arm 3 ($p=0.002$). Treatment on arm 1 improved PFS (p>0.001) and CR rates (20.7% versus 7%) and molecular responses compared with arm 2. Infusion-related reactions were more common on arm 1 compared with arm 2 but there was no difference in the risk of infection.

Anti-CD52

Alemtuzumab

This is a recombinant, fully humanized, anti-CD52 MAb, which showed 33–53% ORR in patients with advanced CLL who had previously failed alkylating agents and fludarabine therapy [34–36]. It has proven to be significantly more effective in high-risk CLL (*del11q*, *del17p*, and *TP53* mutations) compared with chlorambucil alone [37] and received US FDA approval as first-line therapy in CLL. Combination studies with fludarabine, FC, and rituximab have also been studied, but this agent was withdrawn from the market in 2012 and is only available on a compassionate use basis currently. Similarly, the European commission had granted approval for its use in CLL (for whom fludarabine treatment is not appropriate) in July 2001 but withdrew approval in August 2012 when the company stopped commercial supply of the product.

Targeted therapies

Bruton tyrosine kinase inhibitor

Ibrutinib

This is a first-in-class, oral, selective, potent, small molecule inhibitor of Bruton tyrosine kinase (BTK) that covalently binds to its target (cysteine-481 residue near the active site of BTK) thereby interrupting B-cell receptor (BCR) signaling and causing apoptosis of B cells. Early phase studies have shown impressive clinical benefit in CLL/SLL patients with an acceptable safety profile [38–40]. In a Phase Ib-II multicenter trial of 85 patients with relapsed/refractory CLL/SLL, two doses (420mg or 840 mg daily) of ibrutinib were tested [39]. The ORR in both groups was 71% with an additional 20% and 15% in each group, respectively exhibiting partial response (PR) with lymphocytosis (PR-L). Responses were independent of any poor prognostic features including del17p. At 26 months, estimated PFS was 75% and OS 83% (median not reached for both). Treatment was well tolerated with predominantly grade 1 and 2 adverse events (AEs), which included (>20% occurrence) diarrhea (usually transient and self-limiting), fatigue, upper respiratory tract infections, cough, arthralgias, rash, pyrexia, and edema. There were 15% grade 3–4 neutropenia events but these did not lead to any treatment discontinuations and were managed with growth factors if needed. Based on the data from the 420 mg group of patients (n=48, ORR 58.3%, no CR), ibrutinib received accelerated US FDA approval in February 2014 in the relapsed/refractory setting. Similarly, in this setting it was granted approval throughout the European Union in October 2014.

Typically, ibrutinib and the other novel targeted agents can lead to rapid reduction in the size of lymphadenopathy and splenomegaly in CLL/SLL, often in conjunction with a simultaneous increase in peripheral blood lymphocytosis due to redistribution [41]. This phenomenon should not be mistaken for disease progression if all other signs and symptoms of CLL/SLL are improving because it is asymptomatic and transient, although it can take several months to resolve typically. It has led to the revision of iwCLL response criteria in which PR-L has been added as a new response criterion to account for this treatment-related redistribution lymphocytosis.

Recently, a Phase III, randomized, controlled, open label, multicenter RESONATE trial of 391 patients with relapsed/refractory CLL/SLL was reported [42]. Patients were randomized between ibrutinib and ofatumumab treatment arms. The ORR was significantly higher in the ibrutinib arm compared with ofatumumab (42.6% versus 4.1%, $p<0.001$), and PFS ($p<0.001$) and OS ($p=0.005$) were significantly improved as well regardless of the presence of poor prognostic indicators. This further confirmed ibrutinib's place in the second-line setting for this disease.

A Phase II trial of ibrutinib in 144 CLL/SLL patients with *del17p* has recently been completed utilizing the 420 mg daily dose [43]. The ORR was 82.6%, including 17.4% PR-L. Median duration of response and median PFS had not been reached at 13 months follow-up. This study has secured ibrutinib's place in frontline and subsequent management of patients with del17p CLL/SLL.

Also recently completed is the Phase III randomized, open label, multicenter RESONATE-2 clinical trial of ibrutinib versus chlorambucil in previously untreated CLL/SLL patients aged ≥65 years [44]. Among 269 randomized and treated patients, the ORR was 86% in the ibrutinib arm and 35% in the chlorambucil arm ($p<0.001$) by independent review. There was significant improvement in EFS, PFS, and OS with single agent ibrutinib compared with chlorambucil. Based on these results, ibrutinib was approved by the US FDA in the frontline treatment of patients with CLL/SLL in March 2016. It is now also being evaluated in combination with various novel targeted agents as well as chemoimmunotherapy to see if further improvements in outcomes can be made in a tolerable fashion.

Ibrutinib can lead to some side effects that one should be aware of as they can affect management decisions: (i) atrial fibrillation – this can occur in up to 10% patients and should be managed with dose hold and beta blockers. In most cases, ibrutinib can be restarted safely (often at lower doses) once the atrial fibrillation is optimally managed. (ii) Bleeding risk – concurrent management with warfarin was contraindicated in most clinical trials due to some episodes of major hemorrhage, including life threatening cerebral hemorrhage, in early trials. The exact mechanism of action of the bleeding risk of ibrutinib is still unknown but there is thought to be some effect on platelets. Many patients have been treated successfully in conjunction with low molecular weight heparin products such as aspirin, clopidogrel, and novel oral anti-coagulants (direct thrombin inhibitors), but some caution should still be exercised in patients requiring warfarin. (iii) Reactivation of viral hepatitis B – certain resistance mutations have also emerged, albeit uncommon thus far [42].

PI3K-delta inhibitor
Idelalisib

This is an oral, selective, PI3K-delta inhibitor that promotes apoptosis of B cells. Early phase clinical trials have shown promising anti-tumor activity and an acceptable safety profile in CLL/SLL and other indolent NHL patients [45,46]. A Phase III, randomized, double blind, placebo-controlled trial of idelalisib + rituximab versus placebo + rituximab enrolled 220 medically unfit patients with relapsed/refractory CLL/SLL [47]. The idelalisib arm had a significantly better ORR compared with the placebo arm (81% versus 13%, $p<0.001$) as well as OS (92% versus 80% at 12 months, $p=0.02$) regardless of the presence of poor prognostic factors including del17p. Most AEs were grade 1–2. There were reports of ≥grade 3 diarrhea, transaminitis, and rash on the idelalisib arm in some patients. Severe diarrhea (colitis) from idelalisib seems to be a late effect and requires management with drug cessation and systemic steroids (including budesonide). Idelalisib-induced transaminitis can be managed with drug-hold and then successful re-challenge upon resolution of transaminitis [48]. Based on these results, in July 2014, the US FDA approved idelalisib in combination with rituximab for the treatment of patients with relapsed/refractory CLL where rituximab alone would be considered appropriate therapy due to the patient's comorbidities. For relapsed/refractory SLL, the US FDA granted approval for single-agent idelalisib in patients who have received at least two prior lines of therapy. In Europe, idelalisib received approved for previously treated CLL in September 2014. Combination trials with other novel agents as well as with chemoimmunotherapy are ongoing. However, over recent months, a number of studies involving idelalisib have been closed due to concerns of frequent infectious deaths.

A recent report of idelalisib plus ofatumumab in frontline CLL treatment demonstrated 50% grade 3 and 38% grade 4 toxicities including 54% severe transaminitis episodes among 24 patients and these required dose hold and steroids for management [49]. The etiology is thought to be immune related as previously untreated CLL/SLL patients may still have a more intact immune system than patients with relapsed/refractory disease. In the frontline setting, another Phase II trial evaluating the combination of idelalisib plus rituximab in patients 65 years of age or older, enrolled 64 patients and showed 67% transaminitis of any grade (23% grade ≥3) among other known side effects such as 64% diarrhea/colitis, but with excellent responses (ORR 97% and CR 19%) [50].

BCL2 inhibitor
Venetoclax
This is a potent, selective, second generation, small molecule inhibitor of BCL2 family proteins. It tilts the balance of these proteins towards apoptosis in CLL cells. Navitoclax was the first generation inhibitor with this mechanism of action (BH3 mimetic) but caused the significant, undesirable, dose-limiting side effect of thrombocytopenia due to the additional inhibition of Bcl-XL on platelets. Therefore, venetoclax was developed instead due to its higher selectivity.

In a Phase I dose escalation trial, following early events of serious tumor lysis syndrome, a weekly ramp up period was implemented in order to reach the full dose over a gradual 5-week period [51]. Among the enrolled 116 patients with CLL/SLL, the ORR was 79% (20% CR) with an estimated 15 month PFS of 69% for the 400 mg dose group. Even in patients with poor risk features such as del17p, fludarabine resistance, and unmutated IgV_H, the ORR was high (71–79% range, with 16–17% having CR). Six (35%) of 17 evaluated CR patients achieved MRD negativity by multicolor flow cytometry (5% of all patients). Combination trials are underway now and this agent received FDA approval in the US as of April 2016 for relapsed/refractory CLL patients with *del17p* based on Phase II data from a multicenter trial of 107 patients showing an ORR of 79.4% [52]. In Europe, venetoclax was granted conditional approval in this setting in December 2016. Across trials, toxicities appear to be manageable and are primarily hematologic and infectious. A handful of cases of Richter's transformation have emerged in the progressing patients and this will need to be monitored in the future.

Immunomodulatory agents
Lenalidomide
This is a second generation thalidomide analog and immunomodulatory agent that has shown encouraging results in CLL/SLL patients with del17p [52]. The ORR in different studies has been 32–54% with monotherapy [51,53] and is better (66%) in combination with rituximab [54]. A tumor flare reaction can occur in up to 58% of patients from the lenalidomide [6]. Grade 3–4 neutropenia, infection, and febrile episodes can occur as well.

Cellular therapeutics
Chimeric antigen receptor-T cells
A powerful way to harness the cytotoxic potential of T cells is the use of genetically engineered autologous T cells that express chimeric antigen receptor (CAR)-T cells targeting CD19 specifically. A CAR is a fusion protein expressing an extracellular moiety to redirect antigen specificity (such as CD19) linked to an intracellular CD3-zeta T-cell signaling

domain via a hinge region and a transmembrane domain. Newer generations of CAR design also add co-stimulatory domains like CD28 and/or 4-1BB. The first reports of this technology were in three multiply relapsed/refractory CLL patients [55,56]. In a recent update, among 14 such patients treated with CTL019 CAR-T cells, at a median follow-up of 9.4 months an ORR of 57% was reported including a CR rate of 21% [57]. There were no infusional toxicities higher than grade 2. Two of the PR patients progressed after 4 months but none of the CR patients relapsed. All responders experienced some reversible signs and symptoms of cytokine release syndrome (CRS) such as fever, nausea, anorexia, myalgia, hypotension, and hypoxia that corresponded to peak T-cell expansion and cytokine (including interleukin 6 [IL-6] and interferon gamma) levels. Five patients required intervention with corticosteroids and/or tocilizimuab (anti-IL-6 antibody). There was no obvious association between cell dose and responses. All patients demonstrated B-cell aplasia but not unusual infectious complications were reported. A Phase II trial with CTL019 is currently ongoing in CLL patients and other centers such as City of Hope are also investigating their own CAR-T cell products as well.

Allogeneic hematopoietic cell transplantation

The role of allogeneic hematopoietic cell transplantation (alloHCT) in CLL/SLL is less well-defined currently. Previously, it was recommended for patients with del 17p cytogenetic abnormality due to the lack of other efficacious treatment options. In the current era of novel therapeutics however, this no longer is the case. Therefore, alloHCT should be reserved for fit patients with multiply relapsed, high-risk disease who have progressed despite novel therapies and have available donors.

Sequencing of systemic treatment

Frontline therapy, no *del17p*/*TP53* mutations

If a clinical trial option is not available, the choice of initial CLL/SLL therapy depends on various factors as outlined in Figure 4.1. For young patients in good physical condition as defined by normal creatinine and a low score on the CIRS, FCR combination chemoimmunotherapy remains the first choice. However, a discussion with each patient prior to initiation of therapy is important in order for them to be aware of the potential risk of MDS/prolonged cytopenias, severe infections, and other toxicities. Benadmustine and rituximab (BR) combination chemoimmunotherapy is another possible option especially for older patients or those with increased risk of infections. If patients have a somewhat impaired physical condition but are otherwise candidates of some therapy, and if no appropriate clinical trial of a novel agent or novel combination therapy is available, then chlorambucil in combination with an anti-CD20 monoclonal antibody (preferably obinutuzumab rather than ofatumumab or

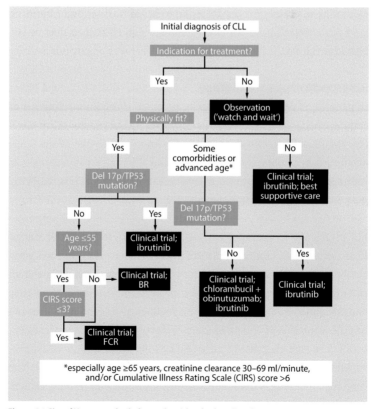

Figure 4.1 City of Hope standard of care algorithm for frontline therapy. BR, bendamustine and rituximab; CIRS, Cumulative Illness Rating Scale; CLL, chronic lymphocytic leukemia; FCR, fludarabine, cyclophosphamide, and rituximab.

rituximab) may be the best treatment option. Single-agent ibrutinib has been recently demonstrated to be a better frontline option for patients 65 years or older than chlorambucil alone.

Frontline therapy, *del17p/TP53* mutations present

If a clinical trial option is unavailable, then single-agent ibrutinib may be the best frontline option. Previously, alemtuzumab was used primarily for any reasonably fit patient with del17p, but ibrutinib has become the new standard of care. Patients with high-risk genetic features should also be considered for alloHCT if deemed eligible candidates because the disease can progress aggressively once ibrutinib fails. If ibrutinib cannot be tolerated, for instance due to atrial fibrillation or bleeding type toxicities, then venetoclax, idelalisib +/– rituximab may be the best alternatives.

Relasped/refractory therapy

In general, frontline therapy can be repeated if the initial duration of response lasted more than 2 years. However, in the current era of novel therapeutics, it may be safer and better to switch to one of the novel agents/novel combinations in any relapsed situation when treatment is indicated. The best approach is enrollment in a clinical trial studying novel agents or novel combinations (Figure 4.2).

For physically fit patients without high-risk cytogenetic features

If no appropriate clinical trials are available or patients are not good candidates to participate in trials, for physically fit patients without high risk cytogenetic features BR can be considered depending on what they had responded well to previously. This regimen gives good responses and has the attraction of a finite amount of therapy followed by a treatment break. The best alternatives include ibrutinib, idelalisib +/– rituximab, venetoclax, or lenalidomide among others, and these agents need to be continued indefinitely until they stop working or patients develop unmanageable toxicities. Studies are underway to determine stopping points of treatment for novel agents, especially in the setting of CR (particularly MRD-negative CR). The role of alloHCT is less well-defined now in CLL patients without poor risk cytogenetic features given the numerous effective new agents available already and more coming down the pipeline.

For physically unfit patients without high-risk cytogenetic features

If no appropriate clinical trial option is available, then for physically unfit patients without high-risk cytogenetic features chlorambucil in combination with one of the anti-CD20 monoclonal antibodies (obinutuzumab preferred over ofatumumab or rituximab) is recommended if not used in the frontline setting recently already. Alternatives include ibrutinib, idelalisib +/– rituximab, lenalidomide, among others.

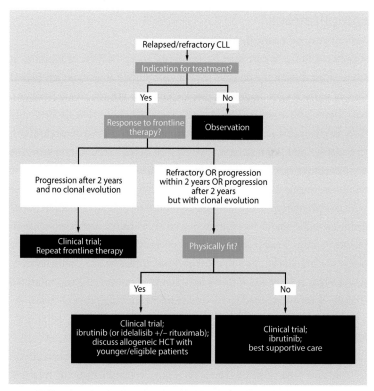

Figure 4.2 City of Hope standard of care algorithm for relapsed/refractory disease. CLL, chronic lymphocytic leukemia; HCT, hematopoietic stem cell transplantation.

For patients with high-risk cytogentics such as *del17p/TP53* or *del11q* mutation

For patients with high-risk cytogentics such as the *del17p/TP53* or *del11q* mutations, ibrutinib is preferred. Venetoclax is also an excellent option now. Alemtuzumab may still be an option if needed and discussion of alloHCT should be conducted with eligible patients. Allogeneic HCT has been utilized in high-risk situations to seek a cure but may come with a heavy price of potential complications such as severe graft versus host disease, life-threatening infections, and transplant-related morbidity and mortality. In addition, most patients with CLL requiring HCT are not eligible for it due to advanced age and/or presence of comorbidities.

Management of associated conditions and complications

Autoimmune complications

A positive Coombs test may be observed in up to 30% of patients at some point during the disease course, although it is uncommon (<5%) during early stages. Autoimmune phenomena are relatively frequent, with hemolytic anemia (lifetime risk approximately 10% to 20%) and thrombocytopenia (lifetime risk approximately 5% to 10%) occurring most commonly. Autoimmune neutropenia and other autoimmune sequelae are infrequent but more common than in the general population. These autoimmune phenomena occur more commonly with advanced disease or with purine analog treatment and generally respond to corticosteroids/immunosuppression. Rituximab is also very useful. Retreatment with purine analogs is not recommended especially if they cause autoimmune hemolytic anemia as this can recur and sometimes be fatal. If the autoimmune event is resistant to these treatments, more specific CLL-directed therapy is recommended to try and stop the inciting process.

Infections

Infections are the most important cause of morbidity and mortality in CLL patients especially infections like sinusitis, pneumonia, and shingles. Immunosuppression due to CLL itself as well as with chemo-, immuno-, and targeted-therapies (especially with agents such as fludarabine and alemtuzumab historically and now with ibrutinib) is the cause of recurrent, lingering or life threatening viral, bacterial, and fungal infections. We recommend the use of pneumocystis jiroveci pneumonia and herpes simplex virus/varicella zoster virus prophylaxis routinely. We also recommend the treatment of therapy-induced neutropenia with granulocyte-colony stimulating factor and prophylactic antibiotics. In addition, CLL patients benefit greatly from intravenous immunoglobulin (IVIG) infusions especially when their IgG levels are less than 400 mg/dL. If they experience recurrent/lingering infections, routine use of IVIG every 1–3 months is recommended prophylactically even if their IgG levels are not very low. This can help prevent life threatening infections in our experience. Vaccinations are also an important source of prophylaxis, especially against streptococcus pneumonia and influenza. We generally avoid live virus vaccines in patients with poor immune systems, so varicella zoster/shingles vaccines may need to be avoided.

Richter's transformation

Transformation to an aggressive large cell B-cell lymphoma variety from CLL is called Richter's transformation and this can occur in <10% cases. Rarely, transformation to HL or another aggressive NHL can also be seen such as PLL or T-cell NHL. Overall, the prognosis is poor with median survival less than 1 year as responses to treatment are generally short-lived. Features include rapid growth of a lymph node group that appears very active on FDG-PET scan, significant elevation of LDH, and B-symptoms. Aggressive combination chemoimmunotherapy such as rituximab, ifosfamide, carboplatin, and etoposide (R-ICE), rituximab, etoposide phosphate, prednisone, vincristine sulfate, cyclophosphamide, doxorubicin hydrochloride (R-EPOCH), or rituximab, doxorubicin hydrochloride, vincristine, and prednisolone (R-CHOP) can be tried and if a remission is achieved and the patient is a candidate for alloHCT, and has an identified donor, they should go to alloHCT, which can sometimes lead to long-term remission. There are ongoing clinical trials currently evaluating the use of programmed death-ligand 1 (PD-L1) antibodies and other checkpoint inhibitors alone and in combination with other agents such as ibrutinib for the treatment of Richter's transformation, and these treatment appear to be promising [59]. Richter's transformation patients should therefore consider clinical trials especially if more standard aggressive chemoimmunotherapy is not effective.

Conclusions

There is a rapid evolution of therapeutics in CLL/SLL currently and each year brings more novel agents/therapies to the forefront so an up-to-date review of the latest data and recommendations should be done regularly for management options.

For his progressing disease, our case patient was offered a frontline clinical trial comparing bendamustine plus rituximab verus ibrutinib versus ibrutinib plus rituximab. He was randomized to the ibrutinib alone arm and remains on study more than 1 year later having achieved a good partial remission.

References

1   Muller-Hermlink HK, et al. In: Jaffe ES, Harris NL, Stein H, Vardiman JW, eds. World Health Organization Classification of Tumours: Pathology and Genetics of Tumours. In *Haematopoietic and Lymphoid Tissues.* Lyon, France. IARC press, 2001: 95-96.

2   National Cancer Institute, Surveillance, Epidemiology, and End Results Program (SEER). SEER clinical statistics review, 1975-2009. https://seer.cancer.gov/archive/csr/1975_2009_pops09/. Accessed March 7, 2017.

3   Brown JR, Neuberg D, Phillips K, et al. Prevalence of familial malignancy in a prospectively screened cohort of patients with lymphoproliferative disorders. *Br J Haem.* 2008;143:361-368.

4   Strati P, Shanafelt T. Monoclonal B-cell lymphocytosis and early-stage chronic lymphocytic leukemia: diagnosis, natural history, and risk stratification. *Blood.* 2015;126:454-462.

5   Hallek M, Cheson BD, Catovsky D, et al. Guidelines for the diagnosis and treatment of chronic lymphocytic leukemia: a report from the International Workshop on Chronic Lymphocytic Leukemia updating the National Cancer Institute-Working Group 1996 guidelines. *Blood.* 2008;111: 5446-5456.

6   Hallek M. Chronic lymphocytic leukemia: 2015 update on diagnosis, risk stratification, and treatment. *Am J Hematol.* 2015; 90: 447-460.

7   Lopez-Guerra M, et al. The γ-secretase inhibitor PF-03084014 combined with fludarabine antagonizes migration, invasion and angiogenesis in NOTCH1-mutated CLL cells. *Leukemia.* 2015;29:96-106.

8   Rossie D. IX. Chronic lymphocytic leukaemia: new genetic markers as prognostic factors. *Hematol Oncol.* 2014;31:57-59.

9   [No authors listed]. Chemotherapeutic options in chronic lymphocytic leukemia: a meta-analysis of the randomized trials. CLL Trialists' Collaborative Group. *J Natl Cancer Institute.* 1999;91:861-868.

10   Knauf WU, Lissichkov T, Aldaoud A, et al. Phase III randomized study of bendamustine compared with chlorambucil in previously untreated patients with chronic lymphocytic leukemia. *J Clin Oncol.* 2009;27:4378-4384

11 Fischer K, et al. Bendamustine combined with rituximab in patients with relapsed and/or refractory chronic lymphocytic leukemia: a multicenter phase II trial of the German Chronic Lymphocytic Leukemia Study Group. *J Clin Oncol.* 2011;29:3559-3566.

12 Fischer K, et al. Bendamustine in combination with rituximab for previously untreated patients with chronic lymphocytic leukemia: a multicenter phase II trial of the German Chronic Lymphocytic Leukemia Study Group. *J Clin Oncol.* 2012;30:3209-3216.

13 Rai KR, et al. Fludarabine compared with chlorambucil as primary therapy for chronic lymphocytic leukemia. *N Engl J Med.* 2000;343:1750-1757.

14 Leporrier M, Chevret S, Cazin B, et al. Randomized comparison of fludarabine, CAP, and ChOP in 938 previously untreated stage B and C chronic lymphocytic leukemia patients. *Blood.* 2001; 98:2319-2325.

15 Hallek M, Eichhorst BF. Chemotherapy combination treatment regimens with fludarabine in chronic lymphocytic leukemia. *Hematol J.* 2004;5:S20-S30.

16 Bosch F, Ferrer A, López-Guillermo A, et al. Fludarabine, cyclophosphamide and mitoxantrone in the treatment of resistant or relapsed chronic lymphocytic leukaemia. *Br J Haematol.* 2002;119:976-984.

17 Eichhorst BF, Busch R, Hopfinger G, et al. Fludarabine plus cyclophosphamide versus fludarabine alone in first-line therapy of younger patients with chronic lymphocytic leukemia. *Hematol J.* 2006;107:885-891.

18 Flinn IW, Neuberg DS, Grever MR, et al. Phase III trial of fludarabine plus cyclophosphamide compared with fludarabine for patients with previously untreated chronic lymphocytic leukemia: US Intergroup Trial E2997. *J Clin Oncol.* 2007; 25: 793-798.

19 Catovsky D, Richards S, Matutes E, et al. Assessment of fludarabine plus cyclophosphamide for patients with chronic lymphocytic leukaemia (the LRF CLL4 Trial): a randomised controlled trial. *Lancet.* 2007;370:230-239.

20 Reynolds C, Di Bella N, Lyons RM, et al. A Phase III trial of fludarabine, cyclophosphamide, and rituximab vs. pentostatin, cyclophosphamide, and rituximab in B-cell chronic lymphocytic leukemia. *Invest New Drugs.* 2012;30:1232-1240.

21 Robak T, Bloński JZ, Kasznicki M, et al. Cladribine with prednisone versus chlorambucil with prednisone as first-line therapy in chronic lymphocytic leukemia: report of a prospective, randomized, multicenter trial. *Blood.* 2000; 96:2723-2729.

22 Montillo M, Tedeschi A, O'Brien S, et al. Phase II study of cladribine and cyclophosphamide in patients with chronic lymphocytic leukemia and prolymphocytic leukemia. *Cancer.* 2003;97:114-120.

23 Robak T, Blonski JZ, Gora-Tybor J, et al. Cladribine alone and in combination with cyclophosphamide or cyclophosphamide plus mitoxantrone in the treatment of progressive chronic lymphocytic leukemia: report of a prospective, multicenter, randomized trial of the Polish Adult Leukemia Group (PALG CLL2). *Blood.* 2006;108: 473-479.

24 Tam CS, Keating MJ. Selection of rituximab dosage in chronic lymphocytic leukemia: where is the evidence? *Leuk Lymphoma.* 2013;54:934-939.

25 Hallek M, Fischer K, Fingerle-Rowson G, et al. Addition of rituximab to fludarabine and cyclophosphamide in patients with chronic lymphocytic leukaemia: a randomised, open-label, phase 3 trial. *Lancet.* 2010;376:1164-1174.

26 Fischer K, Bahlo J, Fink AM, et al. Long-term remissions after FCR chemoimmunotherapy in previously untreated patients with CLL: updated results of the CLL8 trial. *Blood.* 2016;127:208-215.

27 Robak T, Dmoszynska A, Solal-Céligny P, et al. Rituximab plus fludarabine and cyclophosphamide prolongs progression-free survival compared with fludarabine and cyclophosphamide alone in previously treated chronic lymphocytic leukemia. *J Clin Oncol.* 2010;28:1756-1765.

28 Foon KA, Boyiadzis M, Land SR, et al. Chemoimmunotherapy with low-dose fludarabine and cyclophosphamide and high dose rituximab in previously untreated patients with chronic lymphocytic leukemia. *J Clin Oncol.* 2009;27:498-503.

29 Eichhorst B, Fink AM, Busch R, et al. Frontline chemoimmunotherapy with fludarabine (F), cyclophosphamide (C), and rituximab (R) (FCR) shows superior efficacy in comparison to bendamustine (B) and rituximab (BR) in previously untreated and physically fit patients (pts) with advanced chronic lymphocytic leukemia (CLL): final analysis of an international, randomized study of the German CLL Study Group (GCLLSG) (CLL10 Study). *Blood.* 2014;124:19.

30 Wierda WG, Kipps TJ, Mayer J, et al. Ofatumumab as single-agent CD20 immunotherapy in fludarabine-refractory chronic lymphocytic leukemia. *J Clin Oncol.* 2010;28:1749-1755.

31 Hillmen P, Robak T, Janssens A, et al. Ofatumumab + chlorambucil versus chlorambucil alone in patients with untreated chronic lymphocytic leukemia (CLL): results of the Phase III study Complement 1 (OMB110911). *Blood.* 2013;122:528.

32 Cartron G, de Guibert S, Dilhuydy MS, et al. Obinutuzumab (GA101) in relapsed/refractory chronic lymphocytic leukemia: final data from the phase 1/2 GAUGUIN study. *Blood.* 2014;124:2196-2202.

33 Goede V, Fischer K, Busch R, et al. Obinutuzumab plus chlorambucil in patients with CLL and coexisting conditions. *N Engl J Med.* 2014;370:1101-1110.

34 Osterborg A, Dyer MJ, Bunjes D, et al. Phase II multicenter study of human CD52 antibody in previously treated chronic lymphocytic leukemia. European Study Group of CAMPATH-1H Treatment in Chronic Lymphocytic Leukemia. *J Clin Oncol.* 1997;15:1567-1574.

35 Rai KR, Freter CE, Mercier RJ, et al. Alemtuzumab in previously treated chronic lymphocytic leukemia patients who also had received fludarabine. *J Clin Oncol.* 2002;20:3891-3897.

36 Keating MJ, Flinn I, Jain V, et al. Therapeutic role of alemtuzumab (Campath-1H) in patients who have failed fludarabine: results of a large international study. *Blood.* 2002;99:3554-3561.

37 Hillmen P, Skotnicki AB, Robak T, et al. Alemtuzumab compared with chlorambucil as first-line therapy for chronic lymphocytic leukemia. *J Clin Oncol.* 2007;25:5616-5623.

38 Advani RH, Buggy JJ, Sharman JP, et al. Bruton tyrosine kinase inhibitor ibrutinib (PCI-32765) has significant activity in patients with relapsed/refractory B-cell malignancies. *J Clin Oncol.* 2013;31:88-94.

39 Byrd JC, Furman RR, Coutre SE, et al. Targeting BTK with ibrutinib in relapsed chronic lymphocytic leukemia. *N Engl J Med.* 2013;369:32-42.

40 O'Brien S, Furman RR, Coutre SE, et al. Ibrutinib as initial therapy for elderly patients with chronic lymphocytic leukaemia or small lymphocytic lymphoma: an open-label, multicentre, phase 1b/2 trial. *Lancet Oncol.* 2014;15: 48-58.

41 Siddiqi T, Rosen S. Novel biologic agents for non-Hodgkin lymphoma and chronic lymphocytic leukemia-part 2: adoptive cellular immunotherapy, small-molecule inhibitors, and immunomodulation. *Oncology (Williston Park).* 2015;29:299-308.

42 Byrd JC, Brown JR, O'Brien S, et al. Ibrutinib versus ofatumumab in previously treated chronic lymphoid leukemia. *N Engl J Med.* 2014;371:213-223.

43 O'Brien S, Jones JA, Coutre SE, et al. Ibrutinib for patients with relapsed or refractory chronic lymphocytic leukaemia with 17p deletion (RESONATE-17): a phase 2, open-label, multicentre study. *Lancet Oncol.* 2016;17:1409-1418.

44 Burger JA, et al. Ibrutinib as initial therapy for patients with chronic lymphocytic leukemia. *N Engl J Med.* 2015;373: 2425-2437.

45 Flinn IW, Kahl BS, Leonard JP, et al. Idelalisib, a selective inhibitor of phosphatidylinositol 3-kinase-δ, as therapy for previously treated indolent non-Hodgkin lymphoma. *Blood.* 2014;123:3406-3413.

46 Brown JR, Byrd JC, Coutre SE, et al. Idelalisib, an inhibitor of phosphatidylinositol 3-kinase p110δ, for relapsed/refractory chronic lymphocytic leukemia. *Blood.* 2014;123:3390-3397.

47 Furman RR, et al. Idelalisib and rituximab in relapsed chronic lymphocytic leukemia. *N Engl J Med.* 2014;370:997-1007.

48 Coutre SE, Barrientos JC, Brown JR, et al. Management of adverse events associated with idelalisib treatment: expert panel opinion. *Leuk Lymphoma.* 2015;56:2779-2786.

49 Lampson BL, Kasar SN, Matos TR, et al. Idelalisib given front-line for treatment of chronic lymphocytic leukemia causes frequent immune-mediated hepatotoxicity. *Blood*. 2016;128:195-203.

50 O'Brien SM, et al. A phase 2 study of idelalisib plus rituximab in treatment-naïve older patients with chronic lymphocytic leukemia. *Blood*. 2015;126:2686-2694.

51 Channan-Khan A, Miller KC, Musial L, et al. Clinical efficacy of lenalidomide in patients with relapsed or refractory chronic lymphocytic leukemia: results of a phase II study. *J Clin Oncol*. 2006;24:5343-5349.

52 Stilgenbauer S, Eichhorst B, Schetelig J, et al. Venetoclax in relapsed or refractory chronic lymphocytic leukaemia with 17p deletion: a multicentre, open-label, phase 2 study. *Lancet Oncol*. 2016;17:768-778.

53 Sher T, Miller KC, Lawrence D, et al. Efficacy of lenalidomide in patients with chronic lymphocytic leukemia with high-risk cytogenetics. *Leuk Lymphoma*. 2010;51:85-88.

54 Ferrajoli A, Lee BN, Schlette EJ, et al. Lenalidomide induces complete and partial remissions in patients with relapsed and refractory chronic lymphocytic leukemia. *Blood*. 2008;111:5291-5297

55 Badoux XC, Keating MJ, Wen S, et al. Phase II study of lenalidomide and rituximab as salvage therapy for patients with relapsed or refractory chronic lymphocytic leukemia. *J Clin Oncol*. 2013;13:584-591.

56 Porter DL, Levine BI, Kalos M, Bagg A, June CH. Chimeric antigen receptor-modified T cells in chronic lymphoid leukemia. *N Engl J Med*. 2011;365:725-733.

57 Kalos M, Levine BL, Porter DL, et al. T cells with chimeric antigen receptors have potent antitumor effects and can establish memory in patients with advanced leukemia. *Sci Transl Med*. 2011;3:95ra73.

58 Porter DL. Chimeric antigen receptor modified T cells directed against CD19 (CTL019 cells) have long-term persistence and induce durable responses in relapsed, refractory CLL. *Blood*. 2013;122:4162.

59 Jain N. Nivolumab combined with ibrutinib for CLL and Richter transformation: a Phase II trial. *Blood*. 2016;128:59.

Chapter 5

Follicular lymphoma

Alex F Herrera

Case presentation

A 52-year-old woman presented to her physician with asymptomatic, waxing and waning axillary lymphadenopathy. Excisional biopsy demonstrated grade 2 follicular lymphoma. Computed tomography (CT) of the chest, abdomen, and pelvis, demonstrated multistation lymphadenopathy (>4 areas) above and below the diaphragm, with the largest nodes (retroperitoneal) measuring 3.4 x 2.3 cm. Complete blood count (CBC), lactate dehydrogenase (LDH), and beta-2-microglobulin were normal, and a bone marrow biopsy was negative. The patient was observed for 2 years, but ultimately she developed increasing fatigue, dyspepsia, constipation, and bloating. Repeat imaging demonstrated considerable enlargement of her intra-abdominal lymphadenopathy, with a mesenteric mass now measuring 8.7 x 6.2 cm.

Epidemiology

Follicular lymphoma (FL) is the most common indolent non-Hodgkin lymphoma (NHL), and second most common subtype of NHL overall, accounting for approximately 20% of all NHL [1]. The median age at diagnosis in patients with FL is 60–65 years old, though younger patients can be affected. The incidence of the disease is higher in whites than in blacks, Asians, or Native Americans [2]. There are no specific risk factors for FL beyond the known associations between exposures (eg, autoimmune diseases) and NHL.

© Springer International Publishing AG 2017
J. Zain and L.W. Kwak (eds.), *Management of Lymphomas:
A Case-Based Approach*, DOI 10.1007/978-3-319-26827-9_5

Pathology

It is believed that FL is a malignancy arising from follicular germinal center B cells. Under the microscope, FL has a nodular growth pattern resembling the germinal centers in a normal lymph node, but the neoplastic infiltrate obliterates the normal follicular architecture. In addition, tingible body macrophages usually seen in a healthy follicle are not present, and the usual polarity between dark and light follicular zones is lost. The tumor is composed of smaller, cleaved centrocytes admixed with larger centroblasts, and the grading of FL is based on the relative abundance of large cells in the infiltrate. Grade 1 FL consists of 0–5 centroblasts per high-powered field (hpf), while there are 6–15 centroblasts/hpf in grade 2 and >15 centroblasts/hpf in grade 3 FL. Grade 3 FL is further classified into grade 3A or grade 3B depending on whether centrocytes are present (grade 3A) or not (grade 3B) [3]. Tissue architecture is critical to the diagnosis and grading of FL, therefore, a fine needle aspirate is insufficient for full pathologic characterization of FL. An excisional or core biopsy is recommended for a complete diagnostic evaluation both at diagnosis and in most cases of relapsed disease.

The typical immunophenotype of FL on immunohistochemistry or flow cytometry is consistent with that of germinal center B cells, with expression of CD20, CD19, CD79a, CD21, surface immunoglobulin, and usually CD10 and BCL-6. CD23 expression can be variable. FLs nearly always harbor the t(14;18) chromosomal translocation, resulting in BCL-2 activation and expression. Thus, BCL-2 is almost uniformly expressed in Gr 1-3A FL, whereas some grade 3B FLs lack the characteristic translocation and/or BCL-2 expression [3].

Clinical presentation

FL is classified as an NHL with indolent clinical behavior. Patients with FL typically present with lymphadenopathy that often waxes and wanes in size. Abdominal or retroperitoneal lymph node masses and splenomegaly are common, and symptoms develop gradually. Rapid growth of lymph nodes, B symptoms, elevated LDH, or non-marrow extranodal involvement should raise suspicion for a transformation to diffuse large B-cell lymphoma (DLBCL).

Staging

Staging of patients with FL should include laboratory studies such as a complete blood count with differential, full chemistry panel (including liver function tests and LDH), hepatitis serologies, human immunodeficiency virus (HIV) testing, and beta-2 microglobulin testing, computed tomography (CT) scan of the chest, abdomen, and pelvis or positron emission tomography (PET)/CT scan, a bone marrow aspiration, and a biopsy. When there is concern for transformation to DLBCL, a PET/CT scan should be performed.

Prognosis

The traditional International Prognostic Index for NHL has been modified to improve prognostic accuracy in patients with FL. The Follicular Lymphoma International Prognostic Index (FLIPI) and FLIPI-2 (Table 5.1) divide patients with FL into separate risk groups based on the number of risk factors present, which correspond to different progression-free and overall survival (OS) differences after standard chemoimmunotherapy (Figure 5.1 and 5.2) [4,5]. The advent of next-generation DNA sequencing has allowed for enhanced genetic characterization of FL,

FLIPI	FLIPI-2
Age ≥ 60	Age > 60
Ann Arbor stage III-IV	Bone marrow involvement
Hemoglobin < 12 g/dL	Hemoglobin < 12g/dL
LDH > ULN	Beta-2 microglobulin > ULN
# of nodal sites > 4	Diameter of largest LN > 6cm
Original FLIPI	
Score	Risk Group
0 – 1	Low
2	Intermediate
3 or more	High
FLIPI-2	
Score	Risk Group
0	Low
1 – 2	Intermediate
3 or more	High

Table 5.1 The Follicular Lymphoma International Prognostic Index (FLIPI) and FLIPI-2.
Data from [4,5].

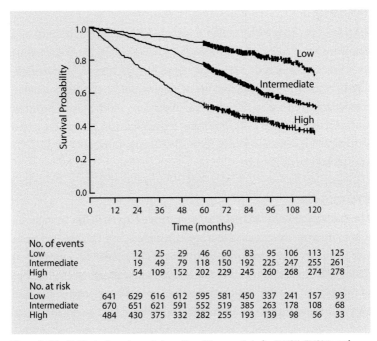

Figure 5.1 The Follicular Lymphoma International Prognostic Index (FLIPI), FLIPI-2, and m7-FLIPI. Overall survival in different FLIPI risk groups. Data from [4].

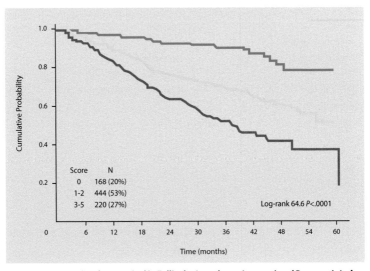

Figure 5.2 Progression-free survival in Follicular Lymphoma International Prognostic Index-2 risk groups. Data from [5].

and the m7-FLIPI incorporates mutation status of 7 genes along with the traditional FLIPI and performance status to improve prognostication for patients with FL (Figure 5.3) [6].

Treatment of limited stage follicular lymphoma

A minority of FL patients (15–30%) present with limited stage (Stage I–II, including IE and IIE) disease. Although spontaneous remissions can occur [7], patients with limited stage FL can potentially be cured [8–10] and should receive treatment. Prospective data defining the optimal treatment of limited stage FL are lacking, but many retrospective studies have demonstrated long-term remissions with radiation therapy (RT) alone. In several retrospective studies, a single course of RT alone resulted in relapse-free survival rates of 40–60% and OS ranging from 60–80% at 10 years, and long-term follow-up studies estimate the median OS at almost 20 years [8,10]. Despite evidence for long-term remission after RT in patients with limited stage FL, RT is underutilized [9,11]. An analysis of the Surveillance, Epidemiology, and End Results (SEER) database compared outcomes in patients with Stage I/II FL who

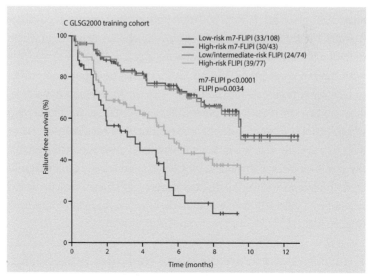

Figure 5.3 Failure-free survival in m7-Follicular Lymphoma International Prognostic Index (FLIPI) risk groups compared to original FLIPI groups. Data from [6].

received an initial course of RT with patients who did not receive RT and demonstrated superior disease-specific and OS at 5, 10, 15, and 20 years. Only one-third of limited stage FL patients in the SEER database received RT [11]. In order to minimize toxicities associated with RT, including myelosuppression, damage to adjacent organs, and increased risk of secondary malignancies involved site RT (ISRT) should be utilized for the treatment of limited stage FL, with a standard RT dose of 24 Gy to the involved lymphoid region. Higher radiation doses of 30–36 Gy should be considered for grade 3 FL. Randomized studies of higher (eg, 40–45 Gy) or lower doses (eg, 4 Gy) of radiation for indolent NHLs have not shown superiority over 24 Gy [12,13]. Bulky disease (>6cm) appears to be a risk factor for failure of RT alone, though there is little data to guide treatment decisions in this population [14].

Although it has not been prospectively studied, the addition of systemic therapy to RT for limited stage FL may improve outcomes [9]. Decision-making in this patient population is further complicated as some patients with limited stage FL who are observed do not require therapy for many years [15].

Because of its potential to induce long-term remissions, we recommend ISRT alone for patients with non-bulky stage I or contiguous stage II grade 1 or 2 FL or patients with bulky disease involvement in whom radiation is feasible without excessive toxicity (see Figure 5.1). Patients with limited stage grade 3A and 3B FL should be treated according to treatment protocols for DLBCL (ie, rituximab, cyclophosphamide, doxorubicin, vincristine, and prednisolone [R-CHOP] plus radiotherapy, when feasible). In select patients who are not ideal candidates for RT or have disease sites that are difficult to irradiate, observation or systemic therapy with rituximab alone or chemoimmunotherapy can be considered. In patients with bulky disease in whom significant toxicity would be expected with RT, chemoimmunotherapy is a reasonable approach (Figure 5.4).

Treatment of advanced stage follicular lymphoma

Most patients with FL present with advanced stage disease, which typically is not cured with standard therapy alone. Asymptomatic

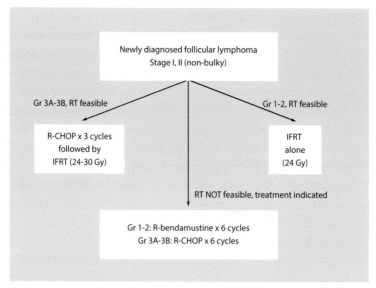

Figure 5.4 City of Hope standard of care treatment algorithm for limited stage follicular lymphoma. IFRT, involved-field radiotherapy; R-CHOP, Rituximab, cyclophosphamide, doxorubicin, vincristine, and prednisolone; RT, radiation therapy.

patients with advanced stage FL should be observed until treatment is necessitated by symptoms or complications of the disease. Patients under observation should have a history, physical exam, and laboratory studies performed every 3 months, with CT imaging performed every 6 months [16]. A randomized study of observation versus systemic therapy in patients with asymptomatic, advanced stage indolent NHL (mostly FL) demonstrated no survival advantage to early therapy, with nearly 20% of patients in the observation group and 40% in the subset of patients older than 70 years of age not requiring therapy at 10 years [17]. A more recent study randomized asymptomatic, low-bulk patients to observation versus single-agent rituximab followed by maintenance and, as expected, the results showed that rituximab-treated patients had a longer interval to the start of new treatment, but no difference in OS [18]. While there appears to be minimal additional toxicity with early rituximab treatment, without the demonstration of a survival benefit, the data are not sufficiently compelling to recommend early treatment for most patients.

Timing of treatment initiation

The timing of treatment initiation in patients with advanced stage FL is often a subjective decision that should be made by the treating physician in conjunction with the patient. There are proposed sets of criteria to guide the decision to treat advanced stage FL, including the Groupe d'Etude des Lymphomes Folliculares (GELF) criteria below, which generally advocate treatment for patients with disease-related cytopenias, significant systemic symptoms, bulky tumors, organ dysfunction or compression caused by lymphomatous lesions, or accelerated disease progression. Systemic therapy should be considered when one or more of the following factors are present [19]:

- tumor mass >7cm in diameter;
- ≥3 lymph node sites involved with diameter >3cm;
- systemic symptoms present (Eastern Cooperative Oncology Group [ECOG] >1);
- substantial splenomegaly;
- pleural or pericardial effusion present;
- organ (eg, ureter, spinal) compression present;
- peripheral blood involvement or cytopenias; and
- LDH or beta-2 microglobulin > upper limit of normal.

Single-agent rituximab

The choice of initial regimen depends on a patient's co-morbidities and the severity of the clinical factor triggering the decision to start therapy. Immunotherapy alone with single-agent rituximab, an anti-CD20 monoclonal antibody, can be utilized in patients with a low tumor burden who require therapy or in patients with co-morbidities that make them poor candidates for combination chemoimmunotherapy. In chemotherapy-naive patients with low grade FL and a relatively low tumor burden, the overall response rate (ORR) observed following a course of weekly rituximab $375mg/m^2$ x four doses ranges from 66–80% [18,20,21]. Studies have examined the use of maintenance rituximab after a course of weekly induction, with improved complete response rates observed. Different maintenance schedules have been evaluated: every 2 months x four doses, every 2 months x 2 years, and every 3 months until progression.

While a short course of maintenance therapy (four doses) was associated with prolonged event-free survival, other schedules did not have a significant impact on time to next treatment or time to cytotoxic therapy [18,20,21]. We recommend induction weekly rituximab alone or a short course of maintenance rituximab (every 2 months x four doses) after induction therapy (Figure 5.5).

First-line chemoimmunotherapy

Most patients with advanced stage FL who require treatment are treated with combined chemoimmunotherapy. The addition of rituximab to chemotherapy confers a clear survival benefit and should be included as part of first-line therapy [22,23]. Bendamustine alone, cyclophosphamide, doxorubicin, vincristine, and prednisone (CHOP), or cyclophosphamide, vincristine, and prednisone (CVP) combined with rituximab (R-) are all acceptable first-line options for advanced stage FL. The overall response rate to these regimens ranges from 88–97%, although fewer complete responses appear to be observed in patients with grade 1–2 disease who are treated with R-CHOP or R-CVP compared with R-bendamustine. When compared head-to-head, R-bendamustine was associated with prolonged progression-free survival and less toxicity as compared with R-CHOP (Figure 5.6) (and a mixed group of patients treated with R-CHOP or R-CVP) [24,25]. In general, we prefer to use R-bendamustine for patients

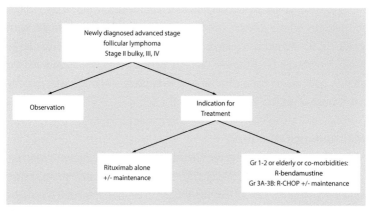

Figure 5.5 City of Hope standard of care treatment algorithm for advanced stage follicular lymphoma. R-CHOP, Rituximab, cyclophosphamide, doxorubicin, vincristine, and prednisolone.

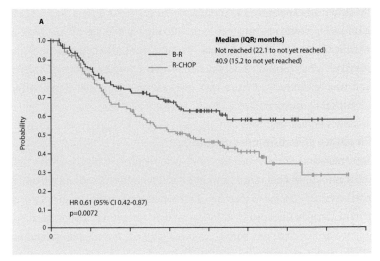

Figure 5.6 Progression-free survival: R-CHOP versus R-bendamustine. R-CHOP, rituximab, cyclophosphamide, doxorubicin, vincristine, and prednisolone Data from [24].

with advanced stage grade 1 or 2 FL due to its improved tolerability and the longer progression-free survival (PFS) observed in studies. The randomized studies above only included grade 1 or 2 FL; therefore, there is limited data regarding the use of bendamustine for grade 3A FL. For patients with grade 3A FL, the choice of regimen should be made based on the clinical behavior of a patient's disease. We typically use R-CHOP for aggressive grade 3A disease, but R-bendamustine could be considered for patients whose disease is not behaving aggressively. Patients with grade 3B FL should be treated similarly to patients with diffuse large B-cell lymphoma (DLBCL; see Chapter 9). R-CVP can be considered for elderly patients or patients with co-morbidities, although we typically use R-bendamustine for these patients.

Maintenance rituximab
Maintenance rituximab after certain combined chemoimmunotherapy regimens has been shown to prolong progression-free survival in patients with advanced stage FL [26,27]. In the PRIMA trial, patients with advanced stage grade 1–3A FL were treated with rituximab plus either CHOP, CVP, or fludarabine, cyclophosphamide, and mitoxantrone (FCM), followed

by either observation or rituximab maintenance (375mg/m^2 every 2 months for a total of 2 years) in patients with at least a partial response to induction therapy. Rituximab maintenance prolonged progression-free survival and improved the depth of responses, but had no impact on OS and was associated with more adverse events, particularly infections (Figure 5.7). Despite this moderate increase in toxicity, the side effects were not severe, and they did not seem to have an impact on quality of life, or result in discontinuation of treatment [27]. Therefore, we typically recommend the use of rituximab maintenance (375mg/m^2 every 2 months for 2 years, starting 8 weeks after the completion of induction) in patients who respond to first-line R-CHOP, R-CVP, or R-FCM. Rituximab maintenance has not been studied after upfront R-bendamustine therapy, and we do not routinely advocate its use in this setting. Studies are currently underway examining the role of rituximab maintenance after R-bendamustine induction therapy.

Surveillance following completion of treatment

Following the completion of upfront therapy for limited or advanced stage FL, patients should have routine surveillance visits, including history and physical examination, laboratory assessment with complete blood count,

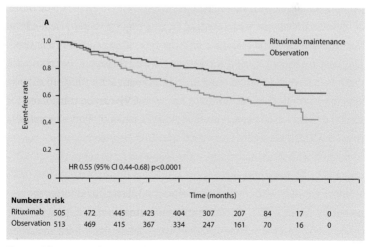

Figure 5.7 Progression-free survival in PRIMA study: rituximab maintenance versus observation after chemoimmunotherapy. Data from [27].

chemistry panel, and LDH. We typically see patients every 3 months in the first 2 years and then every 3–6 months for patients who remain in remission/response. The role of imaging surveillance following initial treatment for FL is not well studied – we typically perform CT scans every 6 months for the first 2 years and then continue expectant management thereafter. Positron emission tomography (PET) scans should be used if there is concern for transformation to DLBCL and are generally not used in routine surveillance [16].

In the case mentioned above, the patient received six cycles of rituximab with bendamustine chemotherapy with a complete remission (CR) at the end of treatment, after which she was subsequently observed.

Treatment of relapsed or refractory follicular lymphoma

Although a proportion of limited stage FL patients are cured with upfront therapy, some limited stage FL patients and the great majority of advanced stage FL patients will either have relapse after an initial response/remission or a minority of patients will have refractory disease. Progression of disease within 2 years of initial chemoimmunotherapy appears to be a particularly poor prognostic sign, with a 5-year OS of 50% observed in these patients compared with 90% in patients with >2-year PFS [28]. The choice of regimen in patients with relapsed FL who require therapy depends on the duration of initial response and the type of initial treatment used. The best treatment option for patients with relapsed FL who require therapy is a well-designed clinical trial. Patients with relapsed disease who are asymptomatic and have a low tumor burden can be observed similar to newly diagnosed, advanced stage FL patients. Typically, patients treated with single-agent rituximab who had durable responses can be re-treated with rituximab alone – the response rates are in the 40–60% range [21,29]. Patients with a short remission duration after rituximab alone or patients who relapse after first-line chemoimmunotherapy are generally treated with an alternative non-crossresistant regimen. For patients who receive upfront R-CHOP, we typically use R-bendamustine, and vice versa. Other options can include fludarabine-based regimens or salvage regimens used for more aggressive lymphomas. Patients with refractory disease to upfront therapy should be considered for clinical trials. If no clinical trial is available or a patient is not a trial candidate, then patients with refractory disease should be treated with an alternative chemoimmunotherapy regimen than was initially utilized (Figure 5.8).

Novel targeted agents for relapsed or refractory follicular lymphoma

Improved understanding of the molecular pathogenesis of lymphoma has led to the development of novel targeted agents that have demonstrated efficacy in the treatment of FL. Novel agents approved for treatment of recurrent FL include: radioimmunotherapy with 90Y ibritumomab tiuxetan, lenalidomide plus rituximab, or idelalisib (Table 5.3). Ibritumomab tiuxetan is composed of anti-CD20 antibody (ibritumomab) linked with a chelator (tiuxetan) that is radiolabeled with 90Yttrium with the goal of delivering radiation directly to the site(s) of lymphoma involvement.

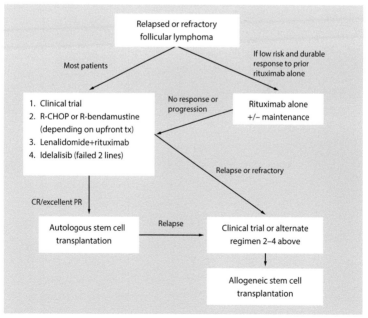

Figure 5.8 City of Hope standard of care treatment algorithm for relapsed or refractory follicular lymphoma. R-CHOP, Rituximab, cyclophosphamide, doxorubicin, vincristine, and prednisolone.

Reference	N	Age in years (range)	Prior treatment; prior regimens (range)	Dose	Response rate	Median duration of response/PFS	Survival
Idelalisib							
Gopal et al 2014 [30]	72	64 (33–87)	4 (2–12)	150 mg BID	57% ORR 6% CR [overall cohort]	12.5 mo DOR 11.0 mo PFS	PFS 47% OS 80% (48 wks)
90Y ibritumomab tiuxetan							
Witzig et al 2007 [31,32]	54	54 (34–73)	4 (1–9)	Rituximab 250 mg/m² days 1 and 8, 90Y ibritumomab tiuxetan 0.4 mCi/kg on day 8	74% ORR 15% CR 59% PR	6.4 mo DOR overall 28.1 mo DOR (in pts with > 12 mo TTP)	Median OS 49.3 mo Median TTP 30.9 mo
Lenalidomide plus rituximab							
Leonard et al 2015 [33]	46	64 (36–89)	4 (2–12)	15mg (C1)/20 mg (C2) on days 1–21 of 28-day cycle, Rituximab 375 mg/m2 days 1, 8, 15, 22	76% ORR 39% CR	24.0 mo PFS	PFS 52% (2 yr) Median OS not reached
Fowler et al 2014 [34]	50	56 (35–84)	0 (only untreated patients enrolled)	20mg on days 1–21 of 28-day cycle, Rituximab 375mg/m² days 1	98% ORR 87% CR	Median PFS not reached	OS 94.4% PFS 78.5% (3 yr)

Table 5.3 Novel agents for relapsed or refractory follicular lymphoma. CR, complete response; DOR, duration of response; ORR, overall response rate; OS, indicates overall survival; PFS indicates progression-free survival, PR, partial response.

Response rates range from 60–80% and the main toxicity is prolonged cytopenias that usually occur 1–2 months after treatment and typically resolve within a month of the nadir [35]. Idelalisib is a is an oral inhibitor of phosphoinositide 3'-kinase delta (PI3Kδ), which is FDA-approved for patients with relapsed FL who have received at least two prior therapies. A 57% ORR was observed in a Phase II study of idelalisib in patients with relapsed indolent NHL, although few CRs were seen (6%) [30]. Hepatotoxicity and gastrointestinal toxicities are the main adverse events observed with therapy. Lenalidomide is an immunomodulatory thalidomide derivative with anti-lymphoma activity, which resulted in an ORR of 76% (39% CR) when combined with rituximab, compared with a 53% ORR (20% CR) when used alone for patients with relapsed FL. The median time to progression was 2 years for lenalidomide plus rituximab [33]. Patients treated with lenalidomide are at risk for thrombotic events, and aspirin or prophylactic anticoagulation should be considered, particularly for patients at high risk for thrombosis. Lenalidomide plus rituximab is becoming more widely used and is a reasonable second-line regimen in patients with relapsed or refractory disease after initial therapy.

In the case study, within 2 years of completing treatment, the patient developed recurrent symptoms with enlarging lymphadenopathy. The patient received six cycles of R-CHOP and again achieved CR at the end of treatment.

Hematopoietic stem cell transplantation for follicular lymphoma

Aside from some patients with limited stage disease, the majority of patients with FL will relapse after initial treatment with a variable duration of response. Subsequent treatments typically lead to shorter remissions. HSCT, including both autologous stem cell transplantation (ASCT) and allogeneic HSCT, can be utilized in patients with relapsed or refractory disease to prolong remission duration and potentially provide durable responses and cures. Consolidative ASCT after upfront therapy prolongs PFS but does not confer OS benefit, and, therefore, is not recommended [36,37]. However, ASCT as consolidation in first relapse after response to chemotherapy prolongs PFS and potentially OS. Multiple retrospective studies and a prospective randomized study have demonstrated improved PFS and OS in patients with relapsed or refractory FL who received ASCT after responding to post-relapse salvage therapy compared with no ASCT (58–93% 5-year OS for ASCT versus 33–70% for no ASCT) [38–41]. Patients who undergo ASCT in second remission appear to have improved survival compared with patients who are transplanted beyond second remission (Figure 5.9) [42].

Although some of these retrospective studies included patients who received prior rituximab, it is important to note that the randomized CUP trial was conducted in the pre-rituximab era, and therefore, it is unclear whether the results are applicable to the current era [40]. However, retrospective studies have shown similar OS benefit of ASCT in relapsed or refractory FL patients that have received prior rituximab [39,41]. In patients with a long response duration after initial therapy (eg, >5 years), the use of second line therapy without consolidative ASCT is a reasonable choice if a patient remains chemosensitive. However, in patients with a short remission duration after initial therapy, consolidative ASCT in second remission should be offered and is preferable to ASCT later in the patient's disease course.

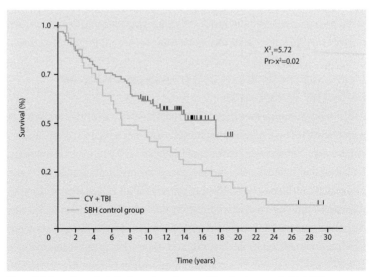

Figure 5.9 Overall survival of relapsed or refractory FL patients treated with ASCT versus chemotherapy alone. CY, cyclophosphamide; SBH, St Bartholomew's Hospital; TBI, total-body irradiation. Data from [42].

Allogeneic stem cell transplantation for follicular lymphoma

Allogeneic HSCT is a potentially curative procedure in patients with FL, and can be considered in selected relapsed or refractory FL patients whose disease remains sensitive to treatment. Initial studies of allogeneic HSCT in NHL using myeloablative conditioning were associated with high rates of transplant-related mortality (TRM) due to graft-versus-host disease, infections, and other complications. Reduced intensity or non-myeloablative (RIC/NMA) conditioning prior to allogeneic HSCT is associated with lower TRM at the expense of increased relapse risk [43], and thus has expanded the use of the procedure to older and frail FL patients. The optimal conditioning regimen for FL patients is unclear, but studies of fludarabine paired with either non-ablative doses of busulfan, cyclophosphamide, melphalan, or bendamustine (+/– rituximab or alemtuzumab) have produced 2–5-year PFS and OS in the range of 43–88% and 52–85%, respectively [44–47]. Studies comparing ASCT and RIC/NMA allogeneic HSCT have shown similar OS but higher TRM and lower relapse risk with the allogeneic approach [48,49]. Despite the curative potential of allogeneic HSCT, we typically reserve the procedure until later in a patient's disease course given the expected long-term survival in FL patients and the relatively high TRM associated with the allogeneic HSCT. We do recommend RIC/NMA allogeneic HSCT for relapsed or refractory FL patients who are young, have relapsed after ASCT, have relapsed or refractory transformed FL, or patients with multiply relapsed FL with diminishing available treatment options.

The patient in the case subsequently underwent high-dose chemotherapy with BEAM followed by autologous HSCT. Two years after her transplant, the patient again developed enlarging cervical and axillary lymphadenopathy. Biopsy again confirmed recurrent FL, grade 3A. As the patient had already received R-bendamustine and R-CHOP, she was treated with lenalidomide and rituximab with an excellent partial response. The patient had a human leukocyte antigen (HLA)-matched sibling and subsequently underwent RIC allogeneic transplantation, and remains in continued CR 4 years later.

Transformed follicular lymphoma

One of the main threats to patients with FL is transformation to a more aggressive lymphoma, typically DLBCL. Transformation typically occurs at a rate of 2–3% per year, and in 10–20% of patients total at 10 years [50,51]. Patients with transformation to DLBCL are typically treated with regimens used for DLBCL. Outcomes for patients with transformed FL after consolidative ASCT appear similar to patients with de novo DLBCL [52]. We treat therapy-naive transformed FL with R-CHOP similar to DLBCL without subsequent ASCT, but for patients who have chemosensitive transformed FL after previous treatment for FL, we typically perform consolidative ASCT in eligible patients. Allogeneic HSCT has been studied in patients with transformed FL, and can be considered in patients who have received prior ASCT or who are chemorefractory but whose disease is controlled with radioimmunotherapy, novel agents, or RT.

Novel agents under development and future directions

Several novel agents are under development for the treatment of FL, including immune therapies and tyrosine kinase inhibitors. Monoclonal antibodies directed against the immune checkpoint, programmed death-1 (PD-1) receptor or its ligand, PD-L1, have demonstrated activity as single agents (ORR 38%) or in combination with rituximab (ORR 66%) in patients with relapsed or refractory FL [53,54]. Idiotype vaccine therapy is a promising approach that produces anti-tumor responses and prolongs PFS as consolidation after initial therapy [55,56]. Bruton's tyrosine kinase inhibitors (eg, ibrutinib) [57], antibody-drug conjugates directed against B-cell antigens (eg, polatuzumab vedotin) [58], novel anti-CD20 antibodies [59], and later generation PI3K inhibitors are among the many therapies under development for FL.

Case conclusion

This patient presented with asymptomatic low tumor-burden disease and was initially observed. She developed symptomatic and progressive disease and was treated with first-line chemoimmunotherapy but relapsed within 2 years of completing treatment, a poor prognostic sign. The patient was able to enter into remission with second-line therapy, and received an autologous stem cell transplantation in CR2, the optimal timing for autologous transplantation in FL patients. Because of the relapse after high-dose chemotherapy, the patient was treated with a novel agent (lenalidomide and rituximab) rather than additional chemotherapy and then subsequently underwent allogeneic stem cell transplantation in their third remission. This case demonstrates the occasionally more aggressive course that is observed with FL, and the potential for novel agents to achieve remissions in chemorefractory patients. This case also highlights the curative potential of allogeneic transplantation for FL.

References

1 Siegel R, DeSantis C, Virgo K, et al. Cancer treatment and survivorship statistics, 2012. *CA Cancer J Clin*. 2012;62:220-241.

2 Morton LM, Wang SS, Devesa SS, Hartge P, Weisenburger DD, Linet MS. Lymphoma incidence patterns by WHO subtype in the United States, 1992-2001. *Blood*. 2006;107:265-276.

3 Harris NL, Jaffe ES, Diebold J, et al. World Health Organization classification of neoplastic diseases of the hematopoietic and lymphoid tissues: report of the Clinical Advisory Committee meeting-Airlie House, Virginia, November 1997. *J Clin Oncol*. 1999;17:3835-3849.

4 Solal-Celigny P, Roy P, Colombat P, et al. Follicular lymphoma international prognostic index. *Blood*. 2004;104:1258-1265.

5 Federico M, Bellei M, Marcheselli L, et al. Follicular lymphoma international prognostic index 2: a new prognostic index for follicular lymphoma developed by the international follicular lymphoma prognostic factor project. *J Clin Oncol*. 2009;27:4555-4562.

6 Pastore A, Jurinovic V, Kridel R, et al. Integration of gene mutations in risk prognostication for patients receiving first-line immunochemotherapy for follicular lymphoma: a retrospective analysis of a prospective clinical trial and validation in a population-based registry. *Lancet Oncol*. 2015;16:1111-1122.

7 Krikorian JG, Portlock CS, Cooney P, Rosenberg SA. Spontaneous regression of non-Hodgkin's lymphoma: a report of nine cases. *Cancer*. 1980;46:2093-2099.

8 Mac Manus MP, Hoppe RT. Is radiotherapy curative for stage I and II low-grade follicular lymphoma? Results of a long-term follow-up study of patients treated at Stanford University. *J Clin Oncol*. 1996;14:1282-1290.

9 Friedberg JW, Byrtek M, Link BK, et al. Effectiveness of first-line management strategies for stage I follicular lymphoma: analysis of the National LymphoCare Study. *J Clin Oncol*. 2012;30:3368-3375.

10 Guadagnolo BA, Li S, Neuberg D, et al. Long-term outcome and mortality trends in early-stage, Grade 1-2 follicular lymphoma treated with radiation therapy. *Int J Radiat Oncol Biol Phys*. 2006;64:928-934.

11 Pugh TJ, Ballonoff A, Newman F, Rabinovitch R. Improved survival in patients with early stage low-grade follicular lymphoma treated with radiation: a Surveillance, Epidemiology, and End Results database analysis. *Cancer*. 2010;116:3843-3851.

12 Lowry L, Smith P, Qian W, et al. Reduced dose radiotherapy for local control in non-Hodgkin lymphoma: a randomised phase III trial. *Radiother Oncol*. 2011;100:86-92.

13 Hoskin PJ, Kirkwood AA, Popova B, et al. 4 Gy versus 24 Gy radiotherapy for patients with indolent lymphoma (FORT): a randomised phase 3 non-inferiority trial. *Lancet Oncology*. 2014;15:457-463.

14 Campbell BA, Voss N, Woods R, et al. Long-term outcomes for patients with limited stage follicular lymphoma: involved regional radiotherapy versus involved node radiotherapy. *Cancer*. 2010;116:3797-3806.

15 Advani R, Rosenberg SA, Horning SJ. Stage I and II follicular non-Hodgkin's lymphoma: long-term follow-up of no initial therapy. *J Clin Oncol*. 2004;22:1454-1459.

16 National Comprehensive Cancer Network. NCCN Clinical Practice Guidelines in Oncology, Non-Hodgkin Lymphoma. https://www.nccn.org/about/nhl.pdf. Accessed March 7, 2017

17 Ardeshna KM, Smith P, Norton A, et al. Long-term effect of a watch and wait policy versus immediate systemic treatment for asymptomatic advanced-stage non-Hodgkin lymphoma: a randomised controlled trial. *Lancet*. 2003;362:516-522.

18 Ardeshna KM, Qian W, Smith P, et al. Rituximab versus a watch-and-wait approach in patients with advanced-stage, asymptomatic, non-bulky follicular lymphoma: an open-label randomised phase 3 trial. *Lancet Oncol*. 2014;15:424-435.

19 Brice P, Bastion Y, Lepage E, et al. Comparison in low-tumor-burden follicular lymphomas between an initial no-treatment policy, prednimustine, or interferon alfa: a randomized study from the Groupe d'Etude des Lymphomes Folliculaires. Groupe d'Etude des Lymphomes de l'Adulte. *J Clin Oncol*. 1997;15:1110-1117.

20 Ghielmini M, Schmitz SF, Cogliatti SB, et al. Prolonged treatment with rituximab in patients with follicular lymphoma significantly increases event-free survival and response duration compared with the standard weekly x 4 schedule. *Blood*. 2004;103:4416-4423.

21 Kahl BS, Hong F, Williams ME, Gascoyne RD, et al. Rituximab extended schedule or re-treatment trial for low-tumor burden follicular lymphoma: eastern cooperative oncology group protocol e4402. *J Clin Oncol*. 2014;32:3096-3102.

22 Marcus R, Imrie K, Solal-Celigny P, et al. Phase III study of R-CVP compared with cyclophosphamide, vincristine, and prednisone alone in patients with previously untreated advanced follicular lymphoma. *J Clin Oncol*. 2008;26:4579-4586.

23 Hiddemann W, Kneba M, Dreyling M, et al. Frontline therapy with rituximab added to the combination of cyclophosphamide, doxorubicin, vincristine, and prednisone (CHOP) significantly improves the outcome for patients with advanced-stage follicular lymphoma compared with therapy with CHOP alone: results of a prospective randomized study of the German Low-Grade Lymphoma Study Group. *Blood*. 2005;106:3725-3732.

24 Rummel MJ, Niederle N, Maschmeyer G, et al. Bendamustine plus rituximab versus CHOP plus rituximab as first-line treatment for patients with indolent and mantle-cell lymphomas: an open-label, multicentre, randomised, phase 3 non-inferiority trial. *Lancet*. 2013;381:1203-1210.

25 Flinn IW, van der Jagt R, Kahl BS, et al. Randomized trial of bendamustine-rituximab or R-CHOP/R-CVP in first-line treatment of indolent NHL or MCL: the BRIGHT study. *Blood*. 2014;123:2944-2952.

26 Vidal L, Gafter-Gvili A, Salles G, et al. Rituximab maintenance for the treatment of patients with follicular lymphoma: an updated systematic review and meta-analysis of randomized trials. *J Natl Cancer Inst*. 2011;103:1799-1806.

27 Salles G, Seymour JF, Offner F, et al. Rituximab maintenance for 2 years in patients with high tumour burden follicular lymphoma responding to rituximab plus chemotherapy (PRIMA): a phase 3, randomised controlled trial. *Lancet*. 2011;377:42-51.

28 Casulo C, Byrtek M, Dawson KL, et al. Early relapse of follicular lymphoma after rituximab plus cyclophosphamide, doxorubicin, vincristine, and prednisone defines patients at high risk for death: an analysis from the National LymphoCare study. *J Clin Oncol*. 2015;33:2516-2522.

29 Davis TA, Grillo-Lopez AJ, White CA, et al. Rituximab anti-CD20 monoclonal antibody therapy in non-Hodgkin's lymphoma: safety and efficacy of re-treatment. *J Clin Oncol*. 2000;18:3135-3143.

30 Gopal AK, Kahl BS, de Vos S, et al. PI3Kdelta inhibition by idelalisib in patients with relapsed indolent lymphoma. *N Engl J Med*. 2014;370:1008-1018.

31 Witzig TE, Molina A, Gordon LI, et al. Long-term responses in patients with recurring or refractory B-cell non-Hodgkin lymphoma treated with yttrium 90 ibritumomab tiuxetan. *Cancer*. 2007;109:1804-1810.

32 Witzig TE, Wiernik PH, Moore T, et al. Lenalidomide oral monotherapy produces durable responses in relapsed or refractory indolent non-Hodgkin's Lymphoma. *J Clin Oncol*. 2009;27:5404-5409.

33 Leonard JP, Jung SH, Johnson J, et al. Randomized trial of lenalidomide alone versus lenalidomide plus rituximab in patients with recurrent follicular lymphoma: CALGB 50401 (Alliance). *J Clin Oncol*. 2015;33:3635-3640.

34 Fowler NH, Davis RE, Rawal S, et al. Safety and activity of lenalidomide and rituximab in untreated indolent lymphoma: an open-label, phase 2 trial. *Lancet Oncol*. 2014;15:1311-1318.

35 Wiseman GA, Gordon LI, Multani PS, et al. Ibritumomab tiuxetan radioimmunotherapy for patients with relapsed or refractory non-Hodgkin lymphoma and mild thrombocytopenia: a phase II multicenter trial. *Blood*. 2002;99:4336-4342.

36 Sebban C, Mounier N, Brousse N, et al. Standard chemotherapy with interferon compared with CHOP followed by high-dose therapy with autologous stem cell transplantation in untreated patients with advanced follicular lymphoma: the GELF-94 randomized study from the Groupe d'Etude des Lymphomes de l'Adulte (GELA). *Blood*. 2006;108:2540-2544.

37 Ladetto M, De Marco F, Benedetti F, et al. Prospective, multicenter randomized GITMO/IIL trial comparing intensive (R-HDS) versus conventional (CHOP-R) chemoimmunotherapy in high-risk follicular lymphoma at diagnosis: the superior disease control of R-HDS does not translate into an overall survival advantage. *Blood*. 2008;111:4004-4013.

38 Brice P, Simon D, Bouabdallah R, et al. High-dose therapy with autologous stem-cell transplantation (ASCT) after first progression prolonged survival of follicular lymphoma patients included in the prospective GELF 86 protocol. *Ann Oncol*. 2000;11:1585-1590.

39 Le Gouill S, De Guibert S, Planche L, et al. Impact of the use of autologous stem cell transplantation at first relapse both in naive and previously rituximab exposed follicular lymphoma patients treated in the GELA/GOELAMS FL2000 study. *Haematologica*. 2011;96:1128-1135.

40 Schouten HC, Qian W, Kvaloy S, et al. High-dose therapy improves progression-free survival and survival in relapsed follicular non-Hodgkin's lymphoma: results from the randomized European CUP trial. *J Clin Oncol*. 2003;21:3918-3927.

41 Sebban C, Brice P, Delarue R, et al. Impact of rituximab and/or high-dose therapy with autotransplant at time of relapse in patients with follicular lymphoma: a GELA study. *J Clin Oncol*. 2008;26:3614-3620.

42 Rohatiner AZ, Nadler L, Davies AJ, et al. Myeloablative therapy with autologous bone marrow transplantation for follicular lymphoma at the time of second or subsequent remission: long-term follow-up. *J Clin Oncol*. 2007;25:2554-2559.

43 Hari P, Carreras J, Zhang MJ, et al. Allogeneic transplants in follicular lymphoma: higher risk of disease progression after reduced-intensity compared to myeloablative conditioning. *Biol Blood Marrow Transplant*. 2008;14:236-245.

44 Armand P, Kim HT, Ho VT, et al. Allogeneic transplantation with reduced-intensity conditioning for Hodgkin and non-Hodgkin lymphoma: importance of histology for outcome. *Biol Blood Marrow Transplant*. 2008;14:418-425.

45 Khouri IF, Saliba RM, Erwin WD, et al. Nonmyeloablative allogeneic transplantation with or without 90yttrium ibritumomab tiuxetan is potentially curative for relapsed follicular lymphoma: 12-year results. *Blood*. 2012;119:6373-6378.

46 Rezvani AR, Storer B, Maris M, et al. Nonmyeloablative allogeneic hematopoietic cell transplantation in relapsed, refractory, and transformed indolent non-Hodgkin's lymphoma. *J Clin Oncol*. 2008;26:211-217.

47 Shea T, Johnson J, Westervelt P, et al. Reduced-intensity allogeneic transplantation provides high event-free and overall survival in patients with advanced indolent B cell malignancies: CALGB 109901. *Biol Blood Marrow Transplant*. 2011;17:1395-1403.

48 van Besien K, Loberiza FR Jr, Bajorunaite R, et al. Comparison of autologous and allogeneic hematopoietic stem cell transplantation for follicular lymphoma. *Blood*. 2003;102:3521-3529.

49 Robinson SP, Canals C, Luang JJ, et al. The outcome of reduced intensity allogeneic stem cell transplantation and autologous stem cell transplantation when performed as a first transplant strategy in relapsed follicular lymphoma: an analysis from the Lymphoma Working Party of the EBMT. *Bone Marrow Transplant*. 2013;48:1409-1414.

50 Casulo C, Burack WR, Friedberg JW. Transformed follicular non-Hodgkin lymphoma. *Blood*. 2015;125:40-47.

51 Link BK, Maurer MJ, Nowakowski GS, et al. Rates and outcomes of follicular lymphoma transformation in the immunochemotherapy era: a report from the University of Iowa/MayoClinic Specialized Program of Research Excellence Molecular Epidemiology Resource. *J Clin Oncol*. 2013;31:3272-3278.

52 Kuruvilla J, MacDonald DA, Kouroukis CT, et al. Salvage chemotherapy and autologous stem cell transplantation for transformed indolent lymphoma: a subset analysis of NCIC CTG LY12. *Blood*. 2015;126:733-738.

53 Westin JR, Chu F, Zhang M, et al. Safety and activity of PD1 blockade by pidilizumab in combination with rituximab in patients with relapsed follicular lymphoma: a single group, open-label, phase 2 trial. *Lancet Oncol*. 2014;15:69-77.

54 Lesokhin AM, Ansell SM, Armand P, et al. Preliminary results of a phase I study of nivolumab (BMS-936558) in patients with relapsed or refractory lymphoid malignancies. *Blood (ASH Annual Meeting Abstracts)*. 2014;124:291.

55 Neelapu SS, Baskar S, Gause BL, et al. Human autologous tumor-specific T-cell responses induced by liposomal delivery of a lymphoma antigen. *Clin Cancer Res*. 2004;10:8309-8317.

56 Schuster SJ, Neelapu SS, Gause BL, et al. Vaccination with patient-specific tumor-derived antigen in first remission improves disease-free survival in follicular lymphoma. *J Clin Oncol*. 2011;29:2787-2794.

57 Advani RH, Buggy JJ, Sharman JP, et al. Bruton tyrosine kinase inhibitor ibrutinib (PCI-32765) has significant activity in patients with relapsed/refractory B-cell malignancies. *J Clin Oncol*. 2013;31:88-94.

58 Palanca-Wessels MC, Czuczman M, Salles G, et al. Safety and activity of the anti-CD79B antibody-drug conjugate polatuzumab vedotin in relapsed or refractory B-cell non-Hodgkin lymphoma and chronic lymphocytic leukaemia: a phase 1 study. *Lancet Oncol*. 2015;16:704-715.

59 Sehn LH, Goy A, Offner FC, Martinelli G, et al. Randomized phase II trial comparing obinutuzumab (GA101) with rituximab in patients with relapsed CD20+ indolent B-cell non-Hodgkin lymphoma: final analysis of the GAUSS study. *J Clin Oncol*. 2015;33:3467-3474.

Chapter 6

Lymphoplasmacytic lymphoma in the era of next generation sequencing

Michelle Afkhami, Tanya Siddiqi, and Steven T Rosen

Case presentation

A 72-year-old Caucasian male was referred to City of Hope in 2015 due to fatigue, malaise, a 12 pound unintentional weight loss over 4 months, and mild normochromic normocytic anemia along with mild thrombocytopenia. His past medical history was significant for an episode of hemolytic anemia and splenomegaly in 2008, which at the time was thought to be due to chronic lymphocytic leukemia (CLL). He was treated with cyclophosphamide, rituximab, and prednisone for eight cycles and achieved a remission although his course was complicated by the development of renal failure resulting in chronic kidney disease. His original bone marrow biopsy was reviewed at City of Hope and a new biopsy was also performed.

Lymphoplasmacytic lymphoma

Lymphoplasmacytic lymphoma (LPL) accounts for approximately 1.5–5% of B-cell lymphoproliferative disorders characterized by a spectrum of small B cells, plasmacytoid lymphocytes, and plasma cells. Plasmacytic differentiation may occur in almost all small B-cell lymphomas therefore the diagnosis of LPL can be difficult. Recently, molecular mutational diagnostic approaches, especially next generation sequencing, have helped

© Springer International Publishing AG 2017   97
J. Zain and L.W. Kwak (eds.), *Management of Lymphomas:
A Case-Based Approach*, DOI 10.1007/978-3-319-26827-9_6

refine the diagnostic criteria for LPL. The utility of molecular testing is not only for diagnosis but can be applied to risk stratification and treatment planning of B-cell lymphomas including LPL. Lymphoplasmacytic lymphoma primarily involves the bone marrow, with less frequent involvement of spleen, lymph nodes, and other tissue sites. Cases with mainly nodal presentation are rarely encountered [1–4].

Work up, diagnosis, and treatment

At the time of initial examination in our clinic, the patient had fatigue, malaise, anorexia, and splenomegaly measuring 2–3 cm below the left subcostal margin. No palpable lymphadenopathy was noted. Laboratory data revealed a normal white blood cell (WBC) count of 5.2 K/μL with a low hemoglobin of 11.3 G/dL (mean corpuscle volume [MCV] 87.9 fL, mean corpuscular hemoglobin concentration [MCHC] 32.7 G/dL), and platelet count of 125 K/μL. Liver functions were normal but lactate dehydrogenase (LDH) was mildly elevated at 677 (reference range 313-618 U/L). Creatinine was at his baseline of 2.25 (reference range 0.7–1.3 mg/dL). His serum free light chains showed a kappa of 17.4 (reference range 3.3–19.4 mg/dL) and lambda 2.59 (reference range 0.57–2.63 mg/dL) with a kappa to lambda ratio of 6.72. His serum IgM level was 674 (reference range 38–271 mg/dL), IgG 981 (reference range 700–1600 mg/dL), and IgA <30 (reference range 70–400 mg/dL). Direct Coombs test and haptoglobin were normal. Computed tomography (CT) imaging of his chest/abdomen/pelvic revealed hepatomegaly and mild splenomegaly. Review of the initial 2008 bone marrow demonstrated a markedly hypercellular bone marrow composed of small B cells with admixed plasma cells. Immunohistochemical stains revealed a population of IgM-/kappa-positive plasma cells infiltrating the bone marrow. The medium-sized lymphocytes in the background were positive for CD20, however the small lymphocytes in the background were negative for CD5 and CD23. This phenotype of the B-cell infiltrate was atypical for CLL and more consistent with involvement by LPL. A bone marrow biopsy was repeated at City of Hope and revealed a hypercellular bone marrow (>95%) infiltrated by a lymphoplasmacytic cell population. Immunohistochemical studies demonstrated a monoclonal plasmacytic infiltrate staining with IgM and kappa light chain (about 10%). These *findings were again consistent with LPL. To confirm this diagnosis, and for risk assessment stratification of the disease process, MYD88 and CXCR4 mutational analysis were performed on the clot section. The molecular testing results were positive for the MYD88 mutation (p.L265P, c.794T>C) as well as the CXCR4 mutation (p.S338*, c.1013G>C). Ibrutinib, a selective oral Bruton's tyrosine kinase (BTK) inhibitor, was initiated at 420 mg daily on 04/01/15 and the patient achieved a hematological remission in three months with normalization of all blood counts. His IgM nadir during this period was 480 mg/dL and his B symptoms had resolved completely.*

Clinical and pathologic diagnosis of lymphoplasmacytic lymphoma

The most frequent symptoms of LPL include weakness, fatigue, and gingival bleeding due to hyperviscosity, and associated impeded flow that can also cause visual impairment, and in some cases even blindness and neurologic problems such as headaches or deafness. The other common clinical presentations are anemia, hepatosplenomegaly, and lymphadenopathy. Most patients are 60 years of age or older, however patients with familial predisposition might present at a younger age [5–8]. LPL is typically but not always associated with an IgM gammopathy. The clinical syndrome of Waldenström's macroglobulinemia (WM) is currently defined as LPL with an associated monoclonal IgM (balanced H or L chains production) protein of any level [1–3]. Most of the cases have been reported to show kappa restriction (>75%). Other small B-cell lymphomas with plasmacytic differentiation such as marginal zone lymphomas or CLL/small lymphocytic lymphoma (SLL) are occasionally associated with IgM paraprotein production as well. In addition, symptomatic WM-like features have been described in association with non-IgM (ie, IgG or IgA) gammopathy [1–4,9]. The pattern of bone marrow infiltration may be diffuse, interstitial, or nodular and is usually intertrabecular. Morphologically the infiltrate in LPL is more monotonous than that in nodal marginal zone lymphoma, with intact and often dilated sinuses. Furthermore, numerous Mott cells with cytoplasmic inclusions are present and the surrounding cells show plasmacytoid features with plasmacytoid lymphocytes most conspicuous adjacent to the sinuses. B-cell proliferation may resemble CLL/SLL but there is plasma cell differentiation with commonly seen Russel and Dutcher's bodies. While Dutcher's bodies (visible cytoplasmic inclusions) are more common in LPL than nodal marginal zone lymphoma, they can be seen in either disease. Increased mast cells and amyloidosis are also reported [2–4,9–12].

Phenotypic marker profiling by immunohistochemistry studies demonstrates the small B lymphocytes in LPL expressing pan B-cell antigens (CD19, CD20, CD22, CD79a, and PAX5) with monotypic surface light-chain restriction. Unlike other subtypes of B-cell lymphoma, there is no specific phenotypically distinct marker profile for LPL. A diagnosis of LPL should not be dismissed in the immunophenotype setting of CD5 or CD23 co-positivity [4,9–11]. Rare examples of LPL with CD10 co-expression are also recognized [6]. In tissue sections, light-chain restriction is usually easily demonstrated in both small lymphocytes and associated plasma cells by immunohistochemistry. The plasma cell component can also be highlighted using antibodies recognizing CD138 or MUM-1 (IRF4) proteins. The majority of LPLs are clearly IgM-positive by heavy chain immunoperoxidase. Recent flow cytometric studies have noted that LPL-associated plasma cells are CD19+, in contradistinction to the plasma cells of multiple myeloma [4,9,11].

Molecular diagnostic features in the era of next generation sequencing

Early genetic associations attributed the presence of a deletion of the long arm of chromosome 6 (6q-) as one of the most common abnormalities in LPL (40% to 60% of cases) with comparable frequency in patients with or without a familial history [5–8,12–16]. In a recent study by Hunter et al [17] whole exome sequencing of 30 WM cases revealed gene losses involved *PRDM2* (93%), *BTG1* (87%), *HIVEP2* (77%), *MKLN1* (77%), *PLEKHG1* (70%), *LYN* (60%), *ARID1B* (50%), and *FOXP1* (37%). Losses in *PLEKHG1, HIVEP2, ARID1B*, and *BCLAF1* constituted the most common deletions within chromosome 6.

Trisomy of chromosome 4 has also been reported in a subset of LPL patients [16]. Cytogenetics findings are relatively nonspecific as a tumor marker in LPL/WM, however IgH rearrangement might be used to clarify the diagnosis of WM from suspected cases of IgM myeloma as 14q32 translocations are a predominant feature of IgM myeloma and are typically absent in WM.

Recent whole-genome sequencing studies revealed diagnostic break-throughs in LPL (WM) by revealing a somatic mutation of *MYD88* in approximately 90–95% of the WM patients [18–45]. The most common variation is a leucine to proline substitution in codon 265 (L265P, c.794T>C), an evolutionarily invariant residue in the hydrophobic core of the Toll/IL1 receptor (TIR) domain of *MYD88*. The L265P-activating mutation triggers interleukin-1 receptor-associated kinase (IRAK) and Bruton's tyrosine kinase (BTK) that in turn activate nuclear factor-kB (NF-kB) and MAPK signalling pathways. Four *IRAK* genes exist in the human genome: *IRAK1, IRAK2, IRAK3,* and *IRAK4*. TLR/IL1R signalling is achieved through differential recruitment of adaptor molecules such as MyD88. These adaptors function in the subsequent recruitment and activation of IRAK family kinases, which end up activating NF-kB pathway.

Although the *MYD88 L265P* alteration might be considered the hallmark of LPL, it can be seen in other B-cell lymphomas. Mutational analysis of primary central nervous system lymphoma (PCNSL) cases in one study reported a *MYD88* mutation in about 38% of PCNSL [25]. A few recent studies reported that about 40% of cases with activated B-cell-like diffuse large B-cell lymphoma (ABC-DLBCL) harbor the *MYD88 L265P* mutation and a few other rare variations of *MYD88*. Three of these rare mutations were in the TIR domain (*S219C, M232T,* and *S243N*) and two variants (*P141T* and *Q143L*) were located between the death and TIR domains [23,24,43]. However, *MYD88 L265P* represents almost the sole *MYD88* mutation in LPL/WM and in 50–60% of patients with the IgM-type monoclonal gammopathy of undetermined significance, which may precede WM. ABC-DLBCL cell lines with *L265P MyD88* mutations reported to exhibit RNAi-mediated knockdown of *MyD88, IRAK4,* or *IRAK1* eliminated NF-kB activation and induced rapid apoptosis. Thus, in this context, sustained *MyD88-IRAK* signaling is necessary for ABC-DLBCL pathogenesis and tumor cell survival. The *MYD88 L265P* mutation has been also reported in (15%) of splenic marginal zone lymphoma cases (SMZL). The mutation was absent from nodal marginal zone lymphoma, extranodal mucosa-associated lymphoid tissue (MALT), [6,21,31] and myeloma, including samples from patients with IgM secreting myeloma [35,36,39]. Thus, detection of this mutation is valuable for the differential diagnosis of WM/LPL from these low-grade B-cell neoplasms [24–26].

The other common somatic variants reported in LPL are the *AT-rich interactive domain 1A gene* (*ARID1A*) alterations. In one study the whole genome sequencing of 30 cases of WM (LPL) revealed that 17% of patients had a mutation in *ARID1A*, including three single-nucleotide variants leading to premature protein truncation (R173, Q547, and Q934), and two frameshift changes (a deletion at position 27057944 and an insertion at position 27107136 in chromosome 1). Patients with both *ARID1A* and *MYD88 L265P* mutations, as compared with patients who did not have *ARIDIA* mutations, had greater involvement of bone marrow disease, a lower hematocrit, and a lower platelet count [13].

Recently, warts, hypogammaglobulinaemia, infections, and mye-lokathexis (WHIM) syndrome-like mutations in *CXCR4* have been described in 28–36% of LPL cases, which involve the carboxyl terminus (C-terminus), the similar location to those observed in the germline of patients with WHIM syndrome, a congenital immunodeficiency disorder characterized by chronic noncyclic neutropenia. This is the first somatic mutation in *CXCR4* described in any human cancer and seems to have an impact on the clinical presentation and response to therapy of the BTK inhibitors, such as ibrutinib [13,46–49,50]. Patients with *MYD88* and *CXCR4* mutations have important differences in disease presentation for patients with WM, including bone marrow (BM) disease burden, presence of extramedullary disease, serum IgM levels, symptomatic status at diagnosis including presentation with hyperviscosity syndrome, and overall survival (OS). These cases showed a higher extent of BM infiltration and lower leukocyte, hemoglobin, and platelet counts [46–49]. These findings are reliable and useful for subtyping small B-cell lymphomas (SBLs) including WM/LPL in BM biopsies and provide a personalized approach to risk stratification and potential therapy for WM/LPL cases [14–49].

Treatment of primary and previously treated disease

Asymptomatic patients are typically observed and therapy is reserved for symptoms associated with disease progression such as fatigue, cytopenias, hyperviscosity, cold agglutinemia, cryoglobulinemia, moderate to severe or advancing paraprotein-related peripheral neuropathy, or extramedullary disease including central nervous system (Bing-Neel syndrome) involvement [13,51]. Treatment initiation should not be based on serum IgM levels per se, although at higher serum IgM levels (>4000 mg/dL), empiric treatment may be appropriate to prevent hyperviscosity-related injury.

For frontline management per the 2014 consensus panels of the International Workshop on WM (IWWM-7), rituximab alone or rituximab combination regimens remain a recommended primary therapy for most patients with WM. Rituximab alone yields an overall response rate (ORR) of 25–40% when given weekly for 4 weeks and 40–60% when this 4 week course is repeated at 3 months [52–54]. The reported median progression free survival (mPFS) of this regimen is 16–29 months. As per the previous recommendations (IWWM-4) dexamethasone, rituximab and cyclophosphamide (DRC) remains a primary consideration for therapy as well with an ORR of 80-90% and mPFS of 3 years [55,56]. However, combinations such as rituximab, cyclophosphamide, doxorubicin, vincristine, and prednisone (R-CHOP) are no longer considered a first-line choice due to poorer tolerance and lower mPFS (29 months) compared with bendamustine-rituximab (BR, mPFS 69 months), which has emerged as a primary treatment option especially for patients with high tumor bulk or extramedullary disease [57,58]. In the current recommendations, the combination of bortezomib (or carflizomib) and rituximab with or without dexamethasone may also be considered a primary option for patients with specific high-risk features like hyperviscosity or in younger patients for whom avoidance of alkylator therapy is a concern. Fludarabine-based combinations are not recommended for primary therapy but remain an option for patients with relapsed/refractory disease with adequate performance status. In patients who may be candidates for single agent oral therapy, oral fludarabine (if available) is recommended over chlorambucil [51,57,59–61]. Of note, rituximab intolerance is common in WM and a switch to ofatumumab may be needed.

Plasmapheresis should be performed for patients with symptomatic hyperviscosity and before treatment with a rituximab-containing regimen in patients with IgM>4000 mg/dL as the occurrence of an IgM flare (defined as a ≥25% increase above the baseline level) is quite common after rituximab therapy in WM patients, with an about 40–50% occurrence rate when rituximab is used as monotherapy. IgM should be monitored closely in these patients thereafter and plasmapheresis should be considered again if symptomatic hyperviscosity occurs or if IgM>4000 mg/dL while on rituximab-containing therapy [51,60,61].

If complete or partial response is achieved with a rituximab-based regimen and the patient is asymptomatic, close monitoring is recommended. Maintenance rituximab given every 2 months for 2 years can prolong survival [62] although prospective confirmation of this is still ongoing [63]. For patients with short remissions (<12 months) or with progressive disease/resistance to a first-line regimen, second-line treatment should include agents of a different class, either alone or in combination. For the patient with a recurrence of disease more than 12 months later, the previous treatment regimen or alternative therapy may be used. In select patients autologous or allogeneic transplantation is a consideration (Figure 6.1) [61]. Adoptive cellular immunotherapy with CD19-specific chimeric antigen receptor (CAR)-T cell therapy is being investigated in WM as well.

Targeted therapies directed against *MYD88* and/or *CXCR4* signaling are emerging as a personalized treatment approach to WM/LPL. *IRAK 1* and *IRAK 4* as well as BTK all signal for *MYD88 L265P* and BTK is activated by CXCR4 [13,18,61,65,66]. Inhibitors to *IRAK* are in clinical development whereas the BTK inhibitor ibrutinib has already shown impressive activity in relapsed and refractory WM patients [48,65,67]. In a recent study by Treon et al, 63 patients with relapsed/refractory WM were treated with ibrutinib 420 mg orally daily. An ORR of 90.5% (73% major response rate, MRR) and an estimated 2-year PFS of 69.1% with an estimated 2-year OS of 95.2% was observed. Major responses were highest in *MYD88 L265P*-mutated and *CXCR4* wild-type patients (*n*=34;

ORR 100%, MRR 91.2%) while those patients with mutated *MYD88/* mutated *CXCR4* were less likely to respond to ibrutinib (*n*=21, ORR 85.7%, MRR 61.9%) and those with wild-type *MYD88/*wild type *CXCR4* had the lowest responses (*n*=7, ORR 71.4%, MRR 28.6%). Ibrutinib was generally well-tolerated, with some events of neutropenia and thrombocytopenia in heavily pre-treated patients especially. Based on these results ibrutinib was approved for the treatment of patients with WM in 2015 both in the US and Europe.

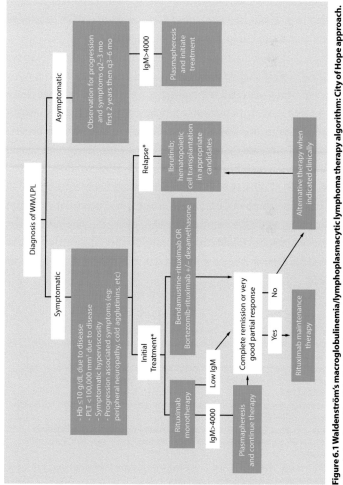

Figure 6.1 Waldenström's macroglobulinemia/lymphoplasmacytic lymphoma therapy algorithm: City of Hope approach. * first choice should be clinical trials with novel agents if available. LPL, lymphoplasmacytic lymphoma; PLT, platelets; WM, Waldenström's macroglobulinemia.

Preclinical studies have also shown that WM cells engineered to express the *S338X CXCR4* NS mutation show resistance to the suppressive effects of ibrutinib on AKT and extracellular signal-regulated kinase 1/2 signaling. In vitro, this could be restored by use of the CXCR4-specific inhibitor plerixafor [65]. Taken together, these studies highlight the importance of understanding both *MYD88* and *CXCR4* mutation status in WM and may provide the basis for a more personalized treatment approach, including the use of relevant inhibitors for *MYD88*-mutated patients and the use of CXCR4 inhibitors in *CXCR4*-mutated WM patients. In addition to plerixafor, several other antagonists to CXCR4 have been developed and are in clinical trials [47,48,65,68].

Prognosis and conclusions

In this era of next generation sequencing, novel molecular changes have been identified in WM, an incurable indolent NHL, and further investigations are bringing even more related changes to light thereby providing the basis of targeted therapeutics in this disease. Novel monoclonal antibodies as well as inhibitors of BTK, PI3K delta, MYD88, CXCR4, IRAK1/4, BCL2, CD27/CD70 and proteosomes are being investigated in clinical trials in search of durable remissions, and potential cures are being sought using CAR-T cell therapy and, in appropriate candidates, allogeneic hematopoietic cell transplantation. Our primary approach to therapy in this disease is to recommend clinical trials with novel agents if available.

References

1   Owen RG, Treon SP, Al-Katib A, et al. Clinicopathological definition of Waldenstrom's macroglobulinemia: consensus panel recommendations from the Second International Workshop on Waldenstrom's Macroglobulinemia. *Semin Oncol.* 2003;30:110-115.

2   Dimopoulos MA, Gertz MA, Kastritis E, et al. Update on treatment recommendations from the Fourth International Workshop on Waldenström's Macroglobulinemia. *J Clin Oncol.* 2009;27:120-126.

3   Dimopoulos MA, Anagnostopoulos A. Waldenström's macroglobulinemia. *Best Pract Res Clin Haematol.* 2005;18:747-765.

4   Swerdlow SH, Campo E, Harris NL, et al (Eds). *World Health Organization Classification of Tumours of Haematopoietic and Lymphoid Tissues.* 4th edn. Lyon, France: IARC Press; 2008. pp 194-195.

5   Treon SP, Hunter ZR, Aggarwal A, et al. Characterization of familial Waldenstrom's macroglobulinemia. *Ann Oncol.* 2006;17:488-494.

6 Kristinsson SY, Björkholm M, Goldin LR, et al. Risk of lymphoproliferative disorders among first-degree relatives of lymphoplasmacytic lymphoma/Waldenstrom macroglobulinemia patients: a population-based study in Sweden. *Blood*. 2008;112:3052-3056.

7 Altieri A, Bermejo JL, Hemminki K. Familial aggregation of lymphoplasmacytic lymphoma with non-Hodgkin lymphoma and other neoplasms. *Leukemia*. 2005;19:2342-2343.

8 Hunter ZR, Xu L, Yang G, et al. The genomic landscape of Waldenstrom macroglobulinemia is characterized by highly recurring MYD88 and WHIM-like CXCR4 mutations, and small somatic deletions associated with B-cell lymphomagenesis. *Blood*. 2014;123:1637-1646.

9 Konoplev S, Medeiros LJ, Bueso-Ramos CE, et al. Immunophenotypic profile of lymphoplasmacytic lymphoma/Waldenstrom macroglobulinemia. *Am J Clin Pathol*. 2005;124:414-420

10 Hunter ZR, Branagan AR, Manning R, et al. CD5, CD10, and CD23 expression in Waldenstrom's macroglobulinemia. *Clin Lymphoma*. 2005;5:246-249.

11 Morice WG, Chen D, Kurtin PJ, et al. Novel immunophenotypic features of marrow lymphoplasmacytic lymphoma and correlation with Waldenstrom's macroglobulinemia. *Mod Pathol*. 2009;22:807-816.

12 Mansoor A, Medeiros LJ, Weber DM, et al. Cytogenetic findings in lymphoplasmatic lymphoma/Waldenstrom's macroglobulinemia. *Am J Clin Pathol*. 2001;116:543-549.

13 Schop RF, Fonseca R. Genetics and cytogenetics of Waldenstrom's macroglobulinemia. *Semin Oncol*. 2003;30:142-145.

14 Schop RF, Kuehl WM, Van Wier SA, et al. Waldenstrom macroglobulinemia neoplastic cells lack immunoglobulin heavy chain locus translocations but have frequent 6q deletions. *Blood*. 2002;100:2996-3001.

15 Chang H, Qi X, Xu W, et al.: Analysis of 6q deletion in Waldenstrom macroglobulinemia. *Eur J Haematol*. 2007;79:244-247.

16 Terre C, Nguyen-Khac F, Barin C, et al. Trisomy 4, a new chromosomal abnormality in Waldenstrom's macroglobulinemia: a study of 39 cases. *Leukemia*. 2006; 20:1634-1636.

17 Treon SP, Tripsas C, Yang G, et al. A prospective multicenter study of the Bruton's tyrosine kinase inhibitor ibrutinib. Patients with relapsed or refractory Waldenstrom's macroglobulinemia. In: Proceedings of the American Society of Hematology. *Blood*. 2013 (abstract 251).

18 Ngo VN, Young RM, Schmitz R, et al. Oncogenically active MYD88 mutations in human lymphoma. *Nature*. 2011;470:115-119.

19 Treon SP, Xu L, Yang G, et al. MYD88 L265P somatic mutation in Waldenström's macroglobulinemia. *N Engl J Med*. 2012;367:826-833.

20 Varettoni M, Arcaini L, Zibellini S, et al. Prevalence and clinical significance of the MYD88 (L265P) somatic mutation in Waldenstrom's macroglobulinemia and related lymphoid neoplasms. *Blood*. 2013;121:2522-2528.

21 Gachard N, Parrens M, Soubeyran I, et al. IGHV gene features and MYD88 L265P mutation separate the three marginal zone lymphoma entities and Waldenström macroglobulinemia/ lymphoplasmacytic lymphomas. *Leukemia*. 2013;27:183-189.

22 Poulain S, Roumier C, Decambron A, et al. MYD88 L265P mutation in Waldenstrom macroglobulinemia. *Blood*. 2013;121:4504-4511.

23 Arcaini L, Rossi D, Lucioni M, et al. The NOTCH pathway is recurrently mutated in diffuse large B-cell lymphoma associated with hepatitis C virus infection. *Haematologica*. 2015;100:246-252.

24 Bohers E, Mareschal S, Bouzelfen A, et al. Targetable activating mutations are very frequent in GCB and ABC diffuse large B-cell lymphoma. *Genes Chromosomes Cancer*. 2014;53:144-153.

25 Bruno A, Boisselier B, Labreche K, et al. Mutational analysis of primary central nervous system lymphoma. *Oncotarget*. 2014;5:5065-5075.

26 Santos Gda C, Saieg MA, Ko HM, et al. Multiplex sequencing for EZH2, CD79B, and MYD88 mutations using archival cytospin preparations from B-cell non-Hodgkin lymphoma aspirates previously tested for MYC rearrangement and IGH/BCL2 translocation. *Cancer Cytopathol*. 2015;123:413-420.

27 Poulain S, Herbaux C, Bertrand E, et al. Genomic studies have identified multiple mechanisms of genetic changes in Waldenström macroglobulinemia. *Clin Lymphoma Myeloma Leuk*. 2013;13:202-204.

28 Braggio E, Fonseca R. Genomic abnormalities of Waldenström macroglobulinemia and related low-grade B-cell lymphomas. *Clin Lymphoma Myeloma Leuk*. 2013;13:198-201.

29 Manasanch EE, Kristinsson SY, Landgren O. Etiology of Waldenström macroglobulinemia: genetic factors and immune-related conditions. *Clin Lymphoma Myeloma Leuk*. 2013;13:194-197.

30 Treon SP, Hunter ZR, Castillo JJ, Merlini G. Waldenström macroglobulinemia. *Hematol Oncol Clin North Am*. 2014;28:945-970.

31 Bruscaggin A, Monti S, Arcaini L, et al. Molecular lesions of signalling pathway genes in clonal B-cell lymphocytosis with marginal zone features. *Br J Haematol*. 2014;167:718-720.

32 Swerdlow SH, Kuzu I, Dogan A, et al. The many faces of small B cell lymphomas with plasmacytic differentiation and the contribution of MYD88 testing. *Virchows Arch*. 2016;468:259-275.

33 Yang G, Zhou Y, Liu X, et al. A mutation in MYD88 (L265P) supports the survival of lymphoplasmacytic cells by activation of Bruton tyrosine kinase in Waldenström macroglobulinemia. *Blood*. 2013;122:1222-1232.

34 Insuasti-beltran G, Gale JM, Wilson CS, Foucar K, Czuchlewski DR. Significance of MYD88 L265P mutation status in the subclassification of low-grade B-cell lymphoma/leukemia. *Arch Pathol Lab Med*. 2015;139:1035-1041.

35 Anderson KC, Alsina M, Bensinger W, et al. Waldenström's macroglobulinemia/ lymphoplasmacytic lymphoma, version 2.2013. *J Natl Compr Canc Netw*. 2012;10:1211-1219.

36 Mori N, Ohwashi M, Yoshinaga K, et al. L265P mutation of the MYD88 gene is frequent in Waldenström's macroglobulinemia and its absence in myeloma. *PLoS ONE*. 2013;8:e80088.

37 Caner V, Sen turk N, Baris IC, et al. MYD88 expression and L265P mutation in mature B-cell non-Hodgkin lymphomas. *Genet Test Mol Biomarkers*. 2015;19:372-378.

38 Wang L, Lawrence MS, Wan Y, et al. SF3B1 and other novel cancer genes in chronic lymphocytic leukemia. *N Engl J Med*. 2011;365:2497-2506.

39 Ondrejka SL, Lin JJ, Warden DW, Durkin L, Cook JR, Hsi ED. MYD88 L265P somatic mutation: its usefulness in the differential diagnosis of bone marrow involvement by B-cell lymphoproliferative disorders. *Am J Clin Pathol*. 2013;140:387-394.

40 Xu L, Hunter ZR, Yang G, et al. MYD88 L265P in Waldenström macroglobulinemia, immunoglobulin M monoclonal gammopathy, and other B-cell lymphoproliferative disorders using conventional and quantitative allele-specific polymerase chain reaction. *Blood*. 2013;121:2051-2058.

41 Jiménez C, Sebastián E, Chillón MC, et al. MYD88 L265P is a marker highly characteristic of, but not restricted to, Waldenström's macroglobulinemia. *Leukemia*. 2013;27:1722-1728.

42 Alley CL, Wang E, Dunphy CH, et al. Diagnostic and clinical considerations in concomitant bone marrow involvement by plasma cell myeloma and chronic lymphocytic leukemia/ monoclonal B-cell lymphocytosis: a series of 15 cases and review of literature. *Arch Pathol Lab Med*. 2013;137:503-517.

43 Kraan W, Horlings HM, Van keimpema M, et al. High prevalence of oncogenic MYD88 and CD79B mutations in diffuse large B-cell lymphomas presenting at immune-privileged sites. *Blood Cancer J*. 2013;3:e139.

44 Braggio E, Philipsborn C, Novak A, Hodge L, Ansell S, Fonseca R. Molecular pathogenesis of Waldenstrom's macroglobulinemia. *Haematologica*. 2012;97:1281-1290.

45 Cao Y, Hunter ZR, Liu X, Yang G, Tripsas CK, Manning R et al. Somatic activating mutations in CXCR4 are common in patients with Waldenstrom's Macroglobulinemia, and their expression in WM cells promotes resistance to ibrutinib. Blood (ASH Annual Meeting Abstracts), December 2013; 4424 2013.

46 Cao Y, Hunter ZR, Liu X, et al. CXCR4 WHIM-like frameshift and nonsense mutations promote ibrutinib resistance but do not supplant MYD88(L265P)-directed survival signalling in Waldenström macroglobulinaemia cells. *Br J Haematol*. 2015;168:701-707.

47 Treon SP, Cao Y, Xu L, Yang G, Liu X, Hunter ZR. Somatic mutations in MYD88 and CXCR4 are determinants of clinical presentation and overall survival in Waldenstrom macroglobulinemia. *Blood*. 2014;123:2791-2796.

48 Nagao T, Oshikawa G, Ishida S, et al. A novel MYD88 mutation, L265RPP, in Waldenström macroglobulinemia activates the NF-κB pathway to upregulate Bcl-xL expression and enhances cell survival. *Blood Cancer J*. 2015;5:e31.

49 Schmidt J, Federmann B, Schindler N, et al. MYD88 L265P and CXCR4 mutations in lymphoplasmacytic lymphoma identify cases with high disease activity. *Br J Haematol*. 2015;169:795-803.

50 Busillo JM, Armando S, Sengupta R, Meucci O, Bouvier M, Benovic JL. Site-specific phosphorylation of CXCR4 is dynamically regulated by multiple kinases and results in differential modulation of CXCR4 signaling. *J Biol Chem*. 2010;285:7805-7817.

51 Treon SP. How I treat Waldenström macroglobulinemia. *Blood*. 2015;126:721-732.

52 Gertz MA, Rue M, Blood E, Kaminer LS, Vesole DH, Greipp PR, et al. Multicenter phase 2 trial of rituximab for Waldenström macroglobulinemia (WM): an Eastern Cooperative Oncology Group Study (E3A98). *Leuk Lymphoma*. 2004;45:2047-2055.

53 Dimopoulos MA, Zervas C, Zomas A, et al. Treatment of Waldenström macroglobulinemia with rituximab. *J Clin Oncol*. 2002;20:2327-2333.

54 Treon SP, Emmanouilides C, Kimby E, et al. Extended rituximab therapy in Waldenström's macroglobulinemia. *Ann Oncol*. 2005;16:132-138.

55 Dimopoulos MA, Anagnostopoulos A, Kyrtsonis MC, et al. Primary treatment of Waldenström macroglobulinemia with dexamethasone, rituximab, and cyclophosphamide. *J Clin Oncol*. 2007;25:3344-3349.

56 Ioakimidis L, Patterson CJ, Hunter ZR, et al. Comparative outcomes following CP-R, CVP-R, and CHOP-R in Waldenström's macroglobulinemia. *Clin Lymphoma Myeloma*. 2009;9:62-66.

57 Dimopoulos MA, Kastritis E, Owen RG, et al. Treatment recommendations for patients with Waldenström macroglobulinemia (WM) and related disorders: IWWM-7 consensus. *Blood*. 2014;124:1404-1411.

58 Rummel MJ et al. Bendamustine plus rituximab versus CHOP plus rituximab as first-line treatment for patients with indolent and mantle-cell lymphomas: an open-label, multicentre, randomised, phase 3 non-inferiority trial. *Lancet*. 2013;381:1203-1210.

59 Gertz M. Waldenström macroglobulinemia: my way. *Leuk Lymphoma*. 2013;54:464-471.

60 Oza A, Rajkumar SV. Waldenstrom macroglobulinemia: prognosis and management. *Blood Cancer J*. 2015;5:e394.

61 Gertz MA. Waldenström macroglobulinemia: 2015 update on diagnosis, risk stratification, and management. *Am J Hematol*. 2015;90:346-354.

62 Treon SP, Hanzis C, Manning RJ, et al. Maintenance rituximab is associated with improved clinical outcome in rituximab naïve patients with Waldenstrom Macroglobulinaemia who respond to a rituximab-containing regimen. *Br J Haematol*. 2011;154:357-362.

63 Rummel MJ, Lerchenmüller C, Greil R, et al. Bendamustin-rituximab induction followed by observation or rituximab maintenance for newly diagnosed patients with Waldenström's Macroglobulinemia: results from a prospective, randomized, multicenter study (StiL NHL 7–2008 –MAINTAIN-; ClinicalTrials.gov Identifier: NCT00877214). *Blood*. 2012;120:abs 2739.

64 Bachanova V, Burns LJ. Hematopoietic cell transplantation for Waldenström macroglobulinemia. *Bone Marrow Transplant*. 2012;47:330-336.

65 Mueller W, Schütz D, Nagel F, Schulz S, Stumm R. Hierarchical organization of multi-site phosphorylation at the CXCR4 C terminus. *PLoS ONE*. 2013;8:e64975.

66 Rhyasen GW, Starczynowski DT. IRAK signalling in cancer. *Br J Cancer*. 2015;112:232-237.

67 Treon SP, Tripsas CK, Meid K, et al. Ibrutinib in previously treated Waldenström macroglobulinemia. *N Engl J Med*. 2015;372:1430-1440.

68 Yang G, Zhou Y, Liu X, et al. A mutation in MYD88 (L265P) supports the survival of lymphoplasmacytic cells by activation of Bruton tyrosine kinase in Waldenström macroglobulinemia. *Blood*. 2013;122:1222-1232.

Aggressive B-cell lymphomas

Chapter 7

Mantle cell lymphoma

Elizabeth Budde

Case presentation

Mr HK is a 67-year-old Caucasian man with a past medical history of hypertension. He presented to his primary care physician's office in June 2014 with 3 months' history of fever, fatigue, and an enlarged cervical lymph node. Excisional biopsy of the cervical lymph node reviewed findings consistent with mantle cell lymphoma. The specific immunophenotype of abnormal cells was CD19+, CD20+, cyclin D1+, CD10-, and CD23-. Cytogenetics and fluorescence in situ hybridization (FISH) studies showed the presence of t(11;14)(q13;q32) translocation and IgH-CCND1 fusion. He was determined to have stage IVB disease based on the results from staging studies including enhanced body computed tomography (CT) scan, positron emission tomography (PET) scan, bone marrow evaluation, and blood work. His simplified mantle cell lymphoma International Prognostic Index (MIPI) score was 3.

Disease overview

Mantle cell lymphoma (MCL) is a rare B-cell non-Hodgkin lymphoma (NHL). It was classified as a distinct lymphoma subtype in 1992. The incidence is approximately 5000 cases per year, representing about 4–7% of all new cases of NHL in the US [1]. It generally affects older adults with the median age at diagnosis of 68 years and is male predominant

© Springer International Publishing AG 2017
J. Zain and L.W. Kwak (eds.), *Management of Lymphomas: A Case-Based Approach*, DOI 10.1007/978-3-319-26827-9_7

with a male to female ratio of 2:1. It is incurable with conventional chemotherapy. The median overall survival is between 4 to 5 years [2].

Clinical presentation

Patients generally have stage III/IV disease at diagnosis and present with extensive lymphadenopathy, blood and bone marrow involvement, and sometimes splenomegaly. Gastrointestinal involvement is common and seen in 15–30% of MCL patients. Other extranodal sites for MCL involvement include the skin, lacrimal glands, and central nervous system. Most patients have an aggressive disease course without immediate anti-lymphoma treatment. A minority of MCL patients (10–15%) with the leukemic variant can have an indolent course and typically present with disease in the bone marrow, blood, and spleen without nodal involvement.

Diagnosis and staging

The pathologic diagnosis is made by histologic examination in combination with immunohistochemistry and cytogenetic/FISH analysis on a biopsy of a lymph node, tissue, bone marrow, or blood. There are 4 histologic subtypes: small cell, mantle zone, diffuse, and the blastoid variant.

Typical MCL cells have an immunophenotype of CD5+, CD20+, CD43+, CD23+/–, cyclin D1+, and CD10+/–. Some cases of MCL may be CD5– or CD23+. Most cases harbor a reciprocal chromosomal translocation t(11:14)(q12;32), leading to aberrant expression of cyclin D1. There are rare cases of cyclin D1– MCL (<5%), which may have overexpression of cyclin D2 or cyclin D3 instead. Recently, overexpression of SOX 11 has been found to be present in majority of MCL cells and represents a useful marker in aiding MCL diagnosis [3]. Staging procedures should include:

1. a complete physical examination and B symptom documentation;
2. complete blood count, comprehensive metabolic panel, a lactic dehydrogenase (LDH), uric acid, hepatitis viral panel, and human immunodeficiency virus (HIV) 1/2 serology;
3. bone marrow evaluation;
4. enhanced body CT with contrast;
5. fluorodeoxyglucose (FDG)-PET/CT;

6. endoscopy/colonoscopy in patients with clinical gastrointestinal symptoms; and

7. lumbar puncture in patients with central nervous system (CNS) symptoms.

Prognosis

The MIPI, established by the European MCL Network [4], has been validated by several groups to separate MCL patients into three risk categories: low risk with the median overall survival (OS) not reached (5-year OS 60%), intermediate risk with a median OS of 51 months, and high risk with a median OS of 29 months. Four independent prognostic factors for OS are used to calculate the score including age, Eastern Cooperative Oncology Group (ECOG) performance status, LDH, and white blood count at diagnosis. For practical matter, a simplified modification of the MIPI has also been developed, which has high concordance to the original MIPI score. Each of the four aforementioned factors is assigned a value between 0 to 3 points. Table 7.1 summarizes the simplified MIPI (sMIPI) calculation. Additionally, high Ki-67 proliferation index also correlates with a worse clinical outcome [5,6]. Using 30% cut-off determined by a standardized immunohistochemistry staining, a higher Ki-67 proliferation index was associated with shorter OS. Use of a modified combination of binary Ki-67 index (30% cut-off) and MIPI (termed combined MIPI (MIPI-c)) stratified patients into four risk groups. However, the generalization of its use for routine clinical practice requires further validation. Gene expression profiling or molecular signature for MCL is still at the exploratory phase and their use is not indicated for clinical application at the moment.

Points	Age (years)	ECOG PS	Ratio of LDH/ ULN	WBC (x 10⁹/L)
0	<50	0–1	<0.67	<6.700
1	50–59	–	0.67–0.99	<6.700–9.999
2	60–69	2–4	1.00–1.49	10.000–14.999
3	≥70		≥1.50	≥15.000

Table 7.1 Simplified MIPI (sMIPI) score calculation. Low risk, 0–3 points; intermediate risk, 4–5 points; high risk, 6–11 points. ECOG, Eastern Cooperative Oncology Group; LDH, lactate dehydrogenase; PS, performance status; ULN, upper limit of normal; WBC, white blood cell count.

Frontline treatment

Whenever possible, clinical trial should be the first choice for all patients as there is no standard of care for patients with newly diagnosed MCL. Several regimens have shown marked activity in clinical trials with CR rates up to 70% although none is curative. A risk-adapted approach is commonly used to decide on a specific treatment regimen based on factors such as a patient's age, performance status, comorbidities, organ function, and transplant eligibility. Early consolidation therapy using high-dose therapy (HDT)/autologous stem cell transplantation (ASCT) has been used as a common strategy to prolong duration of remission and progression-free survival (PFS) [7]. Figure 7.1 summarizes the City of Hope preferred MCL frontline treatment pathway.

Patients with initial clinical presentation consistent with leukemic variant type MCL, can be often managed with the dynamic watch and wait approach [8]. However, the majority of patients would have a more aggressive course requiring anti-lymphoma treatment. Two randomized Phase III trials (StiL and BRIGHT) compared treatment with bendamustine

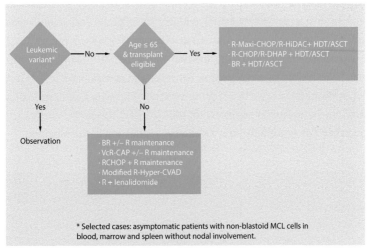

Figure 7.1 City of Hope untreated mantle cell lymphoma frontline therapy pathway. ASCT, autologous stem cell transplantation; BR, bendamustine and rituximab; R-CHOP, rituximab, cyclophosphamide, doxorubicin, vincristine, and prednisone; R-HiDAC, rituximab and high-dose cytarabine; R-HyperCVAD, rituximab, hyperfractionated cyclophosphamide, vincristine, doxorubicin, and dexamethasone.

and rituximab (BR) versus rituximab, cyclophosphamide, doxorubicin hydrochloride, vincristine, and prednisolone (R-CHOP) as first-line induction therapy in patients with indolent or mantle cell lymphoma. For the MCL subgroup analysis, both studies reported similar overall response rate (ORR) in both arms. The complete response rate (CR) was significantly higher in the BR arm: 40% versus 30%, and 50% versus 27%, respectively. A longer PFS (35.4 months) in the BR arm than the R-CHOP arm (22.1 months) was also observed in the StiL study. These together with its well-tolerated toxicity profile have made BR the preferred choice of induction regimen for patients older than 65 years of age. It is also reasonable to offer this treatment to transplant-eligible patients as induction therapy followed by consolidation therapy using HDT/ASCT. Cytarabine-containing regimens such as R-CHOP/rituximab, dexamethasone, cytarabine, and cisplatin (R-DHAP) [9] and the Nordic regimen (R-Maxi-CHOP alternating with R and high-dose cytarabine) [10] followed by HDT/ASCT consolidation have shown robust activity for young (<65 years of age) and otherwise fit patients. The CR rates were 54% and 57%, respectively, and median event-free survival (EFS) was 84 months and 7.4 years, respectively. In addition, the rituximab, cyclophosphamide, vincristine, doxorubicin, and dexamethasone (R-HyperCVAD) [11–13] regimen was tested in a few studies with CR rate ranging between 55% to 72%, although specific attention needs to be paid to its toxicity profiles and its use should be limited to young and fit patients. Given the concern of potential marrow toxicity and the negative impact on stem cell mobilization and collection, this regimen is not one of the preferred regimens at our center for patients who are transplant-eligible.

For transplant-ineligible patients, VR-CAP regimen (bortezomib in place of vincristine in the R-CHOP regimen) is a valid option. In a Phase III randomized study [14], treatment with VR-CAP led to a superior CR rate of 48% and prolonged median PFS of 24.7 months in comparison to that of R-CHOP (41% CR and 14.4 months of median PFS). For medically unfit patients, lenalidomide and rituximab may also provide promising disease control. In a single center Phase II study, this combination led to a CR of 64% and a 2-year PFS of 85% in 35 enrolled patients [15]. It is worth noting that in this regimen rituximab maintenance was given every 8 weeks until disease progression. Using rituximab as maintenance therapy following other induction therapies has also been tested [16,17]. In a Phase III study conducted by the European MCL network, responders who were older than 60 years of age and HDT-/ASCT-ineligible had an impressive 4-year OS rate of 87% after R-CHOP induction followed by rituximab maintenance [16]. Therefore, for patients who are not medically fit or not a candidate for HDT/ASCT, rituximab maintenance after induction may prolong survival with acceptable toxicities and is strongly recommended.

Management of relapsed/refractory mantle cell lymphoma

At relapse, treatment selection should be based on patient's age, co-morbidities, fitness condition, and goal of care. Clinical trials should be considered as the first choice for all patients. Figure 7.2 depicts the preferred treatment pathway for patients with relapsed or refractory MCL at City of Hope.

Many chemotherapy-based regimens have some activity in relapsed or refractory MCL including rituximab ifosfamide, carboplatin, and etoposide (RICE), BR, and fludarabine-based regimens. A Phase II study [18] of bendamustine in combination with rituximab resulted in an ORR of 92% and CR rate of 42% in a subgroup analysis of patients with relapsed or refractory MCL (*n*=12). In a Phase III study, BR led to an ORR of 83.5% and CR rate of 38.5% in a subgroup analysis of 41 patients

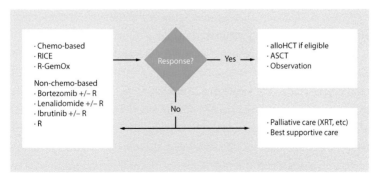

Figure 7.2 City of Hope mantle cell lymphoma relapsed/refractory therapy pathway. alloHCT, allogeneic hematopoietic cell transplantation; ASCT, autologous stem cell transplantation; R-GemOx, rituximab, gemicitabine, oxaliplatin; RICE, rituximab, ifosphamide, carboplatin, and etoposide.

with recurrent MCL. Median PFS was 30 months [19]. However, with the increasing use of BR in the frontline setting, it is expected to be less efficacious in the recurrent MCL setting. The activity associated with other traditional chemotherapy-based salvage treatment is unfortunately limited. It remains a challenge to achieve high CR rate and durable remission. Hence, novel biologics have been tested in this setting. Currently, there are three biologics that have received United States (US) food and Drug Administration (FDA) approval as monotherapy for relapsed MCL including bortezomib, lenalidomide, and ibrutinib (Table 7.2). Ibrutinib is also approved for this indication in Europe.

Bortezomib is a proteinase inhibitor and the first US FDA-approved biologic for patients with relapsed or refractory MCL after failure of at least one prior therapy. As a single agent, it induced an ORR of 33% and CR rate of 8% in the pivotal Phase II PINNACLE trial with 141 evaluable patients that led to its approval [20]. The median duration of response was 9 months. Median time to progression was 6 months. Bortezomib in combination with rituximab was tested in a small 14 patient Phase II study with an ORR of 29% with all responders achieving a CR, suggesting promising activity [21].

Lenalidomide is an imunodulating agent. As a monotherapy it was tested in two Phase II studies before FDA approved it for patients with MCL who had failed bortezomib. The observed ORR was 35% (12% CR/CRu)in a Phase II study with 54 patients [22] and 28% (7.5% CR/CRu) in a larger Phase II study with 134 patients [23]. In the latter study, the

Regimen	N (evaluable)	Phase	ORR%	CR%	Median PFS (months)	Median DOR (months)
Bortezomib	155	II	32	8	6	9
Bortezomib+R	14	II	29	29	2	–
Lenalidomide	134	II	28	8	4	16.6
Lenalidomide+R	52	II	57	36	11	19
Ibrutinib	111	II	68	21	14	17.5
Ibrutinib+R	50	II	88	44	–	–

Table 7.2 Activity of United States FDA-approved biologics in mantle cell lymphoma treatment. CR, complete response; DOR, duration of treatment; FDA, Food and Drug Administration; ORR, overall response; PFS, progression-free survival.

median duration of response was 16.6 months and median PFS was 4 months. Promising results have been observed in a Phase II study testing lenalidomide and rituximab combination in 52 evaluable patients [24]. The ORR was 57% with 36% CR in the Phase II portion. Median duration of response was 19 months. Median PFS was 11 months.

Ibrutinib is a Bruton tyrosine kinase (BTK) inhibitor and is approved in US and Europe for the treatment of patients with MCL who have received at least one prior therapy. In a study of 111 evaluable MCL patients, ibrutinib led to an ORR of 68% and CR rate of 21% [25]. The median duration of response was 17.5 months and median PFS was 14 months. There were no differences in response rate between bortezomib-naive or bortezomib-refractory patients. In a recent Phase II study, ibrutinib in combination with rituximab led to an impressive 88% ORR with 44% CR rate in patients with recurrent MCL [26].

Patients who respond to salvage regimen treatment and are transplant-eligible, are strongly encouraged to move on to ASCT to maximize the chance of cure. HDT/ASCT might be a choice in a subset of patients if a donor is not available and the patient has not had an autologous transplant [27].

Case conclusion

In the case presented at the start of this chapter the patient underwent treatment with bendamustine and rituximab for a total of six cycles. CT scan after two cycles demonstrated a partial response. PET/CT scan after six cycles showed a complete resolution of hypermetabolic activity. Bone marrow study demonstrated absence of any lymphoma cells. He was deemed to achieve a complete response. His autologous peripheral blood stem cells were subsequently mobilized and collected after priming with cyclophosphamide and granulocyte-colony stimulating factor (G-CSF). Two months later, he received high-dose therapy using the BEAM preparative regimen followed by autologous stem cell infusion. Rituximab maintenance was started 4 months after autologous stem cell transplantation. He has remained in complete remission.

References

1   [No authors listed]. A clinical evaluation of the International Lymphoma Study Group classification of non-Hodgkin's lymphoma. The Non-Hodgkin's Lymphoma Classification Project. *Blood.* 1997;89:3909-3918.

2   Herrmann A, Hoster E, Zwingers T, et al. Improvement of overall survival in advanced stage mantle cell lymphoma. *J Clin Oncol.* 2009;27;511-518.

3   Fernàndez V, Salamero O, Espinet B, et al. Genomic and gene expression profiling defines indolent forms of mantle cell lymphoma. *Cancer Res.* 2010;70;1408-1418.

4   Hoster E, Dreyling M, Klapper W, et al. A new prognostic index (MIPI) for patients with advanced-stage mantle cell lymphoma. *Blood.* 2008;111;558-565.

5   Geisler CH, Kolstad A, Laurell A, et al. The Mantle Cell Lymphoma International Prognostic Index (MIPI) is superior to the International Prognostic Index (IPI) in predicting survival following intensive first-line immunochemotherapy and autologous stem cell transplantation (ASCT). *Blood.* 2010;115:1530-1533.

6   Hoster E, Rosenwald A, Berger F, et al. Prognostic value of Ki-67 index, cytology, and growth pattern in mantle-cell lymphoma: results from randomized trials of the European Mantle Cell Lymphoma Network. *J Clin Oncol.* 2016;34:1386-1394

7   Dreyling M, Lenz G, Hoster E, et al. Early consolidation by myeloablative radiochemotherapy followed by autologous stem cell transplantation in first remission significantly prolongs progression-free survival in mantle-cell lymphoma: results of a prospective randomized trial of the European MCL Network. *Blood.* 2005;105;2677-2684.

8   Martin P, Chadburn A, Christos P, et al. Outcome of deferred initial therapy in mantle-cell lymphoma. *J Clin Oncol.* 2009;27;1209-1213.

9   Delarue R, Haioun C, Ribrag V, et al. CHOP and DHAP plus rituximab followed by autologous stem cell transplantation in mantle cell lymphoma: a phase 2 study from the Groupe d'Etude des Lymphomes de l'Adulte. *Blood.* 2013;121:48-53.

10 Geisler CH, Kolstad A, Laurell A, et al. Long-term progression-free survival of mantle cell lymphoma after intensive front-line immunochemotherapy with in vivo-purged stem cell rescue: a nonrandomized phase 2 multicenter study by the Nordic Lymphoma Group. *Blood.* 2008;112;2687-2693.

11 Bernstein SH, Epner E, Unger JM, et al. A phase II multicenter trial of hyperCVAD MTX/Ara-C and rituximab in patients with previously untreated mantle cell lymphoma; SWOG 0213. *Ann Oncol.* 2013;24:1587-1593.

12 Merli F, Luminari S, Ilariucci F, et al. Rituximab plus HyperCVAD alternating with high dose cytarabine and methotrexate for the initial treatment of patients with mantle cell lymphoma, a multicentre trial from Gruppo Italiano Studio Linfomi. *Br J Haematol.* 2012;156;346-353.

13 Romaguera JE, Fayad L, Rodriguez MA, et al. High rate of durable remissions after treatment of newly diagnosed aggressive mantle-cell lymphoma with rituximab plus hyper-CVAD alternating with rituximab plus high-dose methotrexate and cytarabine. *J Clin Oncol.* 2005;23:7013-7023.

14 Robak T, Huang H, Jin J, et al. Bortezomib-based therapy for newly diagnosed mantle-cell lymphoma. *N Engl J Med.* 2015;372:944-953.

15 Ruan J, Martin P, Shah B, et al. Lenalidomide plus rituximab as initial treatment for mantle-cell lymphoma. *N Engl J Med.* 2015;373:1835-1844.

16 Kluin-Nelemans HC, Hoster E, Hermine O, et al. Treatment of older patients with mantle-cell lymphoma. *N Engl J Med.* 2012;367:520-531.

17 Kenkre VP, Long WL, Eickhoff JC, et al. Maintenance rituximab following induction chemo-immunotherapy for mantle cell lymphoma: long-term follow-up of a pilot study from the Wisconsin Oncology Network. *Leuk Lymphoma.* 2011;52;1675-1680.

18 Robinson KS, Williams ME, van der Jagt RH, et al. Phase II multicenter study of bendamustine plus rituximab in patients with relapsed indolent B-cell and mantle cell non-Hodgkin's lymphoma. *J Clin Oncol.* 2008;26;4473-4479.

19 Rummel M, Kaiser U, Balser C, et al. Bendamustine plus rituximab versus fludarabine plus rituximab for patients with relapsed indolent and mantle-cell lymphomas: a multicentre, randomised, open-label, non-inferiority phase 3 trial. *Lancet Oncol.* 2016;17:57-66.

20 Fisher RI, Bernstein SH, Kahl BS, et al. Multicenter phase II study of bortezomib in patients with relapsed or refractory mantle cell lymphoma. *J Clin Oncol.* 2006;24;4867-4874.

21 Baiocchi RA, Alinari L, Lustberg ME, et al. Phase 2 trial of rituximab and bortezomib in patients with relapsed or refractory mantle cell and follicular lymphoma. *Cancer.* 2011;117:2442-2451.

22 Zinzani PL, Vose JM, Czuczman MS, et al. Long-term follow-up of lenalidomide in relapsed/refractory mantle cell lymphoma: subset analysis of the NHL-003 study. *Ann Oncol.* 2103;24:2892-2897.

23 Goy A, Sinha R, Williams ME, et al. Single-agent lenalidomide in patients with mantle-cell lymphoma who relapsed or progressed after or were refractory to bortezomib: phase II MCL-001 (EMERGE) study. *J Clin Oncol.* 2013;31:3688-3695.

24 Wang M, Fayad L, Wagner-Bartak N, et al. Lenalidomide in combination with rituximab for patients with relapsed or refractory mantle-cell lymphoma: a phase 1/2 clinical trial. *Lancet Oncol.* 2012;13;716-723.

25 Wang ML, Rule S, Martin P, et al. Targeting BTK with ibrutinib in relapsed or refractory mantle-cell lymphoma. *N Engl J Med.* 2013;369;507-516.

26 Wang ML, Lee H, Chuang H, et al. Ibrutinib in combination with rituximab in relapsed or refractory mantle cell lymphoma: a single-centre, open-label, phase 2 trial. *Lancet Oncol.* 2016;17;48-56.

27 Cassaday RD, Guthrie KA, Budde EL, et al. Specific features identify patients with relapsed or refractory mantle cell lymphoma benefitting from autologous hematopoietic cell transplantation. *Biol Blood Marrow Transplant.* 2013;19:1403-1406.

Chapter 8

Burkitt lymphoma

Auayporn Nademanee

Case presentation

The patient is a 61-year-old female with a past history of hypertension who presented with a few days' history of severe abdominal pain and nausea/vomiting. Abdominal X-ray showed partial small bowel obstruction. Computed tomography scan showed thickened cecal wall and bilateral adnexal masses. She underwent exploratory laparotomy with partial colectomy, total abdominal hysterectomy, bilateral salphingo-oophorectomy, omentectomy, and colostomy. Pathology showed an omental mass measured 32 x 14 cm, right adnexa mass 7 x 3.5 cm, left adnexa mass 7.5 x 3.5 cm, and a mass in the small bowel 3.5 cm. All the specimens were high-grade B-cell lymphoma. There was a diffuse infiltrate of monomorphic medium-sized lymphoid cells with high mitotic activity and 'starry-sky' pattern. Immunohistochemical studies were positive for CD20, CD43, CD10, and kappa light chain restriction. Ki-67 was 100%. Fluorescence in situ hybridization (FISH) analysis was positive for MYC and IGH translocation. A diagnosis of Burkitt lymphoma was made and she was transferred to us for further treatment. Laboratory tests were notable for white count 21,500/cm, hemoglobin 8.9 gm/dl, lactate dehydrogenase (LDH) 2467 (normal 313-618) U/L, and uric acid 9 mg/dl. Bone marrow biopsy showed extensive involvement (80%). Lumbar puncture was negative.

© Springer International Publishing AG 2017
J. Zain and L.W. Kwak (eds.), *Management of Lymphomas: A Case-Based Approach*, DOI 10.1007/978-3-319-26827-9_8

Introduction

Burkitt lymphoma (BL) is a highly aggressive B-cell non-Hodgkin lymphoma (NHL) that frequently presents with extranodal involvement and rarely as leukemia. There are three clinical variants: endemic, sporadic, and immunodeficiency-associated. Endemic BL, which is uniformly Epstein-Barer virus (EBV)-positive, is highly prevalent with approximately three to six cases per 100,000 children per year in equatorial Africa. Sporadic BL is rare, accounting for 30% of pediatric lymphomas and 1–2% of adult NHLs in the United State and Europe. It is more common in young individuals and the median age of occurrence in adults is 30 years of age. Immunodeficiency-associated BL is prevalent among patients with human immunodeficiency virus (HIV) infection regardless of the CD4 count. In general, treatment is similar in all three clinical forms [1].

Pathology

BL is characterized by deregulation of the gene encoding MYC as a result of a chromosomal translocation involving the *MYC* gene locus on chromosome eight and the immunoglobulin heavy chain (IgH) locus on chromosome 14, t(8;14).

Biopsies of BL show complete effacement by sheets of atypical lymphocytes, which are medium-sized and highly monomorphic with round nuclei, multiple prominent nucleoli, and basophilic cytoplasm. Interspersed among these lymphocytes are benign histiocytes that are large and irregular shaped and have ingested apoptotic tumor debris, which gives the classic 'starry-sky' appearance. The proliferative index as measured by Ki-67 is closed to 100%. BL cells are positive for IgM surface immunoglobulin and surface light chains (κ>λ), B-cell-associated antigens CD19, CD20, CD22, and PAX5, and are also positive for germinal center-associated antigens CD10 and BCL6. They are negative for CD5, BCL-2, TdT, and CD23. *MYC* gene rearrangement is detected in 95% of BL with 80% of cases harboring a t(8;14) at 14q32 breakpoint. Fifteen percent and 5% of cases demonstrate translocation involving either the κ light chain gene on chromosome 2, t(2;8) or the λ light chain gene on chromosome 22, t(8;22), respectively. Five percent of BL do not harbor a *MYC* gene rearrangement [2].

Differential diagnosis

The distinction between BL and diffuse large B-cell lymphoma (DLBCL) is important as treatment with rituximab, cyclophosphamide, vincristine, adriamycin, and prednisone (R-CHOP) is not appropriate for patients with BL who may be cured with intensified chemotherapy regimens including intrathecal or central nervous system (CNS) prophylaxis. The histopathology and immunohistochemical profile of BL is distinct from DLBCL and B-cell lymphoma unclassifiable between BL and DLBCL (see Table 8.1).

Clinical presentation

Patients with BL typically present with rapidly enlarging masses and evidence of spontaneous tumor lysis syndrome (TLS) and high serum LDH levels. Sporadic BL typically present with abdominal involvement both nodal and extranodal sites including bowel, ovary, ascites, and pleural effusion as well as pharyngeal and sinus involvement. Bone marrow and central nervous system (CNS) involvement occurs in 30% and 15%, respectively [3].

	DLBCL	Gray zone	BL
Morphology	Variable, ranging from medium-sized to large, pleiomorphic nuclei with a large morphological range	BL-morphology with or without large cells	Cohesive, starry-sky, medium-sized, round nuclei with multiple small nucleoli
Immunophenotype	BCL-2, CD10, BCL-6, MUM-1 highly variable Ki-67 30->95%	BCL-2 often strong, CD10 mostly +, BCL-6 mostly +, MUM-1 variable Ki-67 50->95%	BCL-2 –, CD10 +, BCL-6 +, MUM-1 variable Ki-67 >95%
MYC translocation	5–15%	80%	90–100%
Non/G partner in *MYC* translocation	40%	40%	None
BCL-2 translocation	20–30%	45%	No
BCL-6 translocation	30%	9%	No
Simple karyotype	Rarely	Rarely	Typical
Complex karyotype	Generally	Generally	No

Table 8.1 Diagnostic features of diffuse large B-cell lymphoma (DLBCL), Burkitt lymphoma (BL) and B-cell lymphoma unclassifiable with features intermediate between DLBCL and BL ('gray zone').

Initial evaluation

The following steps should be taken when a patient presents with symptoms of BL:

1. Pathologic diagnosis should be confirmed by an experienced hematopathologist expert in lymphoma, given the overlap between BL and other aggressive DLBCL as treatment and prognosis differ.

2. Laboratory evaluation includes complete blood count with differential, comprehensive metabolic panel including LDH and uric acid, and human immune deficiency virus (HIV) and hepatitis panel.

3. Radiologic evaluation includes computed tomography (CT) scan of neck, chest, abdomen and pelvis. In addition, if clinical condition permits, a positron emission tomography (PET) scan should be done.

4. Bone marrow aspiration and biopsy and cytogenetic study.

5. Lumbar puncture and cerebral spinal fluid (CSF) for cytology, and flow cytometry, often with administration of intrathecal therapy.

6. Cardiac evaluation with either echocardiogram or multigated acquisition (MUGA) scan.

7. Men and women of child-bearing potential should be counseled for potential effect of treatment on their fertility and if time permits consider sperm banking for men. Options for women are limited due to urgent need for treatment.

Treatment

The patient presented above had recent surgery, high tumor burden and marked elevated LDH level. She was given rusburicase, cyclophosphamide, and prednisone. Once recovered, she received rituximab, cyclophosphamide, vincristine doxorubicin, and methotrexate (R-CODOX-M)/ ifosfamide, cytarabine, and etoposide (IVAC) for two cycles each along with IT chemotherapy. She has achieved complete remission and has remained in remission now for 4 years. Her treatment highlights the management approach for patients with Burkitt lymphoma, which will be discussed below.

The following steps are recommended when treatment is initiated for patients with BL:

1. Prevention and treatment of tumor lysis syndrome (TLS). Start allopurinol, IV fluid, and alkalinization. If there is evidence of

spontaneous TLS with elevated LDH level, hyperuricemia, and hyperphosphatemia, rusburicase should be given prior to initiation of chemotherapy.

2. The optimal initial therapy has not been clearly defined but there are several intensive regimens that demonstrate excellent activity in BL. The choices of regimens are dependent on the patient age, patients' physical conditions, and co-morbidity as well as the physician/center experiences and preferences. However, it is critical that a more intensive regimen, not R-CHOP, is given along with CNS prophylaxis. There are three common regimens used at our center for adults with BL (see Figure 8.1). The regimens and dosing schedules are presented at the end of the chapter.

3. The choice of regimens includes:

A. CODOX-M/IVAC was developed by Magrath et al [4]. Patients with low-risk disease defined as a single mass <10 cm with normal LDH level or completely resected abdominal disease received three cycles of CODOX-M. All other patients were considered high-risk and received two cycles each of CODOX-M and IVAC. Forty-nine patients including 20 adults, with a

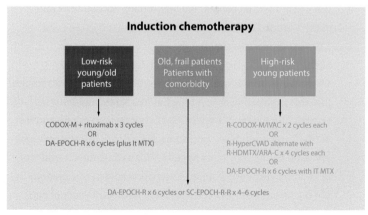

Figure 8.1 Standard of care algorithm for the treatment of Burkitt lymphoma at City of Hope.
ARA-C, cytarabine; DA/SC-EPOCH-R, dose-adjusted/short-course etoposide, doxorubicin, cyclophosphamide, vincristine, prednisone, and rituximab; IVAC, ifosfamide, cytarabine, and etoposide; R-CODOX-M, rituximab, cyclophosphamide, vincristine doxorubicin, and methotrexate; R-HDMTX, rituximab plus high-dose methotrexate; R-HyperCVAD, rituximab, cyclophosphamide, vincristine, doxorubicin, and dexamethasone.

median age of 25 years, were treated and the 2-year event-free survival (EFS) was 92%. The same regimen was used in 52 adult patients, median age 35 years. The 2-year overall survival (OS) was 82% and 70% in low- and high-risk patients, respectively. However, CODOX-M/IVAC is toxic with risk of severe myelosuppression and infection. In a subsequent study, the dose of methotrexate (MTX) was reduced to 3 gm/m^2 for patients <65 years of age and 1 gm/m^2 for older patients >65 years of age. The dose of cytarabine was also reduced to 1 gm/m^2 in older patients. This trial included 11 low-risk and 42 high-risk patients. The 2-year progression-free survival (PFS) was 85% and 64% for low- and high-risk patients, respectively [5]. When rituximab was added to CODOX-M/IVAC, there were fewer relapses and a trend in improved 3-year PFS (74% versus 61%) and 3-year OS (77% versus 66%) [6]. Due to toxicity of CODOX-M/IVAC, most patients require a prolonged inpatient hospitalization and blood transfusion support. We usually recommend rituximab plus CODOX-M/IVAC for young fit patients with high-risk disease. For patients with low-risk disease defined as early stage, non-bulky, normal LDH and good performance status, I would recommend three cycles of CODOX-M plus rituximab.

B. Hyper-fractionated cyclophosphamide, vincristine, doxorubicin and dexamethasone (hyper-CVAD) plus rituximab [7]: this regimen was developed at MD Anderson. Patients receive four cycles of hyper-CVAD alternating with four cycles of MTX and high-dose cytarabine. Rituximab 375 mg/m^2 was given on days 1 and 11 of hyper-CVAD and on days 1 and 8 of MTX and cytarabine course. Thirty-one adults, at a median of 46 years of age were treated; 29% were ≥60 years of age. The CR rate was 86%. The 3-year OS and disease-free survival (DFS) were 89%, and 88%, respectively. For elderly patients, the 3-year OS was 89%. Thus this regimen can be used in both younger and older patients. In addition, CNS prophylaxis can be achieved with both MTX and high-dose cytarabine

(HDAC) as they do penetrate blood brain barrier. This regimen is associated with severe myelosuppression, therefore prophylactic antibiotic, acyclovir, fluconazole and PCP prophylaxis with bactrim must be given in addition to growth factor support. I would use this regimen in young patients <60 years of age with high-risk disease, stage IV, extranodal involvement, and CNS involvement.

C. Dose-adjusted etoposide, prednisone, vincristine, cyclophosphamide, and doxorubicin (EPOCH) and rituximab (DA-EPOCH-R) [8]: this regimen was designed to preserve efficacy by prolonging infusion of chemotherapy to maximize the killing activities of lymphoma cells while reducing toxicity. Etoposide was substituted for MTX and the cycle repeated every 3 weeks. HIV-negative patients received two cycles after complete remission (six to eight cycles). A lower-dose short course combination with a double dose of rituximab (SC-EPOCH-RR) to reduce toxicity was given in HIV-positive BL patients for a total of three to six cycles (1 cycle beyond CR). Prophylaxis intrathecal (IT) MTX 12 mg was administered on days 1 and 5 every 3 weeks beginning in cycle three for eight doses with DA-EPOCH-R and for six doses with SC-EPOOCH-R. Patients with evidence of CSF involvement received treatment with IT MTX 12 mg or 6 mg via Ommaya reservoir twice weekly for 4 weeks, then once weekly for 6 weeks, and then once a month for 4 months. Thirty patients were treated; 19 received DA-EPOCH-R and 11 received SC-EPOCH-RR. The median age was 33 years; 73% had intermediate risk and only 10% had high-risk. With a median follow-up of 86 months, the freedom from progression (FFP) and OS were 95% and 100% with DA-EPOCH-R and 100% and 90%, respectively with SC-EPOCH-RR. Fever and neutropenia were low and no treatment-related deaths were recorded. Although the results are excellent, the patients treated in this study were quite favorable. Nevertheless, this combination is effective and can be given in the outpatient setting. I recommend this regimen for older patients who are not able to tolerate more intensive regimens and also in younger patients with low-risk disease.

D. There are other regimens that have proven to be effective. The German Multicenter Study Group for Adult ALL (GMALL) adopted a regimen from the pediatric ALL (BFM), B-NHL90 using a pre-phase with cyclophosphamide and prednisone followed by six alternating cycles A (ifosfamide, teniposide, vincristine, cytarabine, dexamethasone, and high dose [HD] MTX) and cycle B (cyclophosphamide, doxorubicin, vincristine, dexamethasone and high dose HD MTX). Both adult Burkitt-acute leukemia (B-AL) and BL were included but overall survival was not improved and there was significant toxicity. In the next trial GMALL-B-ALL/NHL2002 enrolled 363 patients with B-AL and BL. Treatment consisted of six 5-day chemotherapy cycles; rituximab was added before each cycle for a total of 8 doses and HD MTX doses were reduced [9]. CR rate was 88% and OS and PFS at 5 yrs were 80% and 71%, respectively. Age >55 years, high-risk IPI, and male sex predict poor survival. Since some of the drugs are not available, this regimen is not commonly used in US. A modified B-NHL 90 was conducted by CALGB with the addition of rituximab in 105 patients, the CR rate was 82% and 2-year EFS and OS were 74% and 79%, respectively. However, toxicity was significant with seven therapy-related deaths [10].

Central nervous system prophylaxis

CNS involvement at diagnosis is frequent and there was a high rate of CNS relapse if no CNS prophylaxis was given. If there is evidence of lep-tomeningeal involvement at diagnosis, intrathecal chemotherapy should be given twice a week until the CSF is clear then once a week. We usually recommend MTX but triple combination consisting of MTX, Ara-C and hydrocortisone can be given if CSF remains positive. Regimens containing high-dose MTX/and or HDAC can also provide CNS prophylaxis. Severe toxicities were reported when liposomal cytarabine was given in combination with hyper-CVAD but was reported to be feasible with CODOX-M/IVAC regimen. It is unclear whether liposomal cytarabine is better for CNS prophylaxis than conventional IT MTX or cytarabine. Cranial irradiation is not routinely recommended but may be considered in selected patients with parenchymal brains lesions if symptomatic.

Stem cell transplantation

Several studies have evaluated the role of autologous stem cell transplant (auto-SCT) during first remission. These studies were done before the era of rituximab and more intensive regimens outlined above. For patients who underwent upfront auto-SCT in first CR, the OS of 72% are comparable to aggressive chemotherapy alone [11]. However, auto-SCT is recommended in patients who fail to achieve remission or relapse after induction chemotherapy. Disease status at transplant predicts outcome. In one study, 3-year OS was 37% for chemo-sensitive relapse and only 7% for chemo-resistant relapse. There are limited experiences of allogeneic stem cell transplant for BL but it is usually performed in patients with persistent bone marrow (BM) involvement or chemo-resistant disease.

Relapse or refractory disease

The prognosis of patients with relapse/refractory disease is extremely poor as they have already received the most active agents and regimens with very intensive combination chemotherapy. Patients should be referred to clinical trials and those with chemo-sensitive disease should be referred for stem cell transplant evaluation. There is no standard treatment for relapsed/refractory BL. The choices of salvage chemotherapy are usually the regimens used for relapsed DLBCL such as EPOCH-R, RICE, R-DHAP, R-gemcitabine-based regimen, or R-high-dose MTX/cytarabine.

Human immunodeficiency virus-positive Burkitt lymphoma

Recent studies have shown that patients with HIV-related BL have similar outcomes when treated with the same intensive chemotherapy regimens used for HIV-negative BL as demonstrated by DA-EPOCH-R outlined above. The AIDS malignancy Consortium treated 34 patients (32 high risk) with HIV-positive BL with modified CODOX-IVAC plus rituximab [12]. Median CD 4 count was 195 cells/μl and highly active antiretroviral therapy (HARRT) therapy was given in 26 patients. The 1-year PFS and OS was 69% and 72%, respectively. The PATHEMA (Programa espiñol de Tratamiento en Hematología) group compared the outcome of 80 HIV-negative with 38 HIV-positive BL patients who were treated with an intensive chemotherapy regimen (modified B-ALL/NHL2002 called BURKIMAB) [13]. Patients with non-bulky stage I–II received four cycles, the remainder received six cycles, and dose modification was done in patients >55 years of age. There were no significant differences in CR rate (82% and 87%), 4-year disease-free survival (DFS; 77% versus 3%), and OS (80% versus 78%).

Special considerations

1. For patients with high white count due to circulating lymphoma cells, high tumor burden, and elevated LDH level, the first dose of rituximab should be delayed for at least 3–7 days to minimize the risk of TLS and infusional reaction.

2. Patients with hyperbilirubinemia due to liver involvement or biliary obstruction who cannot receive adriamycin or vincristine, we would recommend using pre-phase cyclophosphamide 200 mg/m^2 daily x 5 days and prednisone 60 mg/m^2/d day 1–5 (GMALL/CALGB) first then start the planned regimen when liver function improves.

Conclusion

BL is highly aggressive lymphoma which is curable with intensive multi-agent chemoimmunotherapy with CNS prophylaxis. For young and fit patients, we favor R-CODOX-M/IVAC as treatment is brief and the inclusion of HD-MTX and HD-cytarabine also provides excellent CNS prophylaxis. DA-EPOCH-R can be given in both older patients and younger patients especially those with low-risk disease. There is no role for auto-SCT during first remission. Patients with relapsed disease have extremely poor prognosis and should be referred for clinical trials. The regimens and dosing schedules discussed earlier in the chapter are now presented in Tables 8.2–8.5.

R-CODOX-M (cycles 1 and 3) [14–17]

Rituximab 375 mg/m^2 IV on day 1

Cyclophosphamide 800 mg/m^2 IV on day 1

Cyclophosphamide 200 mg/m^2 IV on days 2 through 5

Doxorubicin 40 mg/m^2 slow IV push on day 1

Vincristine 1.5 mg/m^2 (maximum 2 mg) IV on days 1 and 8 (cycle 1) and days 1, 8, and 15 (cycle 3)

Methotrexate:

Age 65 years or younger: 300 mg/m^2 IV loading dose over one hour on day 15, followed by 2700 mg/m^2 IV infusion administered over the next 23 hours; leucovorin rescue begins 36 hours from the start of the methotrexate infusion

Age 65 years: 100 mg/m^2 IV loading dose over one hour on day 15, followed by 900 mg/m^2 IV infusion administered over the next 23 hours; leucovorin rescue begins 36 hours from the start of the methotrexate infusion

Granucolate colony-stimulating factor begins 24 hours after leucovorin rescue is started and continues until the absolute neutrophil count is >1000/microL

Intrathecal medications:

Intrathecal cytarabine 70 mg (if >3 years of age) on days 1 and 3

Intrathecal methotrexate 12 mg (if >3 years of age) on day 15

Oral leucovorin 15 mg/dose on day 16, 24 hours after intrathecal methotrexate

Enhanced CNS directed therapy for patients with CNS disease at presentation: Cytarabine 70 mg/dose (if >3 years of age) intrathecal (or 15 mg if via Ommaya reservoir) on day 5 and methotrexate 12 mg (if >3 years of age) intrathecal (or 2 mg if via Ommaya reservoir) on day 17 in cycle 1 [15]

R-IVAC (cycles 2 and 4) [14–17]

Rituximab 375 mg/m^2 IV on day 1

Ifosfamide:

Age 65 years or younger: 1500 mg/m^2 IV on days 1 through 5 with mesna uroprotection

Age >65 years: 1000 mg/m^2 IV on days 1 through 5 with mesna uroprotection

Etoposide 60 mg/m^2 IV on days 1 through 5

Cytarabine:

Age 65 years or younger: 2 g/m^2 IV every 12 hours on days 1 and 2 (four doses)

Age >65 years: 1 g/m^2 IV every 12 hours on days 1 and 2 (four doses)

Granulocyte colony-stimulating factor begins 24 hours the completion of IV chemotherapy and continues until the absolute neutrophil count is >1000/microL

Intrathecal medications:

Intrathecal methotrexate 12 mg (if >3 years of age) on day 5

Oral leucovorin 15 mg on day 6, 24 hours after intrathecal methotrexate

Enhanced CNS directed therapy for patients with CNS disease at presentation: cytarabine 70 mg (if >3 years of age) intrathecal (or 15 if via Ommaya reservoir) on days 7 and 9 in cycle 2 [15]

Table 8.2 R-CODOX-M/IVAC (Magrath) regimen for Burkitt lymphoma. The R-CODOX-M/IVAC regimen is composed of four cycles, each cycle lasting until the absolute neurophil count returns to >1000/microL and the platelet count >100,000/microL. Cycles 1 and 3 are R-CODOX-M and cycles 2 and 4 are R-IVAC. Three cycles of R-CODOX-M are sufficient for patients with low-risk disease (ie, a single focus of disease <10 cm in diameter and a normal serum lactate dehydrogenase level). IVAC, ifosfamide, cytarabine, and etoposide; R-CODOX-M , rituximab, cyclophosphamide, vincristine doxorubicin, and methotrexate. Data from [14–17].

Regimen A: CODOX-M[a]													
Day	1	2	3	4	5	6	7	8	9	10	11	12	13
Cyclophosphamide 800 mg/m²	X	X											
Vincristine[b] 1.4 mg/m²	X									X			
Doxorubicin 50 mg/m²	X												
Methotrexate 3 gm/m²										X			
Leucovorin											X		
IT cytarabine 50 mg			X[c]										
G-CSF[d]	X	X	X	X	X	X						X	X
Regimen B: IVAC													
Day	1	2	3	4	5	6	7	8	9	10	11	12	13
Ifosfamide 1500 mg/m²	X	X	X	X	X								
Mesna	X	X	X	X	X								
Etoposide 60 mg/m²	X	X	X	X	X								
Cytarabine 2 gm/m²[e]	X	X	X	X									
IT methotrexate 12 mg					X								
G-CSF						X	X	X	X	X	X	X	X

[a]Low-risk patients receive 3 cycles of regimen A (A-A-A). High-risk patients receive 4 alternating cycles of regimens A and B (A-B-A-B); [b]Vincristine maximum 2 mg dose; [c]High-risk only; [d]ANC <1000 on day 12, restart G-CSF; [e]Cytarabine 2g/m² q 12 hr x 4 doses

Changes from original Magrath regime (all in regimen A)

Change cyclophosphamide from 800 mg/m² d1 and 200 mg/m² d2–5 to 800 mg/m² d 1 and 2 only

Cap vincristine at 2 mg total dose

Increase doxorubicin from 40 mg/m² to 50 mg/m²

Decrease IV methotrexate from 6.7 gm/m² to 3 gm/m²

Decrease IT cytarabine from 70 mg to 50 mg

Table 8.3 Modified Magrath regimen for Burkitt lymphoma. All low-risk patients received three cycles of regimen A (CODOX-M). High-risk patients received alternating cycles of regimen A and B (IVAC) for a total of four cycles (A-B-A-B). G-CSF support was used with all cycles. Several modifications were made to regimen A (CODOX-M) from the previously reported Magrath regimen. Cyclophosphamide was changed from 800 mg/m² day 1 followed by 200 mg/m² days 2–5 to 800 mg/m² days 1 and 2 to reduce myelosuppression. Vincristine was capped at 2 mg total and the dose of intracathecal cytarabine was reduced from 70 mg to 50 mg to reduce the incidence of neurotoxicity. The systemic dose of intravenous methotrexate was decreased from 6720 mg/m² to 3,000 mg/m² to reduce toxicity while maintaining adequate CNS penetration. Doxorubicin dose was increased from 40 mg/m² to 50 mg/m². Data from [17].

DA-EPOCH (dose-adjusted)-rituximab

Rituximab: IV: 375 mg/m^2 day 1 (total dose/cycle = 375 mg/m^2)

Etoposide: IV: 50 mg/m^2/day continuous infusion days 1 to 4 (total dose/cycle = 200 mg/m^2)

Vincristine: IV: 0.4 mg/m^2/day continuous infusion days 1 to 4 (total dose/cycle = 1.6 mg/m^2)

Doxorubicin: IV: 10 mg/m^2/day continuous infusion days 1 to 4 (total dose/cycle = 40 mg/m^2)

Cyclophosphamide: IV: 750 mg/m^2 day 5 (total dose/cycle = 750 mg/m^2)

Prednisone: Oral: 60 mg/m^2/day (given once daily or in 2 divided doses) days 1 to 5 (some centers may use 60 mg/m^2 twice daily days 1 to 5) (total dose/cycle = 300 mg/m^2 or 600 mg/m^2)

DA-EPOCH dose-adjustment

Filgrastim: SubQ: 5 mcg/kg/day beginning day 6; continue until ANC recovery

Repeat cycle every 21 days (for at least 2 cycles beyond best response; minimum of 6 cycles and maximum of 8 cycles) with etoposide, doxorubicin, and cyclophosphamide dose adjustments (based on CBC 2 times/week) according to the following schedule:

- Nadir ANC ≥500/mm^3: 20% increase (above previous cycle) for etoposide, doxorubicin, and cyclophosphamide
- Nadir ANC <500/mm^3 (on 1 or 2 measurements): Same doses as previous cycle
- Nadir ANC <500/mm^3 (on ≥3 measurements): 20% decrease below previous cycle for etoposide, doxorubicin, and cyclophosphamide (dosing adjustments below starting dose levels only apply to cyclophosphamide

Table 8.4 DA-EPOCH regimens for Burkitt lymphoma. ANC, absolute neutrophil count; CBC, complete blood count; DA-EPOCH, dose-adjusted/short course etoposide, doxorubicin, cyclophosphamide, vincristine, prednisone, and rituximab; IV, intravenous.

Hyper-CVAD (courses 1, 3, 5, and 7)			
Cyclophos-phamide	IV	300 mg/m² over 2–3 hrs every 12 hrs for 6 doses	Days 1–3
Mesna	IV	600 mg/m²/day adminstered as a continuous infusion starting with cyclophosphamide and ending 6 hours after last dose of cyclophosphamide	Days 1–3
Vincristine	IV	2 mg per day	Days 4 and 11
Doxorubicin	IV	If LVEF ≥ 50%: 50 mg/m² over 24 hrs	Day 4
Dexanethasone	PO/IV	40 mg per day	Days 1–4 and days 11–14
High dose methotrexate plus cytarabine (courses 2, 4, 6, and 8)			
Methotrexate	IV	200 mg/m² administered over the first 2 hours then 800 mg/m² administered over 24 hours (total dose per cycle of 1 gram/m²)	Day 1
Leucovorin	IV	50 mg IV 12 hours after end of methotrexate; then 15 mg IV every 6 hours for 8 doses or until methotrexate level <0.1 micromol/L. Dose modifications made based upon methotrexate levels.	Day 2
Cytarabine	IV	For patients<60 years old: 3 g/m² administered over 2 hours every 12 hours for 4 doses	Day 2 and 3
		For patients >60 years old: 1 g/m² administered over 2 hours every 12 hours for 4 doses	
Rituximab (courses 1, 2, 3, 4)			
Rituximab	IV	375 mg/m² over 2–6 hours	Days 1 and 11 of Hyper-CVAD and days 2 and 8 of high dose methotrexate plus cytarabine
CNS prophylaxis: total number of intrathecal treatment varies based upon risk factors*			
Methotrexate	IT	12 mg (6 mg if through Ommaya)	Day 2 of each cycle
Cytarabine	IT	100 mg	Day 8 of each cycle

Table 8.5 Rituximab plus hyperfractionated cyclophosphamide, vincristine, doxorubicin, and dexamethasone (hyper-CVAD) regimen for Burkitt lymphoma . Dose intensive phase: the dose intensive phase consists of 8 courses of therapy administered at 21-day intervals. The drugs used in each course alternate such that Hyper-CVAD is used for courses 1, 3, 5, and 7 while high-dose methotrexate plus cytarabine is given for courses 2, 4, 6, and 8. Details on dose of medication, prophylactic antibiotics, growth factor support, can be found in the original articles. Data from [18].

References

1. Magrath I. Epidemiology: clues to the pathogenesis of Burkitt lymphoma. *Br J Haematol*. Mar 2012;156:744-756.

2. Slack GW, Gascoyne RD. MYC and aggressive B-cell lymphomas. *Adv Anat Pathol*. 2011;18: 219-228.

3. Blum KA, Lozanski G, Byrd JC. Adult Burkitt's leukemia and lymphoma. *Blood*. 2004;104: 3009-3020.

4. Magrath I, Adde M, Shad A, et al. Adults and children with small non-cleaved-cell lymphoma have a similar excellent outcome when treated with the same chemotherapy regimen. *J Clin Oncol*. 1996;14:925-934.

5. Mead G, Barrans SL, Qian W et al. A prespective clinicopathologic study of dose-modified CODOX-M/IVAC in patients with sporadic Burkitt lymphoma defined using cytogenetic and immunophenotypic criteria (MRC/NCRI LY10 trial). *Blood*. 2008;112;2248-2260.

6. Barnes JA, LaCasce AS, Feng Y, et al Evaluation of the addition of rituximab to CODOX-M/IVAC for Burkitt's lymphoma: a retrospective analysis. *Ann Oncol*. 2011;22:1859-1864.

7. Thomas DA, Faderl S, O'Brien S, et al. Chemoimmunotherapy with hyper-CVAD plus Rituximab for the treatment of adult Burkitt and Burkitt type lymphoma or acutelymphoblastic leukemia. *Cancer*. 2006;106:1569-1580.

8. Dunleavy K, Pittaluga S, Shovlin M et al. Low-intensity therapy in adults with Burkitt's lymphoma. *N Engl J Med*. 2013;369:1915-1925.

9. Hoelzer D, Walewski J, Dohner H, et al. Improved outcome of adult Burkitt lymphoma/leukemia patients with rituximab and intensive chemotherapy: report of a large prospective multicenter trial. *Blood*. 2014;124:3870-3879.

10. Rizzieri DA, Johnson JL, Byrd JC, et al. Improved efficacy using rituximab and brief duration, high intensity chemotherapy with filgrastim support for Burkitt or aggressive lymphomas: cancer and Leukemia Group B study 10 002. *Br J Haematol*. 2014;165:102-111.

11. Sweetenham JW, Pearce R, Taghipour G, Blaise D, Gisselbrecht C, Goldstone AH. Adult Burkitt's and burkitt-like non-Hodgkin's lymphoma-outcome for patients treated with high-dose therapy and autologous stem-cell transplantation in first remission or at relapse: results from The European Group for Blood and marrow Transplantation. *J Clin Oncol*. 1996;14:2465-2472.

12. Noy A, Kaplan L, Lee J. A modified dose intensive R-CODOX-M/IVAC for HIV-associated Burkitt and atypical Burkitt lymphoma (BL) demonstrates high cure rates and low toxicity: prospective multicenter phase II trial of the AIDS Malignancy Consortium. *Blood*. 2012;122:639.

13. Ribera JM, García O, Grande C, et al. Dose-intensive chemotherapy including rituximab in Burkitt's leukemia or lymphoma regardless of human immunodeficiency virus infection status: final results of phase 2 study. *Cancer*. 2012;119:1660-1668.

14. Magrath I, Adde M, Shad A, et al. Adults and children with small non-cleaved-cell lymphoma have a similar excellent outcome when treated with the same chemotherapy regimen. *J Clin Oncol*.1996;14:925.

15. Mead GM, Sydes MR, Walewski J, et al. An International evaluation of CODOX-M and CODOX-m alternating with IVAC in adult Burkitt's lymphoma: results of Unites Kingdom Lymphoma Group LY06 Study. *Ann Oncol*. 2002;13:1264.

16. Mead GM, Barrans SL, Qian W, et al. A prospective clinicopathologic study of dose-modified CODOX-M/IVAC in patients with sporadic Burkitt lymphoma defined using cytogenetic and immunophenotypic criteria (MRC/NCRI LY10 Trial). *Blood*. 2008;112:2248.

17. Lacasce A, Howard O, Lib S, et al. Modified magrath regimens for adults with Burkitt and Burkitt-like lymphomas: preserved efficacy with decreased toxicity. *Leuk Lymphoma*. 2004;45:761.

18. Thomas DA, Faderl S, O'Brien S, et al. Chemoimmunotherapy with Hyper-CVAD plus rituximab for the treatment of adult Burkitt lymphoma or acute lymphoblastic leukemia. *Cancer*. 2006;106:1568-1580.

Chapter 9

Diffuse large B-cell lymphoma
Leslie Popplewell

Case presentation

A 56-year-old Chinese-American man previously in excellent health presented with symptoms of abdominal bloating, ascites, drenching night sweats, fatigue, and weight loss of 40 pounds over a period of 2 months. Computed tomography (CT) scan demonstrated several masses in the liver, up to 10 cm in size. Fluorodeoxyglucose (FDG)-positron emission tomography (PET)/CT scan also demonstrated intensely FDG-avid uptake in midline nasopharynx and in nodes at left neck level 1 and left submandibular area, lower posterior mediastinum, upper abdomen, and retroperitoneal locations as well as bilateral pleural effusions and moderate ascites. Biopsy of a representative liver mass was consistent with diffuse large B-cell lymphoma, not otherwise specified (DLBCL-NOS), which was positive for CD20, CD10, BCL-6, and Bcl-2 by immunohistochemistry, consistent with a germinal center B-cell-like (GCB) origin based on the Hans algorithm. The proliferation index was 30–40% seen with Ki-67 staining. A bone marrow biopsy did not show any evidence of lymphoma and was otherwise normal. He was given a diagnosis of stage IVB DLBCL, GCB-subtype. An acute hepatitis panel was suggestive of chronic hepatitis B infection confirmed by a positive polymerase chain reaction (PCR) for hepatitis B.

© Springer International Publishing AG 2017
J. Zain and L.W. Kwak (eds.), *Management of Lymphomas:*
A Case-Based Approach, DOI 10.1007/978-3-319-26827-9_9

Pathologic features

DLBCL accounts for about a quarter to one-third of cases of non-Hodgkin lymphoma (NHL) [1,2]. Median age is 64 years. It is a heterogeneous group of tumors composed of large B cells growing in sheets. The recent 2016 WHO classification [3] recognizes several types of DLBCL as distinct clinicopathologic entities as described in Table 9.1. A pathologic diagnosis needs to include the subtype in the final report.

Gene expression profiling led to the recognition of three different subtypes of DLBC, NOS: germinal center (GC), activated B-cell-like (ABC), and the unclassifiable group [4]. A retrospective analysis identified the 5-year overall survival of patients with GC subtype to be 70% versus only 12% for patients with the ABC subtype highlighting the clinical differences between entities [5]. All patients were treated with cyclophosphamide, doxorubicin, vincristine, and prednisone (CHOP)-based regimens. Immunohistochemical categorization of the GCB and non-GCB subtypes based on expression of CD10, BCL6, and IFR4/MUM1 is the clinically recognized method to classify these neoplasms, with the Hans

Diffuse large B-cell lymphoma (DLBCL), not otherwise specified (NOS)
- Germinal center B-cell type*
- Activated B-cell type*

T-cell/histiocyte-rich large B-cell lymphoma

Primary DLBCL of the central nervous system

Epstein-Barr virus (EBV)+ DLBCL, NOS*

EBV+ mucocutaneous ulcer*

Primary cutaneous DLBCL, leg type

DLBCL associated with chronic inflammation

ALK+ large B-cell lymphoma

Plasmablastic lymphoma

Primary effusion lymphoma

Human herpes virus 8+ DLBCL, NOS*

Burkitt-like lymphoma with 11q aberration*

High-grade B-cell lymphoma, with *MYC* and *BCL2* and/or *BCL6* rearrangements*

High-grade B-cell lymphoma, NOS*

B-cell lymphoma, unclassifiable, with features intermediate between DLBCL and classical Hodgkin lymphoma

Table 9.1 Diffuse large B-cell lymphoma subtypes based on the 2016 World Health Organisation classification. * denotes changes from the 2008 classification. Data from [3].

algorithim being the most common format [6]. Immunohistochemical categorization is considered an essential component of the pathology report (Figure 9.1) and it correlates with patient outcomes.

Molecular studies that can evaluate genetic alterations and translocations are becoming increasingly important in DLBCL. Chromosomal rearrangements of the C-*MYC* gene (8p24) in conjunction with translocations of *BCL-2*, usually t(14;18), and/or *BCL-6* on chromosome 3, define a DLBCL subgroup – 'double-hit' or 'triple-hit' lymphomas – associated with an aggressive phenotype, poor prognosis independent of the International Prognosis Index (IPI), and dismal outcomes with standard chemoimmunotherapy [7–13]. Concurrent overexpression of the MYC and BCL-2 proteins in DLBCL cells is associated with a similarly poor prognosis [14–16].

Some of the distinctive entities of DLBCL include primary DLBCL of the central nervous system (CNS; discussed in Chapter 14), including primary mediastinal large B-cell lymphoma – commonly associated with

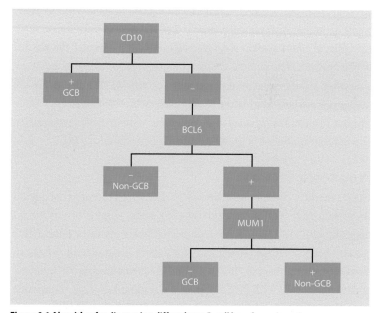

Figure 9.1 Algorithm for diagnosing diffuse large B-cell lymphoma based on histochemical staining. GCB, germinal center B-cell-like. Adapted from © American Society of Hematology, 2004. All rights reserved. Hans et al [6].

a clinical syndrome of mediastinal lymphoma in young women (median age 37), T-cell histiocyte-rich large B-cell lymphoma, intravascular large B-cell lymphoma, and Epstein-Barr (EBV)-positive DLBCL of the elderly. Unique treatment approaches are being developed for each of these entities. High grade lymphomas with *MYC* and *BCL2/BCL6* rearrangements will be discussed later in this chapter.

Staging and workup

In accordance with the Ann Arbor staging system [17], this patient has disease both above and below the diaphragm based on imaging studies, with liver involvement but a negative marrow. An 18 FDG-PET scan is used to delineate areas of disease involvement, and gives further information in intensity of uptake of the radiolabeled glucose. Of note, this patient did have abnormal uptake in the nasopharynx. Occult involvement of the CNS (5–25%) at diagnosis is more common in patients who have a high lactate dehydrogenase (LDH) level, more than one extranodal site, or specific site involvement in the Waldeyer's ring (including the nasopharynx), testicle, breast, or kidney involvement confers a high risk of CNS involvement [18]. Therefore, in addition to the staging workup already performed, this patient should have a lumbar puncture with evaluation of fluid cytology, and even if negative should have prophylaxis with intrathecal (IT) chemotherapy (we suggest methotrexate 12 mg IT with each cycle of chemotherapy). Some advocate the administration of moderate-to-high dose systemic methotrexate as a superior approach to prevent future CNS involvement [19].

Prognostic factors

The IPI predicts patient outcomes with CHOP-based therapy based upon the patient's age, performance status (PS), stage, number of extranodal sites, and LDH level [20]. A revised International Prognostic Index (rIPI) has also been developed specifically for patients treated with rituximab plus CHOP chemotherapy (R-CHOP), and is a better predictor of outcome in patients treated with R-CHOP than the standard IPI [21]. Using this revised IPI, four-year OS for the very good (IPI=0), good (IPI 1 or 2), and poor (IPI 3 or more) risk groups is 94, 79, and 55%, respectively. Remember the acronym 'APLES' (apples with one 'p': age, PS, LDH, Eastern

Cooperative Oncology Group PS, and extra nodal site). However, the use of molecular markers in the diagnosis of DLBCL may prove to be a more reliable predictor of outcomes than clinical factors alone.

Fluorodeoxyglucose-positron emission tomography

The use of FDG-PET scanning to assess for disease staging and response evaluation has moved into the standard of care as per Cheson's revised response criteria [22] – patients are considered in complete remission (CR) if the FDG-PET shows a normal FDG uptake. Patients with a positive interim FDG-PET after four cycles of CHOP or R-CHOP were seen to have a poorer outcome in a study by Haioun et al [23]. Additional cycles of the same chemotherapy were not sufficient to cure these patients. However, positive PET findings need confirmation by biopsy as inflammation and post-chemotherapy changes can lead to false positives. Moskowitz et al reviewed results of 98 patients with DLBCL treated with four cycles of R-CHOP14 [24,25]. After four cycles, a PET scan was performed and patients with negative scans were treated with consolidation with ifosfamide, carboplatin, and etoposide (ICE) x 3 followed by observation. Patients with a positive interim PET scan were first biopsied, and if positive for residual NHL on biopsy, received consolidation B, including ICE x 2, rituximab plus ICE (R-ICE) x 1, followed by autologous stem cell transplant (ASCT). Of the patients with a positive interim scan (n=38) only 5 patients had a positive interim biopsy and received ASCT. Three of the five patients remained alive and free of disease, while all 33 patients with positive interim PET and negative biopsy received ICE without ASCT, and 26 of those patients remain alive without any subsequent relapse. The negative biopsies found in the PET-positive patients demonstrated signs of inflammation.

Initial therapy

Multi-agent chemotherapy has been the backbone of therapy for DLBCL. The CHOP regimen was first introduced in 1990s and remains the mainstay of systemic therapy, having proven to be more effective than three other more intensive regimens [26]. The addition of rituximab, a recombinant anti-CD20 antibody to chemotherapy, has resulted in a 10–15%

increase in overall survival as compared with chemotherapy alone [27] and this difference has been maintained after a follow-up of more than 10 years in clinical trials where patients were randomized to R-CHOP versus CHOP alone. Using a combination of R-CHOP in 200 patients over 65 years of age, the 10 year OS was reported to be 44%, while patients younger than 60 years of age had an event-free survival (EFS) of 79% after 3 years with 93% overall survival (OS) rates at 6 years [28]. Based on this data, R-CHOP has become the standard regimen for most cases of DLBCL. The majority of trials use six to eight cycles of therapy given at an interval of every three weeks. Rituximab therapy does impose a risk of hepatitis B reactivation among patients positive for hepatitis B surface antigen (HBsAg) or hepatitis B surface antibody (anti-HBc). Patients should be screened for evidence of past or present hepatitis B infection and monitored during therapy, and treated with appropriate antiviral therapy.

The patient in the case presented above was started on treatment with CHOP chemotherapy, initially without rituximab due to a finding of hepatitis B with positive PCR. His transaminases were normal and the liver did not appear to be cirrhotic on scan. The patient was put on entecavir and subsequently rituximab was added to his chemotherapy. The patient had a total of six cycles of chemotherapy. An interim PET scan after cycle three showed resolution of all FDG-avid disease. The ascites had almost completely resolved.

Given the heterogeneity in the diagnosis and prognosis of DLBCL, newer treatment approaches are being investigated to tailor therapies to particular subtypes of disease. Already it is clear that the use of R-CHOP in the ABC subgroup results in a markedly decreased survival as opposed to the GC subtype. Other regimens that have been tested are discussed below.

The addition of bortezomib to R-CHOP in a 40 patient Phase II trial resulted in an overall response rate (ORR) of 88% with 75% achieving a complete response (CR). At a median follow-up of 51 months, two-year rates of progression-free (PFS) and OS were 64 and 70%, respectively. The addition of bortezomib was associated with higher than usual rates of peripheral neuropathy. Of interest, there was no survival difference observed between patients with GCB or ABC gene expression profiles

(GEP) suggesting that the inferior outcomes normally seen in patients with ABC DLBCL may be abrogated with the addition of bortezomib [29].

Two Phase II trials have evaluated the addition of lenalidomide to R-CHOP. The open-label, single arm, multicenter trial (REAL07) and another similar study evaluated the use of R-CHOP plus lenalidomide (R2-CHOP) in patients with previously untreated advanced stage DLBCL or grade 3b follicular lymphoma. In REAL07, the OR and CR were 92 and 86%, respectively. After a median follow-up of 28 months, the estimated 2-year PFS and OS were 80 and 92%, respectively. Results were similar among those with GCB and ABC subtypes [30]. In a separate Phase II trial the ORR was 98% (80% CR). Estimated event-free survival (EFS) and OS rates at 24 months were 59 and 78%, respectively. EFS rates were similar for those with GCB and ABC subtypes. Hematologic toxicity was universal. Three patients developed a second malignancy (acute myeloid leukemia [AML], glioblastoma, and metastatic colon cancer). Both of these trials suggest that the addition of lenalidomide appears to mitigate a negative impact of non-GCB phenotype on patient outcome [31].

Treatment of specific subtypes

For primary mediastinal B-cell lymphoma (PMBCL), R-CHOP followed by involved field radiation therapy has shown a 3-year EFS of 78% but there are long-term sequences to chest radiotherapy including second tumors and the acceleration of atherosclerosis and anthracycline-mediated cardiac events [32]. Use of dose-escalated rituximab, etoposide, vincristine, anthracycline, and prednisone (R-EPOCH) without involved field radiation therapy has shown a 5-year OS of 93–100% [33] and is now the preferred approach for newly diagnosed PMBCL. The treatment of PCNS lymphoma will be discussed in Chapter 14 in this book. The approach to double hit (DH) lymphoma will be discussed later in this chapter.

Management of relapsed disease

Approximately 30% of those with newly diagnosed DLBCL will eventually relapse and another 10% will fail to achieve a state of remission after initial therapy (refractory disease) [26]. These patients have a poor prognosis with a life expectancy of 3–4 months if left untreated [34].

However, it is essential that the patients undergo a diagnostic biopsy to confirm relapse and then they should be restaged. Bone marrow biopsy should be performed as well as imaging studies and lumbar puncture in patients with neurologic-related symptoms. An IPI should be determined again at relapse [35].

Patients who relapse after first line therapy or fail upfront therapy should be evaluated for high dose therapy and ASCT but need salvage chemotherapy prior to transplant in order to demonstrate chemosensitivity and achieve disease control. Survival benefit with high dose therapy and ASCT is only demonstrated with chemosensitive disease. Common salvage regimens include combinations of rituximab with ICE [36], dexamethasone, high dose cytosine arabinoside, and cisplatin (DHAP) [37], carmustine, etoposide, arabinoside, and melphalan [mini-BEAM], and gemcitabine-based regimens [38]. The ORR varies between 55 and 70% with CR rates of 25–55%. The CORAL study [39] was the only randomized study to compare two regimens: R-ICE versus R-DHAP. With long-term follow-up it was established that the GCB subtype appeared to benefit more from R-DHAP as compared with R-ICE but this difference was not sustained for the non-GCB subtype. This study also established that patients relapsing within 12 months after diagnosis but who had been treated with an upfront rituximab-containing regimen had a poor prognosis with 3-year survivals of 20%. PET negativity after salvage therapy is the most important prognostic factor to predict positive outcomes after ASCT [40]. Patients who fail to achieve an adequate PET response after salvage therapy should be considered for investigational agents and targeted therapies, which is discussed later in this chapter. Use of novel salvage regimens is needed to improve response rates [39,41].

High-dose therapy and autologous stem cell transplant

Patients with relapsed DLBCL should be evaluated for high dose chemotherapy and ASCT if they are found to be responsive to salvage chemotherapy and meet criteria for transplantation. The PARMA trial (1995) established the superiority of high dose therapy followed by ASCT in chemosensitive patients with relapsed DLBCL as compared with salvage therapy alone with ASCT [42]. This was a randomized, multi-center trial that compared ASCT with consolidation therapy in 215 patients with chemotherapy-sensitive NHL. All patients had achieved a first remission with an anthracycline-containing chemotherapy regimen. All patients received DHAP, with harvesting of autologous bone marrow, followed by a second cycle of DHAP. Patients were then randomized to 4 more cycles of DHAP versus ASCT using a BCNU, etoposide, cytarabine, and cyclophosphamide (BEAC)-conditioning regimen. There were no differences in prognostic factors between the groups. After a median follow-up of 63 months, the response rate was 84% after bone marrow transplantation versus 44% after conventional therapy. At five years, EFS was 46% in the transplantation group and 12% in the group receiving chemotherapy without transplantation ($P=0.001$), and the OS was 53 and 32%, respectively ($P=0.038$). Subsequent studies of the PARMA outcomes reported that patients with a longer initial remission fared better (relapse after >1 year versus <1 year) with higher response to DHAP x 2 (69 versus 40%) and OS at 8 years of 29 versus 13%, and that survival advantages were only seen in patients with an IPI of greater than zero at the time of relapse. In the post-rituximab era, while upfront cure rates have improved, salvage rates have decreased. The Centers for International Bone Marrow Transplant Registry (CIBMTR) have reported that amongst the 8373 patients who received an ASCT for DLBCL between 2002 and 2012, the 3 year probability of survival was 65% +/− 1% and 41% +/− 2% for patients with chemosensitive and chemoresistant disease, respectively. Besides chemosensitivity, patients are considered suitable candidates for ASCT if they have adequate organ function (as assessed by pre-transplant left ventricular ejection fraction [LVEF], diffuse capacity of the lung for carbon monoxide [DLCO], 24-hour creatinine clearance, and appropriate social support. It is important to confirm the presence of stem cells without morphologic or cytogenetic evidence of early myelodysplastic changes prior to collection of stem cells. Marrow free of involvement with lymphoma is highly desirable. Post-transplantation maintenance with immunomodulatory agents such as immune checkpoint inhibitors is being evaluated in order to improve overall outcomes and decrease relapses after ASCT.

Allogeneic stem cell transplantation

The use of allogeneic stem cell transplant in patients with relapsed DLBCL is limited to patients who relapse after an autologous stem cell transplant or fail to meet criteria of stem cell collection prior to ASCT. This approach relies on a graft versus lymphoma effect to provide disease control but the presumed clinical benefit is offset by the toxicity of an allogeneic stem cell transplant and its effect on the patient's quality of life [43]. Retrospective studies comparing autologous and allogeneic transplants for DLBCL have found no difference in survival between the two types of therapy. However, there is an increased risk of relapse with ASCT but higher non-relapse mortality with the allogeneic approach [44]. Nonetheless, it is offered to patients in transplant centers if the patient has an appropriate donor and is otherwise transplant-eligible based on physiologic age and comorbidities. Patients who are transplanted in clinical remission have a better outcome again pointing to a need for more effective salvage regimens.

New therapeutic targets

Use of molecular techniques and gene expression profiling has led to the identification of many molecular targets both in the tumor and the micro-environment including CD22, proteasome inhibition, BCL-2, mechanistic target of rapamycin (mTOR)/AKT, PKC-B, Syk, Bruton's tyrosine kinase (BTK), programmed cell death protein 1 (PD-1) and programmed death-ligand 1 (PD-L1). Some of these agents have been discussed above as part of upfront therapy. However, there is now accumulating evidence of the efficacy of these agents in the relapsed setting as single agents as well as combination therapies. Most promising are the BTK inhibitors such as ibrutinib, which has shown a response rate of 37% in patients with relapsed DLBCL of non-germinal cell type [45]. It is being evaluated in combination with cytotoxic chemotherapy.

High grade B-cell lymphoma with MYC and BCL2 and/or BCL6 rearrangements

High grade B-cell lymphoma, also known as double hit or double expresser lymphomas, are now known to have a worse outcome with standard therapies [46,47]. Hence all patients with suspected DLBCL should be tested for MYC, BCL2, and BCL6 rearrangements or protein expression. The MYC-driven nature also makes these patients more susceptible to CNS involvement. These patients need to be treated with more aggressive upfront therapies. In a retrospective study, DA-R-EPOCH, rituximab, cytoxan, vincristine, doxorubicin, dexamethasone/methotrexate, and high-dose Ara-C (R-hyperCVAD/MA), or rituximab, cyclophosphamide, doxorubicin, vincristine, methotrexate/ifosfamide, etoposide, high-dose cytarabine (R-CODOX-M/IVAC) resulted in a higher median PFS (21.6 months versus 7.8 months) compared with R-CHOP alone [48]. Patients should be encouraged to enroll in a clinical trial but increasingly the standard is to administer DA-R-EPOCH with prophylactic CNS-directed therapy as part of the induction regimen. One approach is to give one cycle of intrathecal methotrexate with each of the six cycles of systemic chemotherapy and then give two to four cycles of systemic high dose methotrexate at the completion of chemotherapy. High dose chemotherapy and ASCT should be considered in patients who achieve a remission even though the data for this approach is not clear [48,49].

There is no clear standard for patients in this group who relapse after upfront therapy. Cuccuini et al indicate that MYC+ DLBCL is not salvaged by classical R-ICE or R-DHAP followed by BEAM plus ASCT [9]. In a subset of patients in the previously mentioned CORAL study [39], of 477 patients enrolled in the study 28 patients (17%) were confirmed to have a MYC rearrangement. Twenty-one of these patients had one or more concurrent translocations, including either bcl2 and in some cases, also bcl6. Patients with the DH markers had a 4-year PFS and OS, which was much lower than those in the MYC-category (18 versus 42%, and 29 versus 62%, respectively). The type of salvage therapy (R-ICE versus R-DHAP) had no impact on survival. This suggests that other treatment, including novel therapies and possibly an allogeneic transplant approach, should be considered in such patients. Outcomes of such an approach are not yet available. Among the 836 patients who underwent a human leukocyte antigen (HLA)-matched sibling hematopoietic SCT for DLBCL from 2002 to 2012, the 3-year probabilities of survival were 50% +/- 2%

and 23% +/– 3% for patients with chemosensitive and chemoresistant disease, respectively.

Case conclusion

Two months after completion of cycle six of chemotherapy, the recurrence of two liver lesions with significant activity was seen on a PET scan as well as two foci of increased activity in the retroperitoneum corresponding to retroperitoneal lymphadenopathy. Biopsy of the lymph node confirmed relapsed disease. The patient underwent salvage chemotherapy and ASCT after achieving a second remission and remains in remission.

This chapter highlights the increasingly nuanced management of DLBCL in the current era. The City of Hope standard of care algorithms for treating DLBCL in the upfront and relapsed setting are included below in Figure 9.2. In addition, there is a large portfolio of clinical trials available for patients evaluating the efficacy of novel targeted agents in various stages and subtypes of disease that will ultimately move the treatment paradigms of treating DLBCL beyond standard therapies to a more personalized and precision based approach.

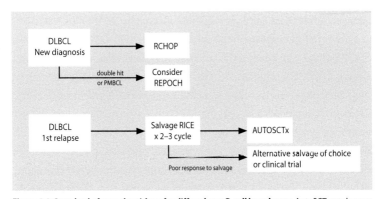

Figure 9.2 Standard of care algorithms for diffuse large B-cell lymphoma. AutoSCT, autologous stem cell transplant; DLBCL, diffuse large b-cell lymphoma; R-CHOP, rituximab, cyclophosphamide, doxorubicin, vincristine, and prednisone; R-EPOCH, rituximab, etoposide, vincristine, anthracycline, and prednisone; R-ICE, rituximab, ifosfamide, carboplatin, and etoposide.

References

1   Sant M, Allemani C, Tereanu C, et al. Incidence of hematologic malignancies in Europe by morphologic subtype: results of the HAEMACARE project. *Blood*. 2010;116:3724-3734.

2   Morton LM, Wang SS, Devesa SS, Hartge P, Weisenburger DD, Linet MS. Lymphoma incidence patterns by WHO subtype in the United States, 1992-2001. *Blood*. 2006;107:265-276.

3   Swerdlow SH, Campo E, Pileri SA, et al. The 2016 revision of the World Health Organization classification of lymphoid neoplasms. *Blood*. 2016;127:2375-2390.

4   Alizadeh AA, Eisen MB, Davis RE, et al. Distinct types of diffuse large B-cell lymphoma identified by gene expression profiling. *Nature*. 2000;403:503-511.

5   Shipp MA, Ross KN, Tamayo P, et al. Diffuse large B-cell lymphoma outcome prediction by gene-expression profiling and supervised machine learning. *Nat Med*. 2002;8:68-74.

6   Hans CP, Weisenburger DD, Greiner TC, et al. Confirmation of the molecular classification of diffuse large B-cell lymphoma by immunohistochemistry using a tissue microarray. *Blood*. 2004;103:275-282.

7   Aukema SM, Siebert R, Schuuring E, et al. Double-hit B-cell lymphomas. *Blood*. 2011;117:2319-2331.

8   Barrans S, Crouch S, Smith A, et al. Rearrangement of MYC is associated with poor prognosis in patients with diffuse large B-cell lymphoma treated in the era of rituximab. *J Clin Oncol*. 2010;28:3360-3365.

9   Cuccuini W, Briere J, Mounier N, et al. MYC+ diffuse large B-cell lymphoma is not salvaged by classical R-ICE or R-DHAP followed by BEAM plus autologous stem cell transplantation. *Blood*. 2012;119:4619-4624.

10 Horn H, Ziepert M, Becher C, et al. MYC status in concert with BCL2 and BCL6 expression predicts outcome in diffuse large B-cell lymphoma. *Blood*. 2013;121:2253-2263.

11 Johnson NA, Savage KJ, Ludkovski O, et al. Lymphomas with concurrent BCL2 and MYC translocations: the critical factors associated with survival. *Blood*. 2009;114:2273-2279.

12 Savage KJ, Johnson NA, Ben-Neriah S, et al. MYC gene rearrangements are associated with a poor prognosis in diffuse large B-cell lymphoma patients treated with R-CHOP chemotherapy. *Blood*. 2009;114:3533-3537.

13 Snuderl M, Kolman OK, Chen YB, et al. B-cell lymphomas with concurrent IGH-BCL2 and MYC rearrangements are aggressive neoplasms with clinical and pathologic features distinct from Burkitt lymphoma and diffuse large B-cell lymphoma. *Am J Surg Pathol*. 2010;34:327-340.

14 Green TM, Young KH, Visco C, et al. Immunohistochemical double-hit score is a strong predictor of outcome in patients with diffuse large B-cell lymphoma treated with rituximab plus cyclophosphamide, doxorubicin, vincristine, and prednisone. *J Clin Oncol*. 2012;30:3460-3467.

15 Hu S, Xu-Monette ZY, Tzankov A, et al. MYC/BCL2 protein coexpression contributes to the inferior survival of activated B-cell subtype of diffuse large B-cell lymphoma and demonstrates high-risk gene expression signatures: a report from The International DLBCL Rituximab-CHOP Consortium Program. *Blood*. 2013;121:4021-4031; quiz 4250.

16 Johnson NA, Slack GW, Savage KJ, et al. Concurrent expression of MYC and BCL2 in diffuse large B-cell lymphoma treated with rituximab plus cyclophosphamide, doxorubicin, vincristine, and prednisone. *J Clin Oncol*. 2012;30:3452-3459.

17 Carbone PP, Kaplan HS, Musshoff K, Smithers DW, Tubiana M. Report of the Committee on Hodgkin's Disease Staging Classification. *Cancer Res*. 1971;31:1860-1861.

18 Fletcher CD, Kahl BS. Central nervous system involvement in diffuse large B-cell lymphoma: an analysis of risks and prevention strategies in the post-rituximab era. *Leuk Lymphoma*. 2014;55:2228-2240.

19 Zahid MF, Khan N, Hashmi SK, Kizilbash SH, Barta SK. Central nervous system prophylaxis in diffuse large B-cell lymphoma. *Eur J Haematol*. 2016;97:108-120.

20 A predictive model for aggressive non-Hodgkin's lymphoma. The International Non-Hodgkin's Lymphoma Prognostic Factors Project. *New Engl J Med*. 1993;329:987-994.

21 Sehn LH, Berry B, Chhanabhai M, et al. The revised International Prognostic Index (R-IPI) is a better predictor of outcome than the standard IPI for patients with diffuse large B-cell lymphoma treated with R-CHOP. *Blood*. 2007;109:1857-1861.

22 Cheson BD, Fisher RI, Barrington SF, et al. Recommendations for initial evaluation, staging, and response assessment of Hodgkin and non-Hodgkin lymphoma: the Lugano classification. *J Clin Oncol*. 2014;32(27):3059-3068.

23 Casasnovas RO, Meignan M, Berriolo-Riedinger A, et al. Early interim PET scans in diffuse large B-cell lymphoma: can there be consensus about standardized reporting, and can PET scans guide therapy choices? *Curr Hematol Malig Reps*. 2012;7:193-199.

24 Moskowitz CH, Zelenetz A, Schoder H. An update on the role of interim restaging FDG-PET in patients with diffuse large B-cell lymphoma and Hodgkin lymphoma. *J Natl Compr Canc Netw*. Mar 2010;8:347-352.

25 Moskowitz CH, Schoder H, Teruya-Feldstein J, et al. Risk-adapted dose-dense immunochemotherapy determined by interim FDG-PET in Advanced-stage diffuse large B-Cell lymphoma. *J Clin Oncol*. 2010;28:1896-1903.

26 Fisher RI, Gaynor ER, Dahlberg S, et al. Comparison of a standard regimen (CHOP) with three intensive chemotherapy regimens for advanced non-Hodgkin's lymphoma. *N Engl J Med*. 1993;328:1002-1006.

27 Coiffier B, Thieblemont C, Van Den Neste E, et al. Long-term outcome of patients in the LNH-98.5 trial, the first randomized study comparing rituximab-CHOP to standard CHOP chemotherapy in DLBCL patients: a study by the Groupe d'Etudes des Lymphomes de l'Adulte. *Blood*. 2010;116:2040-2045.

28 Schmitz N, Zeynalova S, Glass B, et al. CNS disease in younger patients with aggressive B-cell lymphoma: an analysis of patients treated on the Mabthera International Trial and trials of the German High-Grade Non-Hodgkin Lymphoma Study Group. *Ann Oncol*. 2012;23:1267-1273.

29 Ruan J, Martin P, Furman RR, et al. Bortezomib plus CHOP-rituximab for previously untreated diffuse large B-cell lymphoma and mantle cell lymphoma. *J Clin Oncol*. 2011;29:690-697.

30 Vitolo U, Chiappella A, Franceschetti S, et al. Lenalidomide plus R-CHOP21 in elderly patients with untreated diffuse large B-cell lymphoma: results of the REAL07 open-label, multicentre, phase 2 trial. *Lancet Oncology*. 2014;15:730-737.

31 Nowakowski GS, LaPlant B, Habermann TM, et al. Lenalidomide can be safely combined with R-CHOP (R2CHOP) in the initial chemotherapy for aggressive B-cell lymphomas: phase I study. *Leukemia*. 2011;25:1877-1881.

32 Rieger M, Osterborg A, Pettengell R, et al. Primary mediastinal B-cell lymphoma treated with CHOP-like chemotherapy with or without rituximab: results of the Mabthera International Trial Group study. *Ann Oncol*. 2011;22:664-670.

33 Dunleavy K, Pittaluga S, Maeda LS, et al. Dose-adjusted EPOCH-rituximab therapy in primary mediastinal B-cell lymphoma. *N Engl J Med*. 2013;368:1408-1416.

34 Pfreundschuh M, Trumper L, Osterborg A, et al. CHOP-like chemotherapy plus rituximab versus CHOP-like chemotherapy alone in young patients with good-prognosis diffuse large-B-cell lymphoma: a randomised controlled trial by the MabThera International Trial (MInT) Group. *Lancet Oncology*. 2006;7:379-391.

35 Hamlin PA, Zelenetz AD, Kewalramani T, et al. Age-adjusted International Prognostic Index predicts autologous stem cell transplantation outcome for patients with relapsed or primary refractory diffuse large B-cell lymphoma. *Blood*. 2003;102:1989-1996.

36 Kewalramani T, Zelenetz AD, Nimer SD, et al. Rituximab and ICE as second-line therapy before autologous stem cell transplantation for relapsed or primary refractory diffuse large B-cell lymphoma. *Blood*. 2004;103:3684-3688.

37 Vellenga E, van Putten WL, van 't Veer MB, et al. Rituximab improves the treatment results of DHAP-VIM-DHAP and ASCT in relapsed/progressive aggressive CD20+ NHL: a prospective randomized HOVON trial. *Blood*. 2008;111:537-543.

38 El Gnaoui T, Dupuis J, Belhadj K, et al. Rituximab, gemcitabine and oxaliplatin: an effective salvage regimen for patients with relapsed or refractory B-cell lymphoma not candidates for high-dose therapy. *Ann Oncol.* 2007;18:1363-1368.

39 Gisselbrecht C, Glass B, Mounier N, et al. Salvage regimens with autologous transplantation for relapsed large B-cell lymphoma in the rituximab era. *J Clin Oncol.* 2010;28:4184-4190.

40 Sauter CS, Matasar MJ, Meikle J, et al. Prognostic value of FDG-PET prior to autologous stem cell transplantation for relapsed and refractory diffuse large B-cell lymphoma. *Blood.* 2015;125:2579-2581.

41 Crump M, Kuruvilla J, Couban S, et al. Randomized comparison of gemcitabine, dexamethasone, and cisplatin versus dexamethasone, cytarabine, and cisplatin chemotherapy before autologous stem-cell transplantation for relapsed and refractory aggressive lymphomas: NCIC-CTG LY.12. *J Clin Oncol.* 2014;32:3490-3496.

42 Philip T, Guglielmi C, Hagenbeek A, et al. Autologous bone marrow transplantation as compared with salvage chemotherapy in relapses of chemotherapy-sensitive non-Hodgkin's lymphoma. *N Engl J Med.* 1995;333:1540-1545.

43 Bishop MR, Dean RM, Steinberg SM, et al. Clinical evidence of a graft-versus-lymphoma effect against relapsed diffuse large B-cell lymphoma after allogeneic hematopoietic stem-cell transplantation. *Ann Oncol.* 2008;19:1935-1940.

44 Aksentijevich I, Jones RJ, Ambinder RF, Garrett-Mayer E, Flinn IW. Clinical outcome following autologous and allogeneic blood and marrow transplantation for relapsed diffuse large-cell non-Hodgkin's lymphoma. *Biol Blood Marrow Transplant.* 2006;12:965-972.

45 Wilson WH, Young RM, Schmitz R, et al. Targeting B cell receptor signaling with ibrutinib in diffuse large B cell lymphoma. *Nat Med.* 2015;21:922-926.

46 Nitsu N, Okamoto M, Miura I, Hirano M. Clinical significance of 8q24/c-MYC translocation in diffuse large B-cell lymphoma. *Cancer Sci.* 2009;100:233-237.

47 Oki Y, Noorani M, Lin P, et al. Double hit lymphoma: the MD Anderson Cancer Center clinical experience. *Br J Haematol.* 2014;166:891-901.

48 Petrich AM, Nabhan C, Smith SM. MYC-associated and double-hit lymphomas: a review of pathobiology, prognosis, and therapeutic approaches. *Cancer.* 2014;120:3884-3895.

49 Herrera AF. Double-hit lymphoma: practicing in a data-limited setting. *J Oncol Pract.* 2016;12:239-240.

CASE STUDY SECTION THREE

T-cell lymphomas

Chapter 10

Cutaneous T-cell lymphoma
Belen Rubio Gonzalez, Steven T Rosen, and Christiane Querfeld

Case presentation
An 83-year-old female presented with a progressing pruritic cutaneous rash that started 8 years ago. On clinical exam there were numerous coalescing, infiltrated, scaly, and partially crusted erythematous plaques distributed over her trunk and extremities and a large fungating ulcerated nodule on her right thigh covering 75% of her total body surface area (Figure 10.1). Lymphoma-associated alopecia and a left axillary lymphadenopathy were also noted. For the past 3–4 months she reported fatigue, severe pruritus, night sweats, 20 pounds of weight loss, and loss of appetite.

She was diagnosed with mycosis fungoides (cutaneous patches and plaques) 4 years ago per skin biopsy. Work-up included computed tomography (CT) scans and laboratory tests such as flow cytometry for Sézary cells that were all negative for systemic involvement. She was initially treated with psoralen and UV-A phototherapy (PUVA) thrice weekly and/or topical rexinoid inhibitor (bexarotene 1% gel) daily for about 2 years, but discontinued due to development of cutaneous ulcerated tumors and lymphadenopathy. Subsequent regimens included vorinostat and prednisone. She developed intractable pruritus and worsening skin rash for the past 3 months for which she was recently started on topical nitrogen mustard 0.016% gel and oral prednisone (20 mg). Her past clinical history is remarkable for lung adenocarcinoma treated with partial lobectomy plus paratracheal lymph node resection, hypertension, smoking, and chronic obstructive pulmonary disease requiring oxygen.

© Springer International Publishing AG 2017   157
J. Zain and L.W. Kwak (eds.), *Management of Lymphomas:*
A Case-Based Approach, DOI 10.1007/978-3-319-26827-9_10

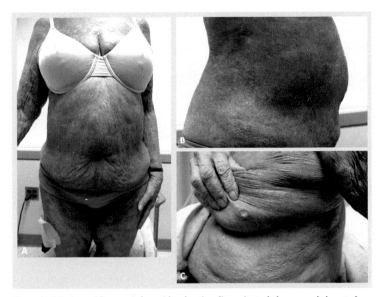

Figure 10.1 Patient with mycosis fungoides showing disseminated plaques and ulcerated tumor lesion on left breast (A–C).

Primary cutaneous T-cell lymphomas (mycosis fungoides and Sézary syndrome)

Primary cutaneous lymphomas represent ~3.9 % of non-Hodgkin lymphomas and are composed of various subtypes encompassing heterogeneous diseases with differences in histopathologic and clinical presentation (Table 10.1) [1]. The most common entities, mycosis fungoides (MF) and Sézary syndrome (SS), account for ~53% of all cases and represent the focus of this case study.

Work up and diagnosis

Recommended staging and work-up for patients with mycosis fungoides and Sézary syndrome is highlighted in Table 10.2 [2]. In the case included above, two skin biopsies were performed from the right thigh (ulcerated tumor nodule) and left thigh (plaque). The biopsy performed on the right thigh showed sheets of large tumor cells consistent with the diagnosis of mycosis fungoides with large cell transformation (MF-LCT) positive for CD30 with expression of cytotoxic markers such as granzyme B, but

Cutaneous T-cell and NK-cell lymphomas	Frequency (%)	5-year survival (%)
Indolent		
Mycosis fungoides (MF)	44	88
MF variants and subtypes		
Folliculotropic MF	4	80
Pagetoid reticulosis	<1	100
Granulomatous slack skin	<1	100
Primary cutaneous CD30+ lymphoproliferative disorders		
Lymphomatoid papulosis	12	100
Primary cutaneous anaplastic large cell lymphoma	8	95
Subcutaneous panniculitis-like T-cell lymphoma	1	82
Primary cutaneous CD4+ small/medium-sized pleomorphic T-cell lymphoproliferative disorder (provisional)	2	75
Aggressive		
Sézary syndrome	3	24
Extranodal NK/T-cell lymphoma, nasal type	<1	–
Primary cutaneous peripheral T-cell lymphoma, unspecified	2	16
Primary cutaneous epidermotropic CD8+ T-cell lymphoma (provisional)	<1	18
Cutaneous γ/δ T-cell lymphoma (provisional)	<1	–
Cutaneous B-cell lymphomas		
Indolent		
Primary cutaneous marginal zone lymphoma	7	99
Primary cutaneous follicular lymphoma	11	95
Intermediate		
Primary cutaneous diffuse large B-cell lymphoma, leg type	4	55
Primary cutaneous diffuse large B-cell lymphoma, other	<1	50
Intravascular large B-cell lymphoma	<1	65
Precursor hematologic neoplasm		
CD4+/CD56+ blastic plasmacytoid dendritic cell neoplasm	–	–

Table 10.1 The revised World Health Organization/European Organization for Research and Treatment of Cancer consensus classification for primary cutaneous lymphomas with relative frequency and 5-year survival. Adapted from © American Society of Hematology, 2005. All rights reserved. Willemze et al [1].

negative for CD56 (Fig 10.2 A–G), while biopsy from the left thigh revealed MF patch/plaque stage without large cell transformation (Fig 10.3 A–C). Both specimens revealed infiltrating the pilosebaceous unit by neoplastic T cells (folliculotropism). A CD4+ T-cell phenotype was seen with a CD4:CD8 ratio of >10:1. An identical monoclonal rearrangement of the gamma T cell receptor (TCR) was detected on both skin biopsies. Laboratory workup and re-staging included a complete blood count with differential, comprehensive chemistry panel, flow cytometry for circulating Sézary

Complete physical examination
Identification of skin burden:
• Percentage of BSA involved of each type of skin lesions (patches, plaques, tumors, erythroderma, and/or any ulcerated, crusted/oozing lesion)
• mSWAT
Identification of any palpable lymph node or organomegaly
Skin biopsy
• Immunophenotyping to include at least the following markers CD3, CD4, CD5, CD7, CD8, and one B-cell marker such as CD20.
• CD30 in large cell transformed MF, or if lymphomatoid papulosis, pcALCL is considered
• T-cell receptor rearrangement analysis
Laboratory work up
• CBC with differential
• Comprehensive metabolic panel
• LDH
• T cell receptor rearrangement analysis (compare to skin if positive)
• Flow cytometry for circulating Sézary cells (CD4+CD7-or CD4+CD26-) (erythrodermic patients)
• HTLV-I/II titers in selected patients
Imaging studies
• No imaging studies are required for stage IA/IB (T1N0M0B0; T2N0M0B0)
• CT scans of chest, abdomen, and pelvis (disseminated stage IB and higher)
• Combined PET/CT scans are recommended
Lymph node biopsy
• Excisional biopsy for lymph nodes ≥1.5 cm and/or firm, irregular, clustered, or fixed nodes
• Biopsy of the largest lymph node draining an involved area or the node with highest standardized uptake value on PET/CTscans
Multidisciplinary assessment by dermatologists, oncologists, pathologists/ dermatopathologists, and social worker is highly recommended

Table 10.2 Recommended ISCL/EORTC initial staging and work up for patients with mycosis fungoides/Sézary syndrome. BSA, body surface area; CBC, complete blood cell count; CMP, comprehensive metabolic panel; CT, computed tomography ;HTLV-I/II, human lymphotropic virus I/II; LDH, lactate dehydrogenase; mSWAT, modified severity-weighted assessment tool; pcALCL, primary cutaneous anaplastic large cell lymphoma; PET, positron emission tomography. Adapted from © American Society of Hematology, 2007. All rights reserved. Olsen et al [2].

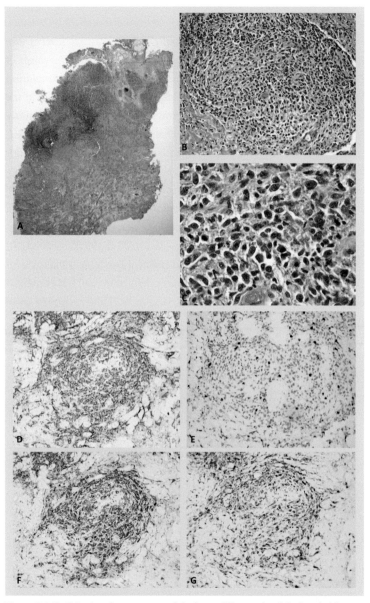

Figure 10.2 (A–C) Sections from a tumor nodule show a diffuse and nodular lymphoid infiltrate consisting of large pleomorphic cells with clumped chromatin. (D–G) The large lymphoid cells are positive for CD2 and negative for CD3 and positive for CD30 and granzyme B.

cells, peripheral blood for TCR rearrangement studies, and PET/CT scans. Results revealed mild anemia (Hbg 10.2 g/dL), an elevated LDH of 938 U/mL (range, 313–618 U/L), a peripheral monoclonal rearrangement of TCR gamma that is identical to skin clone, but no evidence of circulating Sézary cells. PET/CT scans showed enlarged and intensely FDG avid left inguinal lymph node (19 x 17 mm; maximal SUV of 2.8 g/mL) and mildly FDG avid right upper medial thigh lymph node (13 x 8 mm; maximal SUV of 2.8 g/mL). Based on the results the patient was diagnosed with MF with large cell transformation, clinical stage IIB (T3NxM0B0b) according to revised staging guidelines of the European Organisation for Research and Treatment of Cancer (EORTC) cutaneous lymphoma task force and ISCL (Table 10.3) [2], with a formal estimation of skin tumor burden using a modified severity-weighted assessment tool (mSWAT) of 158 (Table 10.4) [3].

The prognosis relies on the type and extent of skin lesions and extracutaneous involvement, which was originally defined in the TNM classification for cutaneous T-cell lymphoma (CTCL) in 1979 and revised in 2007

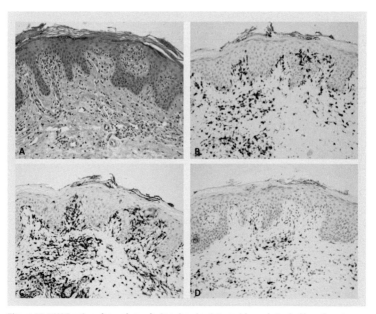

Figure 10.3 (A) Sections from plaque lesion showing intraepidermal atypical lymphocytes and a mild perivascular and interstitial lymphoid infiltrate. (B–D) The T cells are positive for CD3, CD4 and negative for CD8. There is a CD4:CD8 ratio of >10:1.

based on EORTC-ISCL recommendations taking nodal clinicopathologic classification and blood involvement into account [2,4]. Lymph node evaluation is recommended by excisional biopsies of clinically abnormal peripheral lymph nodes (>1.5cm) or any palpable peripheral irregular or firm node on physical examination. Fine needle aspiration may yield inadequate sampling for evaluation. Transformed MF with large cells expressing CD30 is often positive for cytotoxic markers (TIA-1, granzyme, perforin) similar to primary cutaneous anaplastic large cell lymphoma (pcALCL). Both share similar histopathologic features; therefore distinguishing MF-LCT from pcALCL may be difficult. Clinical features, prognosis, and outcome are the most discriminative to differentiate between the two entities [5].

Stage	T	N	M	B
IA	**T1**	N0	M0	0,1
IB	T2	N0	M0	0,1
IIA	**T1,2**	N1,2	M0	0,1
IIB	**T3**	N0–2	M0	0,1
IIIA	T4	N0–2	M0	0
IIIB	T4	N0–2	M0	1
IVA1	T1–4	N0–2	M0	2
IVA2	T1–4	N3	M0	0–2
IVB	T1–4	N0–3	M1	0–2

T	Skin	N	Lymph nodes
T1	Limited patch/plaque (<10% BSA)	N0	LN clinically uninvolved
T2	Generalized patch/plaque (>10% BSA)	N1	Enlarged; histologically uninvolved
T3	Tumors	N2	Clinically uninvolved; histologically involved
T4	Erythroderma	N3	LN enlarged and involved
B	BLOOD	M	VISCERAL
B0	No Sézary cells (≤5% of LC)	M0	No visceral organ involvement
B1	Circulating Sézary cells (>5%) non other B2	M1	Visceral involvement (pathology confirmation)
B2	≥1000/μL Sézary cells with positive clone		*Organ involved should be specified

Table 10.3 Current staging system for mycosis fungoides and Sézary syndrome according to the International Society for Cutaneous Lymphoma/European Organization of Research and Treatment of Cancer, cutaneous lymphoma task force.

Recommended treatment and discussion

Treatment regimens for MF/SS are determined by extent of disease, prognostic factors (folliculotropic type of MF, large cell transformation), age, other comorbidities and the impact on quality of life. Early stage MF (stages IA-IIA) has a favorable prognosis and disease is confined to the skin requiring skin-directed therapies as first-line regimens (Figure 10.4) [6–8]. Advanced stage MF/SS (stages IIB-IVB) is often refractory and results in an unfavorable prognosis; treatment is aimed at reducing the tumor burden, delaying disease progression, and preserving quality of life. Large cell transformation (LCT) is defined by the presence of more

Regions	% TBSA for the region	%TBSA Patch (or flat erythema	% TBSA Plaque (or elevated/ indurated erythema)	%TBSA Tumor/ Ulceration (or erythema w/fissuring, ulceration)
Head	7			
Neck	2			
Anterior trunk	13			
Posterior trunk	13			
Buttocks	5			
Genitalia	1			
Upper arms	8			
Forearms	6			
Hands	5			
Thighs	19			
Lower leg	14			
Feet	7			
% BSA by category	100			
Severity weighting factor				
Skin score subtotal				
TOTAL mSWAT				

Measure the total body surface area (TBSA) by using the patient's palm and fingers to represent 1% BSA. Maximum mSWAT score=400

Table 10.4 Estimation of the skin tumor burden using a modified severity-weighted assessment tool (mSWAT). mSWAT, modified severity-weighted assessment tool; TBSA, total body surface area. Adapted from © American Society of Clinical Oncology, 2011. All rights reserved. Olsen et al [3].

than 25% of large lymphocytes of the infiltrate in skin or lymph nodes and is generally associated with disease progression and advanced stages. When LCT occurs in MF it usually presents as tumor lesions. Most commonly, it develops as new solitary or multiple nodules in patients with long standing MF or Sézary syndrome [9]. LCT has a median survival of 24 months, compared with 163 months for conventional MF. Some studies suggest that the transformation at the time of the initial diagnosis may carry a better prognosis compared with when LCT is diagnosed in the disease course [9,10]. Factors in MF-LCT significantly associated with shorter survival include age ≥60 years, stage III/IV, early onset of transformation (in the first 2 years) and high serum LDH and beta 2 microglobulin [10]. A recently proposed prognostic index for MF-LCT may be helpful in predicting patients who have aggressive or more indolent clinical course. MF-LCT patients with ≥two adverse prognostic factors (advanced age, LCT, folliculotropism, elevated LDH, and peripheral

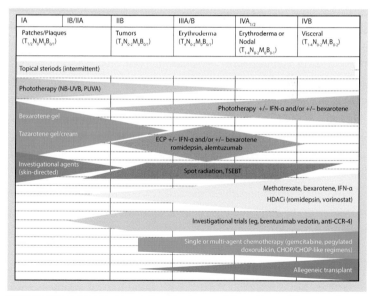

Figure 10.4 Stage-based treatment algorithm for mycosis fungoides and Sézary syndrome.
ECP, extracorporeal photopheresis; HDACi, histone deacetylase inhibitor; IFN-α, interferon-alpha; NB-UVB, narrowband-ultraviolet light B; PUVA, psoralen ultraviolet light A; TSEBT, total skin electron beam therapy; CHOP, cyclophosphamide, doxorubicin, vincristine, prednisone.

blood clone matching skin clone) have a worse prognosis compared with patients with <one adverse prognostic factor [10].

Given the patient's age and comorbidities she was initially treated with a combined skin-directed and systemic regimen with weekly doses of oral methotrexate (20 mg) and topical nitrogen mustard (NM) gel at bedtime. Due to the local irritative potential of NM a mid-potent topical steroid triamcinolone 0.1% ointment was added in the morning.

In general, the presence of LCT does not require a different stage-based treatment compared with classic MF with similar stage. Localized radiation therapy is considered in patients with unifocal transformation.

The ulcerated tumor (right upper thigh) was irradiated and cleared with two fractionated doses of 4 Gy. However, the patient was disabled by her severe pruritus so prednisone was given for short-term symptom relief; it was tapered over weeks and then discontinued. The patient received antihistamines (25 mg hydroxyzine at bedtime) that moderately controlled pruritus. Gabapentin or aprepitant was another consideration; however, the patient opted for hydroxyzine. Mild skin care using unscented mild soaps and emollients was recommended to improve the pruritus, dryness/scaling, and to keep barrier function intact. Weekly bleach baths were implemented to minimize bacterial colonization with Staphylococcus aureus. Her disease was stable with slowly improving plaques over the following 6 months, but she subsequently developed numerous ulcerated plaques and tumor nodules requiring a more aggressive treatment. Given the findings of relapsed/refractory CD30+ transformed MF she was started on brentuximab vedotin (1.8 mg/kg intravenously every 3 weeks). She received four cycles in total achieving complete remission (CR). On repeated PET/CT scans no lymphadenopathy or increased FDG uptake was noted. While on treatment she developed a peripheral neuropathy that has improved, but is persisting.

Outcomes with standard treatment regimens

Early-stage MF is favorably treated with skin-directed regimens with complete response rates ranging between 60–100% (Table 10.5) [7,8,11]. Total skin electron beam therapy (TSEBT) should be reserved for rapidly progressing or refractory widespread plaque and tumor disease. Long-term side effects can lead to cosmetic disfigurement (permanent hair loss, pigmentation) and the development of skin cancers and subsequent radiation is limited or not possible. Current approaches for advanced MF include biologic and targeted therapies with chemotherapy regimens reserved for rapidly progressing or refractory disease (Table 10.6) [6,12–36].

The duration of clinical response is often short. Local radiation therapy is effective for isolated/localized cutaneous tumors, or chronic, painful/ulcerated lesions, with a complete remission rate (CRR) of >90% and a mean time to relapse of 9.25 months (range 5–14 months). A single fraction radiation of 700 cGy–800 cGy provides excellent palliation for CTCL lesions and is cost effective and convenient for the patient [11]. Lower responses are common in transformed MF and lower extremity lesions associated with poor circulation and wound healing.

Biologic agents such as interferon-alpha (IFN-α), retinoids (all-trans retinoic acid, isotretinoin), rexinoids (bexarotene), and methotrexate are commonly used as first-line monotherapy in advanced MF and are also used in low-dose combination with skin-directed agents (narrowband-UVB or PUVA phototherapy, topical steroids, topical NM or spot radiation) [8,14]. IFN-α monotherapy has shown efficacy in all stages, with

Stage	Therapy type	Treatment	Response
Early stage MF (IA–IIA)	Topical/ skin-directed therapy	Steroids	ORR 80–90%; CR 63%(T1), 25% (T2) [6–8]
		Phototherapy	CR 71.4%; CRR 54.2%–91% (hypopigmented MF) [6–8]
		Nitrogen mustard	CR 72%; CRR 76–80% stage IA, CRR 35–68% stage IB [6–8]
		Bexarotene	ORR 63%, CR 21% [19–21]
		Local radiation	CRR>90%, low-dose (7-8 Gy) single or two fractions [11]
		TSEBT	CR 75% (T2), CR47% (T3) [6–8]
Refractory early stage MF (IA–IIA)	Combination therapy	PUVA or nbUVB and IFN-α (low-dose)	CR 70% [14]
		PUVA or nbUVB and bexarotene (low-dose)	CR 50-80% [14]

Table 10.5 Summary of treatments and response for patients with early stage mycosis fungoides (stage IA-IIA). CR, complete response; CRR, complete response rate; IFN-α, interferon-alfa; nbUVB, narrowband ultraviolet B light; MF, mycosis fungoides; ORR, overall response rate; PUVA, psoralen plus ultraviolet A light phototherapy; TSEBT, total skin electron beam therapy.

Therapy type	Treatment	Response
Skin-directed therapy	TSEBT	CR 35% (10–20 Gy) [6–8]
	Interferons (INF-α and INF-γ)	ORR 29–80%; CRR 4–41% [12,13]
Immunomodulators	Retinoid/rexinoid (bexarotene)	ORR 45–55% [19–21]
	ECP	ORR 35–71%, CRR 14–26% [15,16]
Biologic/targeted therapies	Alemtuzumab	ORR 86–100% (erythrodermic MF/SS) [29]
	HDACis (romidepsin and vorinostat)	ORR 36% (romidepsin) [26,27], 24% (vorinostat) [28]
	Antifolates (methotrexate, pralatrexate)	ORR 33–58% (methotrexate, low-dose) [22,23], ORR 45% (pralatrexate, relapse/refractory CTCL) [6]
Combined therapy	IFN-α and phototherapy	CR 70% [14]
	IFN-α and retinoids/rexinoids	CR 50–80% [14]
	Retinoid and phototherapy	CR 38% [6,19,20]
	ECP and INF-α	CR 44% [17,18]
	ECP and retinoids/rexinoids	No data available
Systemic chemotherapy (single-agent)	Pegylated doxorubicin	ORR 40.8–88% [32]
	Purine/pyrimidine analogues (gemcitabine)	ORR 68–75% [31]
Multiagent chemotherapy	CHOP/CHOP-like	Comparable efficacy than single agents, higher toxicity [30–32]
Stem cell transplant	Autologous	CRR 83%, all relapse within median of 6 months [34]
	Allogenic	ORR 68%, CRR 58%; 1/5-year PFS = 65%/60% [34]
Investigational therapy	Lenalidomide	ORR 29% [6]
	Bortezomib	ORR 67% (relapsed/refractory CTCL) [6]
	Brentuximab vedotin (anti-CD30)	ORR 70% [35]
	Anti-CCR4 antibody	ORR 56% [6]
	Anti-PD1/anti-PD-L1 antibodies	No data available
	TLR agonists	ORR 32% [6]
	Interleukin-2	ORR 18% [6]
	PI3-kinase δ/γ inhibitor (Phase I trial)	ORR 27% (37)

Table 10.6 Summary of treatments and responses for patients with advanced stage mycosis fungoides/Sézary syndrome (stage IIB–IVB). CR, complete response; CRR, complete response rate; CTCL, cutaneous T cell lymphoma; ECP, extracorporeal photophoresis; HDACis, histone deacetylase inhibitors; IFN-α: interferon-alfa; MF, mycosis fungoides; ORR, overall response rate; PI3K -δ/γ inhibitor, phosphoinositide-3-kinase-delta/gamma inhibitor; SS, Sézary syndrome; TSEBT, total skin electron beam therapy.

29–80% overall response rates (ORRs) and 4–41% complete response rates (CRRs) [12]. Tumor-stage and transformed MF do not respond well [13]. Combination therapies with retinoids do not have a higher response than IFN-α alone [13] and are inferior to IFN-α plus PUVA (38% CR with non-bexarotene retinoids versus 70% CR with IFN plus PUVA) [15]. Common side effects are dose-related and include headaches, flu-like symptoms, fatigue, anorexia, weight loss, and depression [13]. Extracorporeal photopheresis is primarily effective in erythrodermic MF/SS with low circulating Sézary cells and short duration of disease showing 35–73% ORR [16,17]. Bexarotene or IFN-α may be added for synergy [18,19].

Oral bexarotene was approved by the US Food and Drug Administration (FDA) for refractory CTCL in all stages. In Phase II and III trials of 94 patients with advanced stage MF (IIB-IVB) refractory to ≥two standard therapies, bexarotene showed ORRs of 45% and 55% with daily doses of 300 and 650 mg/m^2, respectively, and the median response duration was 7–9 months [20–22]. A daily dose regimen of 300 mg/m^2 is recommended based on the safety profile. The most common side effects include hypertriglyceridemia, hypercholesterolemia, and central hypothyroidism, requiring dose adjustments, lipid-lowering agents, and thyroid medications. Low-dose weekly methotrexate has an ORR of 33% and 58% for plaque (T2) MF and erythrodermic (T4) MF, respectively with median time to treatment failure of 15 months for patients with stage T2 disease and 31 months for erythrodermic MF [23,24]. An increased ORR was noted at higher doses (60–240 mg/m^2 intravenously) [25]. Common side effects of methotrexate include oral mucositis/stomatitis, gastrointestinal symptoms, bone-marrow suppression, and elevated transaminase levels. Decreased or defective Fas expression by neoplastic T cells has been associated with advanced/aggressive MF and impaired Fas-mediated apoptosis [26]. Methotrexate increases Fas and FasL in MF at least in part by decreasing Fas/FasL promoter methylation, resulting in enhanced Fas pathway apoptosis.

Based on two large Phase II studies, the US FDA approved romidepsin for relapsed/refractory MF/SS [27,28]. Romidepsin showed prolonged clinical responses in a subset of patients, particularly in SS patients with blood involvement with manageable side-effect profile. Reported ORR were 36% for romidepsin and less (24%) for the oral histone deacetylase inhibitor (HDACi) vorinostat with median response duration of 15 months and 6 months, respectively [28,29]. Alemtuzumab is particularly active in erythrodermic MF/SS with ORR of 86–100% and less effective in MF possibly due to distinct T-cell subsets seen for MF and SS. However, median progression free survival was only 6 months [30].

No large comparative studies were done to compare treatment efficacies and outcomes. A recent retrospective study analyzed ~200 MF/SS patients undergoing at least three systemic therapies. Primary endpoint was time to next treatment (TTNT) with median TTNT for IFN-α of 8.7 months, HDACi of 4.5 months, and single/multiagent chemotherapy of 3.9 months [31]. The study highlights that chemotherapy should be reserved if other options are exhausted. Commonly used single chemo-agents are gemcitabine and liposomal doxorubicin [32,33]. Allogenic transplant is the only potential curative treatment option in MF. A proposed graft-versus-lymphoma (GVL) effect is thought to be responsible for higher effectiveness of allogeneic transplants. Autologous transplant has yielded disappointing results with rapid disease relapses. Experiences with allogeneic hematopoietic stem cell transplant (HSCT) with myeloablative, and reduced-intensity conditioning in MF/SS have shown more promising results with treatment-related morbidity and mortality rates of 25–30% [6,34,35].

Case study follow-up

Following 10 months of CR the patient developed new small ulcerated plaques and tumors, which are controlled with topical steroids (plaques) and/or low-dose spot radiation (tumors). The patient was also restarted on low-dose methotrexate (16 mg weekly orally [PO]) for disease palliation. Disease palliation with preserving quality of life is the main goal in this patient. Given the patient's age and comorbidities, more aggressive chemotherapy regimens and allogeneic transplantation is not a consideration.

References

1   Willemze R, Jaffe ES, Burg G, et al. WHO-EORTC classification for cutaneous lymphomas. *Blood.* 2005;105:3768-3785.

2   Olsen E, Vonderheid E, Pimpinelli N, et al. Revisions to the staging and classification of mycosis fungoides and Sezary syndrome: a proposal of the International Society for Cutaneous Lymphomas (ISCL) and the cutaneous lymphoma task force of the European Organization of Research and Treatment of Cancer (EORTC). *Blood.* 2007;110:1713-1722.

3   Olsen EA, Whittaker S, Kim YH, et al. Clinical end points and response criteria in mycosis fungoides and Sezary syndrome: a consensus statement of the International Society for Cutaneous Lymphomas, the United States Cutaneous Lymphoma Consortium, and the Cutaneous Lymphoma Task Force of the European Organisation for Research and Treatment of Cancer. *J Clin Oncol.* 2011;29:2598-2607.

4   Lamberg SI, Bunn PA, Jr. Cutaneous T-cell lymphomas. Summary of the Mycosis Fungoides Cooperative Group-National Cancer Institute Workshop. *Arch Dermatol.* 1979;115:1103-1105.

5   Fauconneau A, Pham-Ledard A, Cappellen D, et al. Assessment of diagnostic criteria between primary cutaneous anaplastic large-cell lymphoma and CD30-rich transformed mycosis fungoides; a study of 66 cases. *Br J Dermatol.* 2015;172:1547-1554.

6   Jawed SI, Myskowski PL, Horwitz S, Moskowitz A, Querfeld C. Primary cutaneous T-cell lymphoma (mycosis fungoides and Sezary syndrome): part II. Prognosis, management, and future directions. *J Am Acad Dermatol.* 2014;70:223.e221-217; quiz 240-222.

7   Horwitz SM, Olsen EA, Duvic M, Porcu P, Kim YH. Review of the treatment of mycosis fungoides and sezary syndrome: a stage-based approach. *J Natl Compr Canc Netw.* 2008;6:436-442.

8   Zelenetz AD GL, Wierde WG, et al. NCCN Clinical Practice Guidelines in Oncology: Non-Hodkin's lymphomas. 2015; v 2.2015. https://www.nccn.org/professionals/physician_gls/f_guidelines.asp. Accessed March 7, 2017.

9   Jawed SI, Myskowski PL, Horwitz S, Moskowitz A, Querfeld C. Primary cutaneous T-cell lymphoma (mycosis fungoides and Sezary syndrome): part I. Diagnosis: clinical and histopathologic features and new molecular and biologic markers. *J Am Acad Dermatol.* 2014;70:205.e201-216; quiz 221-202.

10 Benner MF, Jansen PM, Vermeer MH, Willemze R. Prognostic factors in transformed mycosis fungoides: a retrospective analysis of 100 cases. *Blood.* 2012;119:1643-1649.

11 Thomas TO, Agrawal P, Guitart J, et al. Outcome of patients treated with a single-fraction dose of palliative radiation for cutaneous T-cell lymphoma. *Int J Radiat Oncol Biol Phys.* 2013;85:747-753.

12 Olsen EA, Rosen ST, Vollmer RT, et al. Interferon alfa-2a in the treatment of cutaneous T cell lymphoma. *J Am Acad Dermatol.* 1989;20:395-407.

13 Olsen EA. Interferon in the treatment of cutaneous T-cell lymphoma. *Dermatol Ther.* 2003;16:311-321.

14 Kuzel TM, Roenigk HH Jr, Samuelson E, et al. Effectiveness of interferon alfa-2a combined with phototherapy for mycosis fungoides and the Sezary syndrome. *J Clin Oncol.* 1995;13:257-263.

15 Stadler R, Otte HG. Combination therapy of cutaneous T cell lymphoma with interferon alpha-2a and photochemotherapy. *Recent Results Cancer Res.* 1995;139:391-401.

16 Knobler R, Duvic M, Querfeld C, et al. Long-term follow-up and survival of cutaneous T-cell lymphoma patients treated with extracorporeal photopheresis. *Photodermatol Photoimmunol Photomed.* 2012;28:250-257.

17 Duvic M, Hester JP, Lemak NA. Photopheresis therapy for cutaneous T-cell lymphoma. *J Am Acad Dermatol.* 1996;35:573-579.

18 Dippel E, Schrag H, Goerdt S, Orfanos CE. Extracorporeal photopheresis and interferon-alpha in advanced cutaneous T-cell lymphoma. *Lancet.* 1997;350:32-33.

19 Haley HR, Davis DA, Sams WM. Durable loss of a malignant T-cell clone in a stage IV cutaneous T-cell lymphoma patient treated with high-dose interferon and photopheresis. *J Am Acad Dermatol.* 1999;41:880-883.

20 Duvic M, Hymes K, Heald P, et al. Bexarotene is effective and safe for treatment of refractory advanced-stage cutaneous T-cell lymphoma: multinational phase II-III trial results. *J Clin Oncol.* 2001;19:2456-2471.

21 Duvic M, Martin AG, Kim Y, et al. Phase 2 and 3 clinical trial of oral bexarotene (Targretin capsules) for the treatment of refractory or persistent early-stage cutaneous T-cell lymphoma. *Arch Dermatol.* 2001;137:581-593.

22 Querfeld C, Rosen ST, Guitart J, et al. Comparison of selective retinoic acid receptor- and retinoic X receptor-mediated efficacy, tolerance, and survival in cutaneous t-cell lymphoma. *J Am Acad Dermatol.* 2004;51:25-32.

23 Zackheim HS, Kashani-Sabet M, McMillan A. Low-dose methotrexate to treat mycosis fungoides: a retrospective study in 69 patients. J Am Acad Dermatol. 2003;49:873-878.

24 Zackheim HS, Kashani-Sabet M, Hwang ST. Low-dose methotrexate to treat erythrodermic cutaneous T-cell lymphoma: results in twenty-nine patients. *J Am Acad Dermatol.* 1996;34:626-631.

25 McDonald CJ, Bertino JR. Treatment of mycosis fungoides lymphoma: effectiveness of infusions of methotrexate followed by oral citrovorum factor. *Cancer Treat Rep.* 1978;62:1009-1014.

26 Wu J, Nihal M, Siddiqui J, Vonderheid EC, Wood GS. Low FAS/CD95 expression by CTCL correlates with reduced sensitivity to apoptosis that can be restored by FAS upregulation. *J Invest Dermatol.* 2009;129:1165-1173.

27 Piekarz RL, Frye R, Turner M, et al. Phase II multi-institutional trial of the histone deacetylase inhibitor romidepsin as monotherapy for patients with cutaneous T-cell lymphoma. *J Clin Oncol.* 2009;27:5410-5417.

28 Whittaker SJ, Demierre MF, Kim EJ, et al. Final results from a multicenter, international, pivotal study of romidepsin in refractory cutaneous T-cell lymphoma. *J Clin Oncol.* 2010;28:4485-4491.

29 Olsen EA, Kim YH, Kuzel TM, et al. Phase IIb multicenter trial of vorinostat in patients with persistent, progressive, or treatment refractory cutaneous T-cell lymphoma. *J Clin Oncol.* 2007;25:3109-3115.

30 Querfeld C, Mehta N, Rosen ST, et al. Alemtuzumab for relapsed and refractory erythrodermic cutaneous T-cell lymphoma: a single institution experience from the Robert H. Lurie Comprehensive Cancer Center. *Leuk Lymphoma.* 2009;50:1969-1976.

31 Hughes CF, Khot A, McCormack C, et al. Lack of durable disease control with chemotherapy for mycosis fungoides and Sezary syndrome: a comparative study of systemic therapy. *Blood.* 2015;125:71-81.

32 Duvic M, Talpur R, Wen S, Kurzrock R, David CL, Apisarnthanarax N. Phase II evaluation of gemcitabine monotherapy for cutaneous T-cell lymphoma. *Clin Lymphoma Myeloma.* 2006;7:51-58.

33 Dummer R, Quaglino P, Becker JC, et al. Prospective international multicenter phase II trial of intravenous pegylated liposomal doxorubicin monochemotherapy in patients with stage IIB, IVA, or IVB advanced mycosis fungoides: final results from EORTC 21012. *J Clin Oncol.* 2012;30:4091-4097.

34 Duarte RF, Canals C, Onida F, et al. Allogeneic hematopoietic cell transplantation for patients with mycosis fungoides and Sezary syndrome: a retrospective analysis of the Lymphoma Working Party of the European Group for Blood and Marrow Transplantation. *J Clin Oncol.* 2010;28:4492-4499.

35 Wu PA, Kim YH, Lavori PW, Hoppe RT, Stockerl-Goldstein KE. A meta-analysis of patients receiving allogeneic or autologous hematopoietic stem cell transplant in mycosis fungoides and Sezary syndrome. *Biol Blood Marrow Transplant.* 2009;15:982-990.

36 Kim YH, Tavallaee M, Sundram U, et al. Phase II investigator-initiated study of brentuximab vedotin in mycosis fungoides and Sezary syndrome with variable CD30 expression level: a multi-Institution Collaborative Project. *J Clin Oncol.* 2015;33:3750-3758.

37 Horwitz SM, Porcu P, Flinn I, et al. Duvelisib (IPI-145), a phosphoinositide-3-kinase-δ,γ inhibitor, shows activity in patients with relapsed/refractory T-cell lymphoma [ASH abstract 803]. *Blood.* 2014;124(suppl 21).

Chapter 11

Systemic T-cell lymphoma

Jasmine Zain

Case presentation

A 55-year-old man presents to his primary medical doctor with a 3 week history of fatigue, chills, and a ten pound unintentional weight loss. On examination, he is found to have several palpable nodes in his neck and right axilla. Excisional biopsy and workup including positron emission tomography (PET)/computed tomography (CT) confirms a diagnosis of peripheral T-cell lymphoma not otherwise specified (PTCL-nos), International Prognostic Index score (IPI) =3, and modified Prognostic Index for T-cell lymphoma (mPIT) =2 (+ R pleural effusion, lactate dehydrogenase [LDH] 2x upper limit of normal [ULN], Eastern Cooperative Oncology Group [ECOG] 1, ki67 80%).

Introduction

The term T-cell lymphoma was first introduced in the 1970s with the Lukes and Collins and the Kiel's classification when immunological differences between B- and T-cell lymphomas led to the recognition of different subtypes of non-Hodgkin lymphoma (NHL) [1]. Mature T-cell lymphomas now refer to lymphoid neoplasm arising from post-thymic lymphocytes both from αβ and γδ T cells determined by the T-cell receptor. The current World Health Organization (WHO) 2016 classification of malignant lymphomas recognizes over 24 different histologic subtypes of mature T-cell and NK-cell neoplasms listed in Table 11.1 as pathologically,

© Springer International Publishing AG 2017

J. Zain and L.W. Kwak (eds.), *Management of Lymphomas: A Case-Based Approach*, DOI 10.1007/978-3-319-26827-9_11

functionally, and clinically complex diseases [2]. It incorporates morphologic, immunophenotypic, genetic, and clinical features of these diseases. Clinical features, particularly the site of origin, provide a more practical approach to classification of these tumors and may be more useful to the treating physician in terms of trying to understand the management options for these patients as listed in Table 11.2. Angioimmunoblastic T-cell lymphoma (AITL), anaplastic large cell lymphoma (ALCL), and PTCL-nos are the most common subtypes of PTCL in the US and account for over 50% of all PTCLs. This chapter will focus on a general approach to treating mature T-cell lymphomas with the exception of cutaneous T-cell lymphomas (CTCL), which was discussed separately in Chapter 10.

Mature T-cell and NK-cell neoplasms
T-cell prolymphocytic leukemia
T-cell large granular lymphocytic leukemia
Chronic lymphoproliferative disorder of NK cells
Aggressive NK leukemia
Systemic EBV-positive T-cell lymphoproliferative disease of childhood
Hydroa vacciniforme-like lymphoma
Adult T-cell leukemia/lymphoma
Extranodal NK/T-cell lymphoma, nasal type
Enteropathy-associated T-cell lymphoma
Hepatosplenic T-cell lymphoma
Subcutaneous panniculitis-like T-cell lymphoma
Mycosis fungoides
Sezary syndrome
Primary cutaneous CD30-positive T-cell lymphoproliferative disorders
Lymphomatoid papulosis
Primary cutaneous anaplastic large cell lymphoma
Primary cutaneous γ/δ T-cell lymphoma
Primary cutaneous CD8-positive aggressive epidermotropic cytotoxic T-cell lymphoma
Primary cutaneous CD4-positive small/medium T-cell lymphoma
Peripheral T-cell lymphoma, NOS
Angioimmunoblastic T-cell lymphoma
Anaplastic large cell lymphoma, ALK positive
Anaplastic large cell lymphoma, ALK negative

Table 11.1 World Health Organization classification of mature T-cell neoplasms. EBV, Eppstein-Barr virus; NK, Natural Killer; NOS, not otherwise specified.

The International Peripheral T-cell and Natural Killer/T-cell Lymphoma study is one of the earliest and largest compilations to date of T-cell lymphoma cases in over 22 centers worldwide and has given us a large amount of information about the epidemiology and outcomes of these diverse diseases [3]. Mature T-cell lymphomas comprise about 15–20% of all aggressive NHL and 5–10% of all NHL worldwide [4]. There is geographical variation in the incidence of peripheral T-cell lymphomas with higher frequencies of PTCL (15–20% of all NHL) observed in Asia, Central, and South America. This is postulated to be related to the increased incidence

Nodal	Peripheral T-cell lymphoma, not otherwise specified (PTCL-nos)
	Angioimmunoblastic T-cell lymphoma (AITL)
	Anaplastic large cell lymphoma (ALCL), alk+
	Anaplastic large cell lymphoma (ALCL), alk-
Cutaneous	Mycosis fungoides
	Sezary syndrome
	Primary cutaneous CD30-positive T-cell lymphoproliferative disorders: • lymphomatoid papulosis • primary cutaneous anaplastic large cell lymphoma
	Primary cutaneous γδ T cell lymphoma
	Primary cutaneous CD8-positive aggressive epidermotropic cytotxic T-cell lymphoma
	Primary cutaneous CD4-positive small medium T-cell lymphoma
Extranodal	Extranodal NK-/T-cell lymphoma, nasal type
	Enteropathy associated T-cell lymphoma
	Hepatosplenic T-cell lymphoma
	Subcutaneous panninculitis-like T-cell lymphoma
	Seroma-associated ALCL of breast
Primary leukemic	Aggressive NK leukemia- associated with hemophago cytic syndrome
	T-cell prolymphocytic leukemia
	T-cell large granular lymphcytic leukemia
	Adult T-cell leukemia lymphoma
Varied presentation	Chronic lymphoproliferative disorder of NK cells
	Systemic EBV positive T-cell lymphoproliferative disease of childhood
	Hydroa vacciniforme-like lymphoma
	Systemic EBV+ T-cell lymphoproliferative disease-associated with hemophagocytic syndrome

Table 11.2 Practical classification of mature T and NK/T-cell lymphomas. AITL, angioimmunoblastic T-cell lymphoma; ALCL, anaplastic large cell lymphoma; EBV, Eppstein-Barr virus; NK, Natural Killer; PTCL-nos, peripheral T-cell lymphoma, not otherwise specified.

and prevalence of viruses such as human T-lymphotropic virus 1 (HTLV1) associated with adult T-cell leukemia/lymphoma (ATLL) in Asia and Caribbean islands and Eppstein-Barr virus (EBV)-associated NK-/T-cell neoplasms in Far East Asia. Besides the viral factors, other geographic variables include increased incidence of enteropathy-associated T-cell lymphoma (EATL) associated with celiac disease in Northern European countries mainly Norway, and the angioimmunoblastic type in Europe [5]. In North America, the most common subtype is alk-positive ALCL.

Median age of presentation of T-cell lymphomas is 62 years but the median age is lower in some subtypes alk+ ALCL (33 years), hepatos-plenic T-cell lymphoma (34years) [3]. In the Western hemisphere, the overall incidence rate of PTCL is 0.5–2 per 100,000 per year. In the US, it is 1.8/100,000 per year [5].

Based on Surveillance, Epidemiology, and End Results (SEER) data, the incidence of PTCL increased by 280% between 1992 and 2005, and the incidence increased with age in all race and sex age groups [6]. Age-adjusted incidence rates were higher in males compared with females, and in blacks. The incidence of extra nodal NK/T-cell lymphoma was prominent among Asian or Pacific islanders. The highest rate of PTCL was seen in native Alaskans and Native Americans [6]. Etiology for most mature T-cell neoplasms is unknown other than HTLV1-associated ATLL and the association of EBV virus infection with some of the other subtypes of PTCL including NK/T-cell lymphoma, AITL, and the EBV-associated lymphoproliferative disorders. Outcomes data from the International Lymphoma project outlines the dismal prognosis of these diseases. The data exclude cutaneous T-cell lymphomas (discussed elsewhere) and the few indolent subtypes of PTCL. The best outcomes is seen for alk+ ALCL with a 5-year overall survival (OS) of over 70%. Most other histologies have a 5-year survival of 30% or less. Alk-negative ALCL has a 5-year survival that is intermediate between 55–60%. The worst 5-year outcome is seen with ATLL (14%), EATL (20%), and hepatosplenic T-cell lymphoma (7%) [3].

This case study highlights some of the challenges in taking care of patients with systemic peripheral T-cell lymphomas (PTCL). Detailed clinical and diagnostic workup is needed to establish a full clinical picture and treatment plan (Table 11.3 and 11.4, Figure 11.1 and 11.2).

These are outlined below along with the treatment algorithms that are used by physicians at City of Hope for the treatment of PTCL and extranodal NK/T-cell lymphomas. They are based on the National Comprehensive Cancer Network (NCCN) consensus guidelines and published literature. Salient features of the more common subtypes of PTCL are presented below to highlight the differences between different subtypes of PTCL.

Peripheral T-cell lymphoma-not otherwise specified

This is a nodal PTCL with heterogeneous pathological features considered to be a diagnosis of exclusion. It is the most common subtype of PTCL in the Western world. Histological features are variable and the tumors can sometimes be classified into subtypes. Presence of epitheliod histiocyties is seen in the lymphepitheliod variant [7], small-to-medium-sized cells that involve the paracortical regions of the node are called the T-zone variant [8] and presence of T helper follicular (T_{FH}) cells defines the follicular variant with features that overlap with AITL [9].

Workup for a patient with peripheral T-cell lymphoma

- Physical examination, assess for performance status, B symptoms, extranodal sites of disease especially skin, and any neurological symptoms. Establish risk factors for viral exposures like HTLV1, EBV
- CBC with differential with attention to eosinophil count, lymphocyte percentage and presence of abnormal cells, LDH, serologies for HIV, HTLV1, acute infectious hepatitis, comprehensive profile, and uric acid. Send flow cytometry on peripheral blood if lymphocytosis or presence of atypical cells is noted
- Staging scans including PET/CT from head to toe to capture any skin or extranodal involvement, MRI of brain and spine if clinically indicated
- Bone marrow biopsy and aspiration
- Consider biopsy of suspicious skin lesions
- MUGA scan
- CSF sampling if clinically indicated or if there is high risk of involvement of CNS
- Establish a prognostic score for each patient at diagnosis. IPI (age, LDH, PS, Ann Arbor stage, extra nodal sites) PIT (age> 60, LDH, PS, bone marrow involvement) or modified PIT (m-PIT; age, PS, LDH, Ki-67)
- Collect tissue samples for research and tissue banking including buccal swabs and blood samples
- HLA typing on patient and any siblings may be initiated if the patient has high risk disease
- Stem cell transplant consult

Table 11.3 Workup for a patient with peripheral T-cell lymphoma. CBC, complete blood count; CNS, central nervous system; CSF, cerebrospinal fluid; EBV, Epstein-Barr virus; HIV, human immunodeficiency virus; HLA, human leukocyte antigen; HTLV1, human T-lymphotropic virus 1; IPI, International Prognostic Index; LDH, lactate dehydrogenase; MUGA, multi-gated acquisition; mPIT, modified Prognostic Index for T-cell lymphoma; PIT, Prognostic Index for T-cell lymphoma; PS, performance status.

Diagnostic pitfalls

- Review pathology. All biopsies performed outside to be reviewed. At least one paraffin block representative of the tumor should be reviewed along with biopsies of other sites that may be involved. Re-biopsy if enough tissue is not available. Consent the patient for tissue collection protocols
- An FNA is not sufficient to make the diagnosis
- Immunohistochemical panel: CD20, CD3, CD10, BCL-6, Ki-67, CD5, CD30, CD2, CD4, CD8, CD56,CD57, CD21, CD23, EBER–ISH, ALK
- Cell surface marker analysis by flow cytometry: kappa/ lambda, CD45, CD3, CD5, CD19,CD20, CD30, CD4, CD8, CD7, CD2, TCRaB: TCRgamma
- Molecular analysis to detect TCR gene rearrangements
- Additional immunohistochemical stains to establish the specific sybtype diagnosis like CXCL13, BF1, TCR-C Myc

Table 11.4 Pitfalls in diagnosing peripheral T-cell lymphoma. ALK, anaplastic lymphoma kinase; EBV, Epstein-Barr virus; FNA, fine-needle aspiration; EBER–ISH, EBV-encoded RNA–in situ hybridization; TCR, T-cell receptor.

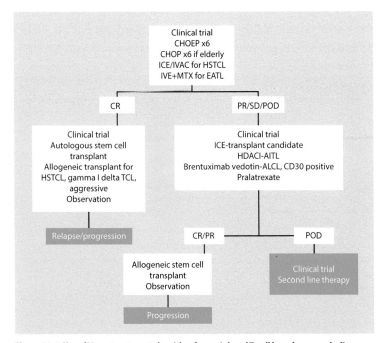

Figure 11.1 City of Hope treatment algorithm for peripheral T-cell lymphoma excluding natural killer-T-cell lymphoma. AITL, angioimmunoblastic T cell lymphoma; CR, complete remission; EATL, enteropathy associated T cell lymphoma; HDACI, histone deacetylase inhibitor; HSTCL, hepatosplenic T cell lymphoma, ICE, ifosfamide, carboplatin, etoposide; IVAC, ifosfamide, etoposide, cytarabine and intrathecal methotrexate; IVE, ifosfamide, epirubicin, etoposide; MTX, methotrexate; PR, partial remission; POD, progression of disease.

In the follicular variant the neoplastic cells are confined to B follicles, may mimic follicular lymphoma, and may express CD10 but are negative for BCL6. None of these subtypes have distinct clinical features or affect prognosis. Immunophenotyping is not helpful in subtyping the tumor. Most cases express CD4 but CD8 expression can also be seen. Loss of one of the other pan T-cell markers is seen in up to 75% of cases mostly CD7. Gene expression profiling shows variable overlap with AITL [10]. Antigen expression can change over time.

PTCL-nos is mostly seen in older adults. Advanced stage disease and extra-nodal involvement is common at the time of presentation. The follicular variant of PTCL may present as localized disease without prominent constitutional symptoms. Treatment recommendations follow the general guidelines for the treatment of PTCL as outlined.

Angioimmunoblastic T-cell lymphoma

AITL, also known as angioimmunoblastic lymphadenopathy with dysproteinemia (AILD), has a nodal presentation with a plethora of additional

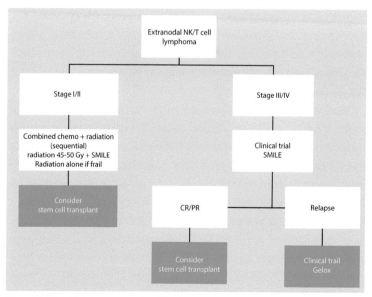

Figure 11.2 City of Hope treatment algorithm for extranodal natural killer-/T-cell lymphoma.
CR, complete remission; Gelox, gemcitabine, asparaginase, oxaliplatin; PR, partial remission; SMILE, dexamethasone, methotrexate, ifosfamide, l-asparaginase, and etoposide.

clinical features that can confuse the diagnosis. These consist of skin rashes, B symptoms, serositis and effusions, arthritis, polyclonal hyper gammaglobulinemia, and a wide spectrum of immunological dysfunction. Histologically, it consists of a polymorphous infiltrate of small-to-medium-sized lymphocytes intermixed with plasma cells and an inflammatory infiltrate with prominent eosinophils that commonly efface the nodal architecture and a striking proliferation of post capillary or high endothelial venules. The aypical T cells have a T follicular helper (TFH) phenotype and are positive for CD3, CD4, CD10 and CD279 (PD-10), and CXCL13 [10]. There is marked B-cell proliferation in the cellular infiltrate and EBV positive B cells are almost always present. The role of EBV in the pathogenesis of AITL is still not defined but progression to EBV-positive diffuse large B-cell lymphoma (DLBCL) has been reported [11]. These EBV-positive B cells may resemble and be confused with Reed-Sternberg cells and may lead to an erroneous diagnosis of Hodgkin disease. Clonal rearrangements of T-cell receptor genes (TCR) are found in most cases of angioimmunoblastic T-cell lymphoma and clonal rearrangements of immunoglobulin genes have been reported in 25–50% of cases [12]. Most common cytogenetic abnormality is trisomy 3, trsisomy 7, and an additional X chromosome. More recently mutations of *IDH2* genes have been described in 20–40% of cases and may be a therapeutic target for this disease [13].

Median age at presentation is 64 years with a slight male predominance. It has an aggressive clinical course but spontaneous regression has been reported on rare occasions. Treatment recommendations follow general guidelines for PTCL treatment. However, it appears that single agent histone deacetylase inhibitors (HDACi) are particularly effective for treating this disease in the relapsed and refractory setting. Romidepsin is reported to have an overall response rate (ORR) of 42% [14] and belinostat had an ORR of up to 66% in the latest pivotal trials [15]. Due to the heavy B-cell infiltrate and the vascularity of these tumors, there have been reports of efficacy of rituximab [17], lenalidomide [18], cyclsoposin/prednisone [19], and low dose methotrexate/prednisone [20]. These agents have been used alone or in combination with chemotherapy and may be combined with more targeted agents in the future.

Anaplastic large cell lymphoma

This subtype is characterized by large lymphoid cells with pleomorphic features and prominent nuclei that tend to grow in a cohesive pattern with a propensity for lymphoid sinuses. There is strong expression of CD30. Most lymphomas are CD2- and CD4-positive but there is a loss of many of the T-cell associated antigens. The cells have a cytotoxic phenotype with positivity for cytotoxic-associated antigens, TIA, granzyme B, clusterin, and perforin. The presence of CD30 has been targeted with the antibody drug conjugate brentuximab vedotin with a response rate of 87% in the relapsed setting. There are many subtypes of this disease with differing prognostic features as described below.

- Alk+ ALCL: Expression of the tyrosine kinase anaplastic lymphoma kinase (alk) defines alk+ ALCL and is more commonly seen in children and young adults with a marked male predominance. Median age at presentation is 35 years and there is a high incidence of extranodal disease with over 75% of patients having advanced stage. The presence of alk as determined by immunohistochemistry (IHC) confers an improved prognosis with a 5-year survival of 79% compared with 46% for alk-negative patients [21,22]. The presence of alk is determined by a characteristic chromosomal translocation t(2:5) involving *NPM/ALK* genes but partners other than NPM have also been identified that lead to over expression of alk [23]. Alk inhibitors are also in clinical trials for relapsed alk+ ALCL with promising results.

- Alk-ALCL: These nodal lymphomas lack the expression of alk but have all other morphological and phenotypical features of a CD30-positive cytotoxic ALCL. They tend to occur in an older age group and in general have a prognosis that is intermediate between alk+ ALCL and other PTCL histologies. Recently genomic sequencing has identified two new genetic lesions DUSP22 and TP63 that seen to have prognostic significance in alk-ALCL [24,25]. A large multicenter study of ALCL cases identified ALK, DUSP22, and TP63 rearrangements as being mutually exclusive. The outcomes of alk-ALCL patients carrying the DUSP22 was similar to patients with ALK + ALCL. However, patients with TP63 rearrangements had the worse prognosis [26].

- Primary cutaneous ALCL is part of the spectrum of CD30-positive cutaneous lymphomas and has histological and clinical features that overlap with lymphomatoid papulosis discussed elsewhere. These lymphomas are alk-negative and have an excellent survival of 100% at 5 years.
- Seroma-associated ALCL of the breast: More than 40 cases of alk-negative ALCL associated with silicone or saline breast implants have been reported and described as seroma-associated ALCL of the breast. The median time to development of these tumors is 8 years from the placement of the implant. The clinical presentation is with a unilateral seroma and a mass in the fibrous capsule surrounding the implant or severe deformity and contracture of the implant. If confined to the seroma, prognosis is excellent although cases have been described with invasion of breast tissue and lymph nodes that portend a worse outcome. Treatment requires removal of the implant and the associated seroma. Further management has not been defined and varies from watchful waiting, local radiation, or systemic therapy depending on the presentation [27–29].

Adult T-cell leukemia/lymphoma

This entity is associated with the retrovirus HTLV1, which is endemic in Japan, the Caribbean basin, and parts of Africa at a prevalence of 6–37% of the population. It is transmitted by cell to cell contact through sexual intercourse blood products containing whole white blood cell, breast milk, shared needles, and vertically via childbirth. The virus gets clonally integrated into the lymphoma cells. HTLV1 encodes three structural genes (pol, gag and tax) and two regulatory genes (tax and rex). These genes play an important part in the pathogenesis and transformation of lymphoma cells [30]. It has a long latency period and only about 2.5% of the infected individuals are at risk for developing ATLL. The median age at presentation is 45 years and there are four clinically distinct forms with variable clinical courses that can be determined as outlined in Table 11.5. Median age at presentation is 45 years. The acute forms of the disease may present as leukemia or lymphoma or both. Other features include hepatosplenomegaly, bone lesion, skin involvement, hypercalcemia and are associated with an aggressive clinical course and a median survival of less than 10 months. Patients with the smoldering form have an indolent course.

The pathologic hallmark of ATLL is a 'flower cell' with a polylobulated nucleus. Peripheral blood involvement can commonly occur without bone marrow involvement. Cells express mature T-cell antigens like CD2, CD3, and CD5 and are typically positive for CD4/CD25 (similar to Tregs). FoxP3 expression can be seen in a minority of tumor cells. Multiple chromosomal abnormalities are found in these tumors. More than six breaks are associated with a poor prognosis and gains of 1q and 4q are more commonly found in aggressive ATLL while gains of 7q are associated with a good prognosis [31] .

The indolent form of the disease can be managed by antiviral approaches mainly zidovudine and interferon [32]. However, more aggressive disease requires aggressive chemotherapy similar to other subtypes of PTCL but relapses are common. Mogamulizumab (KW-0761), a humanized anti-CCR4 antibody, has been shown to be effective for the treatment of relapsed and refractory ATLL with an objective response rate of 50% and

	Healthy carrier	Smoldering ATLL	Chronic ATLL	Acute ATLL	ATLL lymphoma
Anti HTLV-1 serology	+	+	+	+	+
Clonal integration of provirus	– (blood)	+ (blood)	+ (blood)	+ (blood)	+ (lymph nodes)
Lymphocyte count	Normal	Normal	Elevated	Elevated	Elevated
Abnormal cells (%)	<5%	>5%	>5%	>5%	<1%
Hyper-calcemia	–	–	–	+	+
LDH	Normal	<1.5N	<2N	>2N	>2N
Skin and lung involvement	–	+	+	+	+
BM or spleen	–	–	+	+	+
Bone, GI or CNS +	–	–	–	+	+

Table 11.5 Clinical subtypes of adult T-cell leukemia/lymphoma. ATLL, adult T-cell leukemia/ lymphoma; BM, bone marrow; CNS, central nervous system; GI, gastrointestinal; HTLV-1, human T-lymphotropic virus 1; LDH, lactate dehydrogenase.

CR of 30% and an acceptable safety profile, and has been approved for this indication in Japan since 2012 [33]. It is currently being evaluated in the US and is being studied in combination with other T-cell-directed therapies. Autologous stem cell transplant has not been shown to be effective in the treatment of HTLV1-associated ATLL [34] but allogeneic stem cell transplantation in select younger patients with available donors and chemosensitive disease has shown a 3-year survival of 36% noted in a large Japanese study of 586 patients [35,36]. Early use of transplantation in the course of disease is associated with improved outcomes (4-yr OS of 49.3% versus 31%) [37] where early transplant was defined as <100 days for diagnosis in a cohort of 428 patients. Hence an allogeneic stem cell evaluation should be performed early in the course of a diagnosis of acute ATLL and stem cell transplantation performed as soon as remission is achieved. Alternative stem cell sources like cord blood and haploidentical donors should be considered if needed. Attention should be paid to evaluate for and aid prophylaxis against central nervous system (CNS) involvement.

Hepatosplenic T cell lymphoma

This rare form of PTCL arises from γδ T cells of the liver sinuses and splenic red pulp and presents with prominent helaptosplenomegaly without significant adenopathy and pancytopenia. It is commonly seen in young males with a median age of 35 years. There is an association with iatrogenic immunosuppression especially with the use of the anti-tumor necrosis factor (TNF) agent infliximab, purine analogues, patients with Crohn's disease, and recipients of solid organ transplantation [38,39]. The disease is aggressive with a median survival of 16 months.

Pathologically, the cells are medium in size and tend to have a marked pattern of sinusoidal infiltration in the liver and spleen as well as bone marrow. Immunophenotypically the cells are positive for CD56 or CD16 but negative for CD4, CD8 (CD8 + can be seen occasionally). TIA-1 is usually positive but other cytotoxic markers of activation such as granzyme and perforin are negative. The most consistent chromosomal abnormality is isochromosome 7q and trisomy 8. Cases of αβ T-cell derivation are seen with similar immunophenotype that are more common in females and present at an older age.

The disease is aggressive and requires early planning for an allogeneic stem cell transplant for long-term survival. Small series have reported on the poor outcome of traditional cyclophosphamide, doxorubicin, vincristine, and prednisolone (CHOP) or CHOP-like regimens [40,41]. In one small retrospective study, intensive induction regimens such as ifosfamide, carboplatin, and etoposide (ICE) or ifosfamide, etoposide, and high dose cytarabine (IVAC) were more likely to lead to remissions as a bridge to stem cell transplant with a median progression-free survival (PFS) of 13.3 months and OS of 59 months of the 7/14 surviving patients [42].

Enteropathy-associated T-cell lymphoma

Enteropathay-associated T-cell lymphoma or EATL is a rare intestinal lymphoma with an aggressive clinical course that has an intestinal presentation. There are two known variants of the disease EATLI and EATL II based on distinct clinical, morphological, and immunophenotypic features and an even rarer indolent variant. EATL should be distinguished from intestinal involvement of other types of lymphoma including PTCL-nos, EBV-positive NK/T-cell lymphoma, and other γδ T-cell lymphoma that lack epitheliotrism.

EATL1 is associated with either overt or salient celiac disease and is seen in patients of European descent. Serologic markers of celiac disease such as anti-gliadin antibodies are positive. The neoplastic cells show prominent invasion of the intestinal mucosa, are of the αβ subtype, and express the mucosal homing receptor CD103 (HML-1). There may be varied expression of CD30 but typically the surrounding mucosa will show villous atrophy. In comparison, type II EATL is composed of cells that show prominent epitheliotropism but the surrounding mucosa is usually intact. The cells are of γδ orgin and are CD8- and CD56-positive. This subtype is more common in Asia and is rarely associated with celiac disease. Both EATL type I and II are aggressive and present with abdominal symptoms and multifocal intestinal involvement that can lead to perforation and other complications. Outcomes are poor with 5-year survival rates of less than 20% [43,44]. Treatment guidelines are as per general PTCL guidelines with support for early stem cell transplant as consolidation based on several studies. Recently there has been recognition of an indolent T-cell lymphoproliferative disorder of intestinal tract with lesions involving any site from the oral cavity to the colon. The infiltrate is composed of small mature lymphoid cells that are mostly CD8+ with no evidence of *STAT3 SH2* domain mutation or activation seen in other types of CD8-positive large granular lymphocytic leukemia. Unlike EATLs I and II, these indolent disorders do not require aggressive therapy [45].

Subcutaneous panninculitis-like T-cell lymphoma

This rare form of T-cell lymphoma presents with subcutaneous nodules that primarily affect the extremities and trunk and vary from 0.5 centimeters to several centimeters in size. Histologically, the cells consist of atypical lymphoid cells that rim individual fat cells. The surrounding infiltrate can have reactive histiocytes and can show vascular invasion, necrosis and karyorrhexis. Immunophenotyping shows the cells to be positive for CD8 and they are of the αβ type. The γ8 subtype is now considered to be a primary cutaneous γ8 T-cell lymphoma the median age at presentation is 30 years but can be seen in children as well. It can be associated with a hemophagocytic syndrome that confers a poor prognosis and can occur either before, concurrent with or even after the disease has been treated. The patients can present with high fevers, hepatosplenomegaly, skin lesions, pulmonary infiltrates, and coagulation abnormalities.

Subacute panninculitis-like T-cell lymphoma (SCPTCL) needs to be differentiated from lupus and other autoimmune diseases that can also occur concurrently with SCPTCL. The clinical course is usually aggressive but an indolent variant has been described [46].

Epstein-Barr virus-associated T-cell and NK-cell proliferation

These systemic EBV-positive T-cell lymphoproliferative disorders include hydroa vacciniforme-like lymphoma, mosquito bite allergy and systemic EBV-positive lymphoproliferative disease. These have mostly been reported in children in Central and South America, and in Asia:

- Hydroa vacciniforme and mosquito bite allergy is usually confined to the skin and induced by sun exposure. The lesions consist of a CD3+ EBER+ infiltrate that forms vesicles. The infiltrate can lack clonality and cytological atypia but can become dense and more atypical in which case it meets criteria for hydroa vacciniforme-like lymphoma [47].

- Systemic EBV-positive lymphoproliferative disease usually arises in the background of EBV infection and has overlapping features with aggressive NK-cell leukemia/lymphoma. It is associated with hemophagocytic syndrome and can be very aggressive with survival measured in weeks unless the patient can receive an allogeneic stem cell transplant [48].

Extranodal natural killer-/T-cell lymphoma, nasal type, and other Epstein-Barr virus-positive T-/natural killer-cell neoplasms

Extranodal NK-/T-cell lymphoma-nasal type is an aggressive EBV-associated lymphoma that is more common in Asia, Central and South America, and in Native American populations. Median age of presentation is 50 years of age. The most common presentation is a destructive nasal or midline facial lesion but other presenting sites include skin, gastrointestinal tract (GIT), upper respiratory tract, or in other organs. It can be associated with hemophagocytic syndrome, which has a negative prognostic value.

Histologically, tumors are of a polymorphic composition and express CD56 but do not express CD57 or CD16. Most T-cell markers are absent except CD2 and cytoplasmic CD3 but T-cell receptor gene rearrangements are generally absent except for a rare subset that may have a true T-cell derivation [49,50]. EBV-positivity by in situ hybridization is seen in most cases. Gene expression profiling has delineated several oncogenic pathways that are activated in these tumors including Notch-1, Wnt, AKT, NF kappa B, and Jak/STAT. Somatic-activating mutations of the *JAK3* gene have been identified in 35% of cases of NK-/T-cell lymphoma and may provide therapeutic targets for clinical use [51]. Similarly, miRNA signature profiling has also identified a distinct signature for these tumors that results in dysregulation of p53, cell cycle control, and mitogen-activated protein kinase (MAPK) signaling [52]. Plasma EBV DNA levels have been shown to correlate with tumor load and survival [53].

A thorough ear, nose, and throat (ENT) evaluation irrespective of the initial site of presentation is required in the management of these cases. PET/CT is the recommended imaging modality for staging and follow-up purposes. The standard uptake value maximum (SUV max) is lower in NK-/T-cell lymphoma than aggressive B-cell lymphoma so very high SUVs >10 should arouse suspicion for coexisting infection or inflammatory processes. Most nasal tumors are accompanied by bony destruction of sinus walls and can extend into the orbit and other surrounding tissues. Retrospective analysis of multi center studies has identified the following prognostic models that are clinically useful. The IPI (age performance status, stage, LDH, and extranodal sites) designed for DLBCL [54], the Korean prognostic score (B symptoms, stage, LDH, and adenopathy) [55], NK-cell Tumor study group (non-nasal disease, stage, performance status, and number of extra nodal sites) [56].

NK/T-cell lymphoma is radiosensitive and treatment of localized disease with radiation alone results in overall response rates between 77 and 100% with better responses seen in doses >50Gy. However, the risk of systemic failure remains high with this approach: 25–40% [57]. Hence, combined modality chemo radiation regimens are used to treat localized disease either in a concurrent or sequential approach. The choice of chemotherapy in NK-/T-cell lymphoma remains challenging as CHOP and other anthracycline-based regimens have failed to provide optimal control of disease with dismal outcomes [57,58]. NK cells have been shown to have high levels of P-glycoprotein and this is retained in the NK-/T-cell lymphoma cells resulting in a multidrug-resistant phenotype [59]. Incorporation of non-multidrug resistance (MDR) agents for example methotrexate and asparaginase into treatment regimens such as dexamethasone, methotrexate, ifosfamide, etoposide, and l-asparaginase (SMILE), dexamethasone, etoposide, ifosfamide, and carboplatin (DeVic), asparginase, dexamethsone, and methotrexate (AspMet Dex), and gemcitabine, asparaginase, and oxaliplatin (GELOX) have improved the outcome of these patients. The concurrent approach, with external bean radiation (XRT) and three cycles of DeVic resulted in an ORR of 81% and CR was achieved in 77% of cases; 5-year OS and PFS was 70% and 63%, respectively [60]. Similarly, another study reported an ORR of

83% and CR of 80% with a 3-year OS and PFS of 85% with concurrent XRT and cisplatin followed by etoposide, ifosfamide, cisplatin, and dexamethasone (VIPD) [61]. Four cycles of the most intense regimen SMILE with XRT incorporated sequentially between cycle two and three has shown ORR and CR of 89.7%. The remission achieved was durable [62].

However, these regimens have significant morbidity associated with them. Deaths due to infection have been reported. Kwong et al have reported an excellent overview of all therapeutic options in this disease and prefer the sequential approach as the best and least toxic for most patients [63]. Localized NK-/T-cell lymphoma presenting outside the nasal and paranasal areas should be treated with similar regimens and involved field XRT where possible.

Advanced stage and relapsed disease should be treated with L-asparagianse containing regimens as described above. ORR of up to 80% and higher have been reported with CRS in the 40–65% range. In one study the 1-year OS and PFS was 55% and 53%, respectively [64]. Another study reported a 5-year OS of 52.3% [62]. Treatment for patients who relapse after L-asparaginase-contatining regimens remains poorly defined. Recent studies have suggested a role for combination therapy using gemcitabine-like Gem/Ox [65] followed by high-dose therapy and stem cell support. Risk of CNS disease in NK-/T-cell lymphoma has been analyzed in a study of 208 patients and the risk appears to be highest in patients with an high prognostic index and advanced stage disease [66]

The use of autologous stem cell transplant (ASCT) in the treatment of NK-/T-cell lymphoma is poorly defined especially regarding the type of transplant, timing, and conditioning regimen. There are several small studies that have looked at the role of ASCT in NK-/T-cell lymphoma and it seems that the outcomes are better for transplants performed in remission as opposed to refractory disease indicating that high-dose therapy is unlikely to salvage refractory patients who are best served by clinical trials of novel targeted agents. The best outcomes are a 5-year survival of 50–55% [67,68]. In early stage disease the outcomes of combined modality therapy in responding patients are excellent and do not warrant consolidation with this approach. It may be considered in patients with advanced disease who achieve a CR though its role remains unclear with highly effective regimens such as SMILE. Allogeneic transplant can be offered to patients with relapsed/refractory disease with 3–5 year survival reported at 40–55% [69] and therapy-related mortality (TRM) of 8% and up to 40% in another study [70].

Follow-up of patients with NK-/T-cell lymphoma can be challenging especially if disease involves mucosal surfaces and destruction. It may be difficult to differentiate between lymphoma and infection/inflammation based on imaging studies only ie, having sinusitis versus a tumor. Thorough ENT evaluations and biopsy of all suspicious lesions should be used in follow-up. Serial follow-up of EBV DNA quantification can be helpful as well and a rising titer may indicate relapse. Relapses have been reported even after decades of remission.

Treatment guidelines for peripheral T-cell lymphoma

Currently, these are applicable for most nodal PTCL cases and Figure 11.1 outlines the recommendations followed at our institution. For the most part they are derived from the NCCN guidelines [2]. Any specific treatments applicable to specific histologies are discussed in the relevant sections. Treatment guidelines for NK-/T-cell lymphomas are presented separately in Figure 11.2.

First-line therapy

First therapy of choice continues to be a clinical trial. This indicates that there is no 'vetted' standard for the upfront care of these patients that is based on randomized clinical data. There are treatment guidelines that are derived from consensus based on clinical experience, inference, and some retrospective data. The NCCN lists anthracycline-based therapies as initial options including CHOP, cyclophosphamide, doxorubicin, vincristine, prednisone, and etoposide (CHOEP), etoposide phosphate, prednisone, vincristine sulfate, cyclophosphamide, and doxorubicin hydrochloride (EPOCH), cyclophosphamide, vincristine, doxorubicin, dexamethasone, methotrexate, and cytarabine (hyper-CVAD), and other combinations derived from therapy of aggressive B-cell lymphomas. The choice is left to the treating physician and their level of comfort and expertise with the regimen. At City of Hope we have used CHOEP or EPOCH as the first-line regimen where possible.

Attempts have been made to establish if anthracyclins are an essential component of upfront therapy. The data on that are conflicting for most histologies in PTCL except ALCL. The International T-cell lymphoma project retrospectively evaluated data from 22 international centers that treated PTCL and found that >85% of patients received CHOP as frontline therapy. The best outcome was seen in ALk+ ALCL with a 5-year failure free survival of 60%. The 5-year failure-free survival (FFS) outcome was much worse for PTCL-nos (20%), AITL (18%), and ALK-negative ALCL (36%) and there was no difference in OS of patients who received anthracyclin compared with those who did not [71]. The British Columbia Cancer registry (BCCA) reported on their 199 PTCL patients seen over a time period of 20 years in whom clinical histology and treatment data were available and confirmed that CHOP-based regimens given initially resulted in a 5-year survival of 20–35% except in low risk ALCL [72]. On the other hand, another large retrospective study of over 400 (442) PTCL patients evaluated treatment and outcomes of these patients: 65% of patients were treated with anthracyclin-based regimens with CHOP being the most common (93%). Only 9% received nonthathracyclin-based combination treatment (gemcitabine-based, cyclophosphamide, vincristine, prednisone [CVP], ICE, cisplatin, cytarabine, dexamethasone [DHAP], etoposide, methylprednisolone, cisplatin, cytarabine [ESHAP]). In this retrospective study, front-line treatment with anthracycline-based regimen was associated with superior PFS and OS (2-year PFS 39% versus 23%) as compared with non-anthracyclin-containing regimens (median OS 18 months versus <2 months) [73].

There is retrospective data to support the use of etoposide in the upfront regiment either as EPOCH or dose-adjusted (DA)-EPOCH or CHOEP. The German High-Grade Non-Hodgkin Lymphoma Study Group (DSHNHL) retrospectively analyzed the outcome of 289 PTCL patients treated with CHOP or CHOEP and reported that 3-year event-free survival (EFS) and OS were 75.8% and 89.8% (ALK-positive ALCL), 50.0% and 67.5% (AITL), 45.7% and 62.1% (ALK-negative ALCL), and 41.1% and 53.9% (PTCL), respectively. For patients less than 60 years of age, the use of etoposide improved the 3-year EFS: 75% versus 51%, which was most notable for alk+ ALCL [74]. The Nordic Lymphoma Group evaluated the role of upfront ASCT after CHOEP in an intent-to-transplant study in those with chemotherapy-sensitive disease and PTCL subtypes (ALK positive cases were excluded). The 5-year OS and PFS were 51% and 44%, respectively with ALK-negative ALCL having the best outcome with a 5-year PFS and OS of 61% and 70%, respectively [75]. The other prospective study looking at the role of DA-EPOCH comes from the National Institutes of Health in a trial by Dunleavy at el where they established that DA-EPOCH resulted in EFS of 72% in alk+ ALCL and 62% in alk– ALCL, and OS of 78% and 87%, respectively [76] indicating a potential cure. A previous abstract from the same group had reported a PFS of 32% at 5 years for other non-ALCL histolgies of PTCL although the numbers were small [77].

This data indicates that for most histologies of PTCL, there is no clear upfront regimen that can lead to long-term disease control. Several trials are ongoing to study this further either in combination with a CHOP/CHOEP-like back bone (pralatrexate, lenalidomide, belinostat, brentuximab vedotin, and new targeted agents) or without a chemotherapy.

Stem cell transplant as consolidation

There is now a substantial body of literature supporting ASCT in first complete remission (CR1) for PTCL, albeit lacking confirmation by randomized trials. The NCCN guidelines for NHL recommend consideration of ASCT for patients with PTCL who achieve a CR or partial remission (PR) after primary therapy and are eligible based on age and comorbidity [71]. Exceptions to this approach include CTCL (discussed elsewhere, and very aggressive T-cell lymphomas including hepatosplenic T-cell lymphoma (HSTCL), HTLV-1-associated ATLL, extra-nasal NK-/T-cell lymphomas, T-cell prolymphocytic leukemia (T-PLL), and primary cutaneous γδ T-cell lymphoma. These diseases have a very aggressive clinical course due to inherent chemoresistance and patients tend to experience multiple failures of primary therapy; hence ASCT approaches have generally not produced long-term remission in these patients [78,79]. Long-term remission and improved survival has been seen in patients with these highly aggressive variants following allogeneic transplantation in first remission.

The largest study comes from the Nordic Lymphoma group that has conducted a prospective study with an intent to treat analysis of patients undergoing ASCT after receiving induction chemotherapy with CHOEP (or CHOP if >60 years of age) [75]. Out of the initial 160 patients 113 (70%) underwent ASCT and the outcomes varied with histology. The best outcomes were seen in patients with ALK-ALCL with 5-year OS of 70% and PFS of 61%; AITL, OS 52%, PFS 49%; PTCL-nos, OS 47%, PFS 38%; and EATL, OS 48%, disease-free survival (DFS) 38%. Several other trials have shown similar results. The general conclusions are that:

- Current approaches to high-dose therapy and ASCT in CR1 can result in an OS ranging from 34% to 73% and PFS from 30% to 53% depending on histology with best outcomes seen for ALCL. The longest follow up is 3–5 years. There are no randomized trials but the outcome data from ASCT in CR1 shows improvement compared with chemotherapy alone at 5 years.
- Many studies have shown that 41–73% of PTCL patients will progress through initial therapy or are ineligible for ASCT due to comorbidities. Thus many patients fail to benefit from this approach.
- Improved strategies are needed in the upfront setting to increase the response rates and duration of response. In addition, the late treatment failure patterns support the need to better define patients at risk for late relapse through biomarker and minimal residual disease (MRD) evaluation. This could define a subset of patients that would benefit from maintenance therapy post-transplant.

The patient in the case presented above received six cycles of CHOEP. Interim PET/CT scans after four cycles confirmed a CR and he continued to receive another two cycles. During this time he was evaluated by the transplant team with the intention to give him high dose chemotherapy and autologous stem cell transplant in CR1 as consolidation therapy. However, he experienced severe chest pain during stem cell collection and was taken to the emergency room where an electrocardiogram (EKG) showed evidence of ischemia and non-ST segment elevation myocardial infarction (NSTEMI).

Urgent cardiac evaluation revealed multi-vessel disease necessitating a stenting procedure and the need for anticoagulation for at least 30 days. This course was complicated by pneumonia and the transplant was delayed for 2 months. By this time his B symptoms returned and restaging CT scans confirmed new adenopathy confirming relapsed disease after a biopsy was done. Salvage therapy was started with pralatrextate and human leukocyte antigen (HLA) typing initiated on him and his two siblings.

Relapsed disease

Given the dismal outcome of upfront therapies it is estimated that over 70% of patients with PTCL will have relapsed and refractory disease [80]. At present there are four US FDA approved agents for the treatment of relapsed PTCL. Their efficacy is based on Phase II clinical trial data and is summarized in Table 11.6. Mogamulizumab is additionally approved in Japan and chidamide, another HDACi is approved in China. Given the rarity of these diseases, it has been difficult to tease out response rates for individual subtypes of PTCL except for ALCL. For the clinician the selection of an appropriate agent remains a challenge and there is little data to guide this choice. In addition, several non-approved agents and combination chemotherapy approaches used for relapsed aggressive lymphoma in general are used extensively including ICE, DHAP, etoposide, methylprednisolone ara-c, and cisplatin (ESAP), and gemcitabine regimens (Table 11.7). It should be noted that all these treatments are palliative and are not considered curative. If appropriate, the patient should be worked up for a stem cell transplant. The choice of ASCT versus an allogeneic transplant is also a matter of debate and will be discussed in the next section [88].

Allogeneic stem cell transplant for relapsed disease

For PTCL, the rationale for allogeneic transplants is based on the intent of invoking a graft-versus-lymphoma effect to provide long-term disease control. Allogeneic transplant has been used in the setting of relapsed or refractory PTCL, although increasingly transplant physicians are using this modality in the upfront setting for particularly aggressive histologies such as the γ/δ T cell lymphomas or extra-nasal NK-/T-cell lymphomas.

Agent	N	Histological subtypes N	Median prior therapies	ORR/CR	Response by histology ORR/CR	DOR	Comments
Pralatrexate [16]	109	PTCL-nos 59 sALCL 17 AITL 13 tMF 12 Other 10	3 (1–12)	29%/11%	PTCL-nos 32% sALCL 35% AITL 8% tMF- 25% Other 38%	10.1 months (1-22.1)	Numbers are small to make individual deductions about histological subtypes
Romidepsin [14]	130	PTCL-nos 69 AITL 27 ALK-ve ALCL 21 Other 13	2 (1–8)	25%/15%	PTCL-nos 29/14 AITL 30/19 Alk-ve ALCL 24/19 Other 0/0	28 months (1-48)	Median OS 11.3 months Median duration of response not reached for CR patients Time to CR is 3.7 months
Belinostat [15]	129	PTCL-nos 77 AITL 22 ALCL 15 EATL 2 NK/T 2 HSTCL 2	2 (1–8)	26%/11%	PTCL-nos 23% AITL 46%/18% ALCL 15% EATL 0 ENKTCL 50% HSTCL 0	13.6 (4.5–29.4)	Seems to have a higher response rate in AITL
Brentuximab vedotin [81]	58	sALCL	2 (1–6)	86%/59%		13.2 (5.7–26.3)	
Mogamulizumab [33]*	27	ATLL	1–3	50%/31%		Median PFS 5.2 months	

Table 11.6 US Food and Drug Administration-approved agents for relapsed/refractory peripheral T-cell lymphoma. *Approved in Japan.

Agent	N	Histological subtypes N	Median prior therapies	ORR/CR	Response by histology ORR/CR	DOR	Comments
Brentuximab vedotin [82]	35	PTCL-nos 59 sALCL 17 AITL 13 tMF 12 Other 10	2 (1–9)	41%/24%	PTCL-nos 33/14 AITL 54/38	PTCL-nos 7.6 AITL 5.5	
ICE [83]	40	PTCL-nos 69 AITL 27 ALK-ve ALCL 21 Other 13	1	70/35		Median PFS 6 months	68% went to transplant 83% relapsed at 3 years
ESHAP [84]	22	PTCL-nos 77 AITL 22 ALCL 15 EATL 2 NK/T 2 HSTCL 2	1	32/18		Median PFS 2.5 months	
Bendamustine [85]	58	sALCL	1 (1–3)	50/28		Median DOR 3.5 (1–21)	Median OS 6.3 months
Alemtuzumab	14	ATLL	2(1–4)	36/21			
Alemtuzumab	9			89/78		NR	
Crizotinib [86]	50		3 (1–11)	22/11	AITL 31/15 PTCL-nos 20		
Lenalidomide [87]	51			69/19		Median PFS 4 months	72% went to auto or allo transplant

Table 11.7 Other agents used for relapsed/refractory peripheral T-cell lymphoma.

Unfortunately, allogeneic transplant is also associated with a high risk of complications related to continued immunosuppression, graft-versus-host disease (GVHD), and the long-term toxicities of conditioning regimens. The largest study to date includes 77 patients from multiple centers in France and was reported by Le Gouill et al [89]. TRM was high at 33%, and 5-year OS and DFS were 57% and 53%, respectively. Best outcomes were seen for nodal histologies. Several small studies have reported similar outcomes. Patients should be referred for transplant consultation early in the course of their disease. If the patient does not have a suitable donor and has not had a prior auto transplant, an autologous transplant can be considered for chemosensitive disease. However, most patients will ultimately relapse.

References

1   Lukes RJ, Collins RD. Immunologic characterization of human malignant lymphomas. *Cancer.* 1974. 34:suppl:1488-1503.

2   Jaffe ES, Nicolae A, Pittaluga S. Peripheral T-cell and NK-cell lymphomas in the WHO classification: pearls and pitfalls. *Mod Pathol.* 2013;26 Suppl 1:S71-S87.

3   Vose J, Armitage J, Weisenburger D; International T-Cell Lymphoma Project. International peripheral T-cell and natural killer/T-cell lymphoma study: pathology findings and clinical outcomes. *J Clin Oncol.* 2008;26:4124-4130.

4   Anderson JR, Armitage JO, Weisenburger DD. Epidemiology of the non-Hodgkin's lymphomas: distributions of the major subtypes differ by geographic locations. Non-Hodgkin's Lymphoma Classification Project. *Ann Oncol.* 1998;9:717-720.

5   Bellei M, Chiattone CS, Luminari S, et al. T-cell lymphomas in South america and europe. *Rev Bras Hematol Hemoter.* 2012;34:42-47.

6   Abouyabis AN, Shenoy PJ, Lechowicz MJ, Flowers CR. Incidence and outcomes of the peripheral T-cell lymphoma subtypes in the United States. *Leuk Lymphoma.* 2008;49:2099-1107.

7   Rüdiger T, Ichinohasama R, Ott MM et al. Peripheral T-cell lymphoma with distinct perifollicular growth pattern: a distinct subtype of T-cell lymphoma? *Am J Surg Pathol.* 2000;24:117-122.

8   Warnke RA, Jones D, His ED. Morphologic and immunophenotypic variants of nodal T-cell lymphomas and T-cell lymphoma mimics. *Am J Clin Pathol.* 2007;127:511-527.

9   Quintanilla-Martinez L, Fend F, Moguel LR, et al. Peripheral T-cell lymphoma with Reed-Sternberg-like cells of B-cell phenotype and genotype associated with Epstein-Barr virus infection. *Am J Surg Pathol.* 1999;23:1233-1240.

10   de Leval L, Rickman DS, Thielen C, et al. The gene expression profile of nodal peripheral T-cell lymphoma demonstrates a molecular link between angioimmunoblastic T-cell lymphoma (AITL) and follicular helper T (TFH) cells. *Blood.* 2007;109:4952-4963.

11   Dunleavy K, Wilson WH, Jaffe ES. Angioimmunoblastic T cell lymphoma: pathobiological insights and clinical implications. *Curr Opin Hematol.* 2007;14:348-353.

12   Tan BT, Warnke RA, Arber DA. The frequency of B- and T-cell gene rearrangements and epstein-barr virus in T-cell lymphomas: a comparison between angioimmunoblastic T-cell lymphoma and peripheral T-cell lymphoma, unspecified with and without associated B-cell proliferations. *J Mol Diagn.* 2006;8:466-475; quiz 527.

13   Cairns RA, Iqbal J, Lemonnier F, et al. IDH2 mutations are frequent in angioimmunoblastic T-cell lymphoma. *Blood.* 2012;119:1901-1903.

14 Coiffier B, Pro B, Prince HM, et al. Romidepsin for the treatment of relapsed/refractory peripheral T-cell lymphoma: pivotal study update demonstrates durable responses. *J Hematol Oncol*. 2014;7:11.

15 O'Connor OA, Horwitz S, Masszi T, et al. Belinostat in patients with relapsed or refractory peripheral T-cell lymphoma: results of the pivotal phase II BELIEF (CLN-19) study. *J Clin Oncol*. 2015;33:2492-2499.

16 O'Connor OA, Pro B, Pinter-Brown L, et al. Pralatrexate in patients with relapsed or refractory peripheral T-cell lymphoma: results from the pivotal PROPEL study. *J Clin Oncol*. 2011;29:1182-1189.

17 Delfau-Larue MH, de Leval L, Joly B, et al. Targeting intratumoral B cells with rituximab in addition to CHOP in angioimmunoblastic T-cell lymphoma. A clinicobiological study of the GELA. *Haematologica*. 2012;97:1594-1602.

18 Fabbri A, Cencini E, Pietrini A, et al. Impressive activity of lenalidomide monotherapy in refractory angioimmunoblastic T-cell lymphoma: report of a case with long-term follow-up. *Hematol Oncol*. 2013;31:213-217.

19 Advani R, Horwitz S, Zelenetz A, Homing SJ. Angioimmunoblastic T cell lymphoma: treatment experience with cyclosporine. *Leuk Lymphoma*. 2007;48:521-525.

20 Quintini G, Iannitto E, Barbera V, et al. Response to low-dose oral methotrexate and prednisone in two patients with angio-immunoblastic lymphadenopathy-type T-cell lymphoma. *Hematol J*. 2001;2:393-395.

21 Gascoyne RD, Aoun P, Wu D, et al. Prognostic significance of anaplastic lymphoma kinase (ALK) protein expression in adults with anaplastic large cell lymphoma. *Blood*. 1999;93:3913-3921.

22 Savage KJ, Harris NL, Vose JM, et al. ALK- anaplastic large-cell lymphoma is clinically and immunophenotypically different from both ALK+ ALCL and peripheral T-cell lymphoma, not otherwise specified: report from the International Peripheral T-Cell Lymphoma Project. *Blood*. 2008;111:5496-5504.

23 Falini B, Pulford K, Pucciarini A, et al. Lymphomas expressing ALK fusion protein(s) other than NPM-ALK. *Blood*. 1999;94:3509-3515.

24 Boddicker RL, Feldman AL. Progress in the identification of subgroups in ALK-negative anaplastic large-cell lymphoma. *Biomark Med*. 2015;9:719-722.

25 Feldman AL, Dogan A, Smith DI, et al. Discovery of recurrent t(6;7)(p25.3;q32.3) translocations in ALK-negative anaplastic large cell lymphomas by massively parallel genomic sequencing. *Blood*. 2011;117: 915-919.

26 Parrilla Castellar ER, Jaffe ES, Said JW, et al. ALK-negative anaplastic large cell lymphoma is a genetically heterogeneous disease with widely disparate clinical outcomes. *Blood*. 2014;124:1473-1480.

27 Roden AC, Macon WR, Keeney GL, et al. Seroma-associated primary anaplastic large-cell lymphoma adjacent to breast implants: an indolent T-cell lymphoproliferative disorder. *Mod Pathol*. 2008;21:455-463.

28 van der Veldt AA, Kleijn SA, Nanayakkara PW. Silicone breast implants and anaplastic large T-cell lymphoma. *JAMA*. 2009;301:1227; author reply 1227.

29 Santanelli di Pompeo F, Laporta R, Sorotos M, et al. Breast Implant-associated anaplastic large cell lymphoma: proposal for a monitoring protocol. *Plast Reconstr Surg*. 2015;136:144e-151e.

30 Franchini G. Molecular mechanisms of human T-cell leukemia/lymphotropic virus type I infection. *Blood*. 1995;86:3619-3639.

31 Tsukasaki K, Krebs J, Nagai K, et al. Comparative genomic hybridization analysis in adult T-cell leukemia/lymphoma: correlation with clinical course. *Blood*. 2001;97:3875-3881.

32 Bazarbachi A, Plumelle Y, Carlos Ramos J, et al. Meta-analysis on the use of zidovudine and interferon-alfa in adult T-cell leukemia/lymphoma showing improved survival in the leukemic subtypes. *J Clin Oncol*. 2010;28:4177-4183.

33 Ishida T, Joh T, Uike N, et al. Defucosylated anti-CCR4 monoclonal antibody (KW-0761) for relapsed adult T-cell leukemia-lymphoma: a multicenter phase II study. *J Clin Oncol*. 2012;30:837-842.

34 Phillips AA, Willim RD, Savage DG, et al. A multi-institutional experience of autologous stem cell transplantation in North American patients with human T-cell lymphotropic virus type-1 adult T-cell leukemia/lymphoma suggests ineffective salvage of relapsed patients. *Leuk Lymphoma*. 2009;50:1039-1042.

35 Ishida T, Hishizawa M, Kato K, et al. Allogeneic hematopoietic stem cell transplantation for adult T-cell leukemia-lymphoma with special emphasis on preconditioning regimen: a nationwide retrospective study. *Blood*. 2012;120:1734-1741.

36 Hishizawa M, Kanda J, Utsunomiya A, et al. Transplantation of allogeneic hematopoietic stem cells for adult T-cell leukemia: a nationwide retrospective study. *Blood*. 2010;116:1369-1376.

37 Fuji S, Fujiwara H, Nakano N, et al. Early application of related SCT might improve clinical outcome in adult T-cell leukemia/lymphoma. *Bone Marrow Transplant*. 20156;51:205-211.

38 Veres G, Baldassano RN, Mamula P. Infliximab therapy for pediatric Crohn's disease. *Expert Opin Biol Ther*. 2007;7:1869-1880.

39 Herrinton LJ, Liu L, Abramson O, Jaffe ES. The incidence of hepatosplenic T-cell lymphoma in a large managed care organization, with reference to anti-tumor necrosis factor therapy, Northern California, 2000-2006. *Pharmacoepidemiol Drug Saf*. 2012;21:49-52.

40 Belhadj K, Reyes F, Farcet JP, et al. Hepatosplenic gammadelta T-cell lymphoma is a rare clinicopathologic entity with poor outcome: report on a series of 21 patients. *Blood*. 2003;102:4261-4269.

41 Falchook GS, Vega F, Dang NH, et al. Hepatosplenic gamma-delta T-cell lymphoma: clinicopathological features and treatment. *Ann Oncol*. 2009;20:1080-1085.

42 Voss MH, Lunning MA, Maragulia JC, et al. Intensive induction chemotherapy followed by early high-dose therapy and hematopoietic stem cell transplantation results in improved outcome for patients with hepatosplenic T-cell lymphoma: a single institution experience. *Clin Lymphoma Myeloma Leuk*. 2013;13:8-14.

43 Delabie J, Holte H, Vose JM, et al. Enteropathy-associated T-cell lymphoma: clinical and histological findings from the international peripheral T-cell lymphoma project. *Blood*. 2011;118:148-155.

44 van de Water JM, Cillessen SA, Visser OJ, et al. Enteropathy associated T-cell lymphoma and its precursor lesions. *Best Pract Res Clin Gastroenterol*. 2010;24:43-56.

45 Perry AM, Warnke RA, Hu Q, et al. Indolent T-cell lymphoproliferative disease of the gastrointestinal tract. *Blood*. 2013;122:3599-3606.

46 Salhany KE, Macon WR, Choi JK, et al. Subcutaneous panniculitis-like T-cell lymphoma: clinicopathologic, immunophenotypic, and genotypic analysis of alpha/beta and gamma/delta subtypes. *Am J Surg Pathol*. 1998;22:881-893.

47 Gupta G, Man I, Kemmett D. Hydroa vacciniforme: A clinical and follow-up study of 17 cases. *J Am Acad Dermatol*. 2000;42:208-213.

48 Kimura H. [EBV-positive T/NK lymphoproliferative disease in childhood]. *Nihon Rinsho*. 2012;70 Suppl 2:692-696.

49 Pongpruttipan T, Sukpanichnant S, Assanasen T, et al. Extranodal NK/T-cell lymphoma, nasal type, includes cases of natural killer cell and alphabeta, gammadelta, and alphabeta/gammadelta T-cell origin: a comprehensive clinicopathologic and phenotypic study. *Am J Surg Pathol*. 2012;36:481-499.

50 Liang R. Diagnosis and management of primary nasal lymphoma of T-cell or NK-cell origin. *Clin Lymphoma*. 2000;1:33-37; discussion 38.

51 Koo GC, Tan SY, Tang T, et al. Janus kinase 3-activating mutations identified in natural killer/T-cell lymphoma. *Cancer Discov*. 2012;2:591-597.

52 Ng SB, Yan J, Huang G, et al. Dysregulated microRNAs affect pathways and targets of biologic relevance in nasal-type natural killer/T-cell lymphoma. *Blood*. 2011;118:4919-4929.

53 Au WY, Pang A, Choy C, Chim CS, Kwong YL. Quantification of circulating Epstein-Barr virus (EBV) DNA in the diagnosis and monitoring of natural killer cell and EBV-positive lymphomas in immunocompetent patients. *Blood*. 2004;104:243-249.

54 Lee J. Nasal-type NK/T cell lymphoma: clinical features and treatment outcome. *Br J Cancer*. 2005;92:1226-1230.

55 Lee J, Suh C, Park YH, et al. Extranodal natural killer T-cell lymphoma, nasal-type: a prognostic model from a retrospective multicenter study. *J Clin Oncol*. 2006;24:612-618.

56 Suzuki R, Suzumiya J, Yamaguchi M, et al. Prognostic factors for mature natural killer (NK) cell neoplasms: aggressive NK cell leukemia and extranodal NK cell lymphoma, nasal type. *Ann Oncol*. 2010;21:1032-1040.

57 Kim SJ, Kim WS. Treatment of localized extranodal NK/T cell lymphoma, nasal type. *Int J Hematol*. 2010;92:690-696.

58 Kim WS, Song SY, Ahn YC, et al. CHOP followed by involved field radiation: is it optimal for localized nasal natural killer/T-cell lymphoma? *Ann Oncol*. 2001;12:349-352.

59 Yamaguchi M, Kita K, Miwa H, et al. Frequent expression of P-glycoprotein/MDR1 by nasal T-cell lymphoma cells. *Cancer*. 1995;76:2351-2356.

60 Yamaguchi M, Tobinai K, Oguchi M, et al. Concurrent chemoradiotherapy for localized nasal natural killer/T-cell lymphoma: an updated analysis of the Japan clinical oncology group study JCOG0211. *J Clin Oncol*. 2012;30:4044-4046.

61 Kim SJ, Kim K, Kim BS, et al. Phase II trial of concurrent radiation and weekly cisplatin followed by VIPD chemotherapy in newly diagnosed, stage IE to IIE, nasal, extranodal NK/T-Cell Lymphoma: Consortium for Improving Survival of Lymphoma study. *J Clin Oncol*. 2009;27:6027-6032.

62 Kwong YL, Kim WS, Lim ST, et al. SMILE for natural killer/T-cell lymphoma: analysis of safety and efficacy from the Asia Lymphoma Study Group. *Blood*. 2012;120:2973-2980.

63 Tse E, Kwong Y-L. How I treat NK/T-cell lymphomas. *Blood*. 2013;121:4997-5005.

64 Yamaguchi M, Kwong YL, Kim WS, et al. Phase II study of SMILE chemotherapy for newly diagnosed stage IV, relapsed, or refractory extranodal natural killer (NK)/T-cell lymphoma, nasal type: the NK-Cell Tumor Study Group study. *J Clin Oncol*. 2011;29:4410-4416.

65 Ahn HK, Kim SJ, Hwang DW, et al. Gemcitabine alone and/or containing chemotherapy is efficient in refractory or relapsed NK/T-cell lymphoma. *Invest New Drugs*. 2013;31:469-472.

66 Kim SJ, Oh SY, Hong JY, et al. When do we need central nervous system prophylaxis in patients with extranodal NK/T-cell lymphoma, nasal type? *Ann Oncol*. 2010;21:1058-1063.

67 Kwong YL. High-dose chemotherapy and hematopoietic SCT in the management of natural killer-cell malignancies. *Bone Marrow Transplant*. 2009;44:709-714.

68 Lee J, Au WY, Park MJ, et al. Autologous hematopoietic stem cell transplantation in extranodal natural killer/T cell lymphoma: a multinational, multicenter, matched controlled study. *Biol Blood Marrow Transplant*. 2008;14:1356-1364.

69 Murashige N, Kami M, Kishi Y, et al. Allogeneic haematopoietic stem cell transplantation as a promising treatment for natural killer-cell neoplasms. *Br J Haematol*. 2005;130:561-567.

70 Ennishi D, Maeda Y, Fujii N, et al. Allogeneic hematopoietic stem cell transplantation for advanced extranodal natural killer/T-cell lymphoma, nasal type. *Leuk Lymphoma*. 2011;52:1255-1261.

71 National Comprehensive Cancer Network. NCCN Clinical Practice Guidelines in Oncology. Non-Hodgkin lymphoma. https://www.nccn.org/professionals/physician_gls/pdf/nhl.pdf. Accessed March 7, 2017.

72 Savage KJ, Chhanabhai M, Gascoyne RD, Connors JM. Characterization of peripheral T-cell lymphomas in a single North American institution by the WHO classification. *Ann Oncol*. 2004;15:1467-1475.

73 Briski R, Feldman AL, Bailey NG, et al. The role of front-line anthracycline-containing chemotherapy regimens in peripheral T-cell lymphomas. *Blood Cancer J*. 2014;4:e214.

74 Schmitz N, Trümper L, Ziepert M, et al. Treatment and prognosis of mature T-cell and NK-cell lymphoma: an analysis of patients with T-cell lymphoma treated in studies of the German High-Grade Non-Hodgkin Lymphoma Study Group. *Blood*. 2010;116:3418-3425.

75 d'Amore F, Relander T, Lauritzsen GF, et al. Up-front autologous stem-cell transplantation in peripheral T-cell lymphoma: NLG-T-01. *J Clin Oncol*. 2012;30:3093-3099.

76 Dunleavy K, Pittaluga S, Shovlin M, et al. Phase II trial of dose-adjusted EPOCH in untreated systemic anaplastic large cell lymphoma. *Haematologica*. 2016;101:e27-29.

77 Dunleavy K, Shovlin M, Pittaluga S, et al. DA-EPOCH chemotherapy is highly effective in ALK-positive and ALK-negative ALCL: results of a prospective study of PTCL subtypes in adults. *Blood*. 2011;118:1618.

78 Al-Toma A, Verbeek WH, Visser OJ, et al. Disappointing outcome of autologous stem cell transplantation for enteropathy-associated T-cell lymphoma. *Dig Liver Dis*. 2007;39:634-641.

79 Terras S, Moritz RK, Ditschkowski M, et al. Allogeneic haematopoietic stem cell transplantation in a patient with cutaneous gamma/delta-T-cell lymphoma. *Acta Dermato-Venereologica*. 2013;93:360-361.

80 Dreyling M, Thieblemont C, Gallamini A, et al. ESMO Consensus conferences: guidelines on malignant lymphoma. part 2: marginal zone lymphoma, mantle cell lymphoma, peripheral T-cell lymphoma. *Ann Oncol*. 2013;24:857-877.

81 Pro B, Advani R, Brice P, et al. Brentuximab vedotin (SGN-35) in patients with relapsed or refractory systemic anaplastic large-cell lymphoma: results of a phase II study. *J Clin Oncol*. 2012;30:2190-2196.

82 Horwitz SM, Advani RH, Bartlett NL, et al. Objective responses in relapsed T-cell lymphomas with single-agent brentuximab vedotin. *Blood*. 2014;123:3095-3100.

83 Horwitz S. Second line therapy with ICE followed by high dose therapy and autologous stem cell transplantation for relapsed/ refractory peripehral T- cell lymphomas: minimal benefit when analyxed by intent to treat. *Blood*. 2005;106:2679.

84 Kogure Y, Yoshimi A, Ueda K, et al. Modified ESHAP regimen for relapsed/refractory T cell lymphoma: a retrospective analysis. *Ann Hematol*. 2015;94:989-994.

85 Damaj G, Gressin R, Bouabdallah K, et al. Results from a prospective, open-label, phase II trial of bendamustine in refractory or relapsed T-cell lymphomas: the BENTLY trial. *J Clin Oncol*. 2013;31:104-110.

86 Mossé YP, Lim MS, Voss SD, et al. Safety and activity of crizotinib for paediatric patients with refractory solid tumours or anaplastic large-cell lymphoma: a Children's Oncology Group phase 1 consortium study. *Lancet Oncol*. 2013;14:472-480.

87 Morschhauser F, Fitoussi O, Haioun C, et al. A phase 2, multicentre, single-arm, open-label study to evaluate the safety and efficacy of single-agent lenalidomide (Revlimid) in subjects with relapsed or refractory peripheral T-cell non-Hodgkin lymphoma: the EXPECT trial. *Eur J Cancer*. 2013;49:2869-2876.

88 Smith SM, Burns LJ, van Besien K, et al. Hematopoietic cell transplantation for systemic mature T-cell non-Hodgkin lymphoma. *J Clin Oncol*. 2013;31:3100-3109.

89 Le Gouill S, Milipied N, Buzyn A, et al. Graft-versus-lymphoma effect for aggressive T-cell lymphomas in adults: a study by the Société Francaise de Greffe de Moëlle et de Thérapie Cellulaire. *J Clin Oncol*. 2008;26:2264-2271.

Hodgkin lymphoma

Chapter 12

Hodgkin lymphoma

Robert Chen

Case presentation

A 52-year-old male patient presented to a primary care office with shortness of breath and a nonproductive cough of 3 months' duration. In addition, he had also noticed fever, chills, and night sweats for the past 2 months. Upon examination, the primary care physician found right axillary lymphadenopathy about the size of a tennis ball and also right inguinal lymph nodes. This patient underwent a core needle biopsy of the right axillary lymph node, and the pathology results showed classical Hodgkin lymphoma, mixed cellularity type. The patient was then referred to a hematologist, who performed a fluorodeoxyglucose (FDG)-positron emission tomography (PET) scan. The scan showed increased standardized uptake value (SUV) and discrete masses in the anterior mediastinum (about 7 x 6 cm), bilateral axillary lymphadenopathy, bilateral pulmonary nodules, periaoritic lymphadenopathy, increased uptake in the spleen, and right inguinal lymphadenopathy. A bone marrow biopsy was performed, indicating no lymphoma involvement in the bone marrow.

Background

In the US, the age-adjusted incidence of Hodgkin lymphoma (HL) ranges from 1.3–3.2 per 100,000, depending on race. Worldwide, the age-adjusted incidence ranges from 0.5–0.8 per 100,000 in less developed regions, whereas it is 1.9–2.3 in more developed regions [1]. The age

© Springer International Publishing AG 2017
J. Zain and L.W. Kwak (eds.), *Management of Lymphomas:
A Case-Based Approach*, DOI 10.1007/978-3-319-26827-9_12

incidence has a bimodal distribution, with peaks at 15–29 and 75–84 years of age, respectively [2]. At this time, there is no definitive casual relationship between HL and other environmental, genetic, or infectious factors. Risk of HL is increased in patients with compromised immune systems, such as patients with human immune deficiency (HIV) or those who have undergone organ transplantation [3]. A subset of HL patients are known to be Epstein-Barr Virus (EBV)-positive. They have elevated anti-EBV titers compared with controls [4], and the Reed Sternberg (RS) cells in HL tumors can stain for latent membrane protein 1 (MP1) or be positive for EBV-encoded small RNAs (EBERs) by fluorescence in situ hybridization (FISH) [5]. The risk of HL is about 11.5-fold higher in HIV patients compared with the general population [6]. This subset of HL patients are almost uniformly EBV-positive [7].

HL can be divided into classical HL and nodular lymphocyte predominant HL (LPHL). Within classical HL, there are four histologic subtypes: nodular sclerosis, mixed cellularity, lymphocyte-depleted, and lymphocyte-rich [8]. Classical HL is characterized by the presence of the RS cell, which is the classic HL tumor cell. This cell is large with a bilobed nucleus, and eosinophilic nucleoli. It stains positive for CD30 and CD15 and negative for BOB1 and OCT2. RS cells make up a small percentage of the tumor mass (up to 5%), and the remaining tumor is composed of inflammatory cells such as macrophages or T cells. The four histologic subtypes are differentiated by the cellular backgrounds. In nodular sclerosis classical HL, the nodular cellular infiltrate is surrounded by broad collagen bands. In mixed cellularity HL, the cellular infiltrates is usually diffuse or vaguely nodular. Lymphocyte-depleted HL is the rarest subtype of classical HL; it features an increased number of Hodgkin/RS (HRS) cells and depletion of small lymphocytes. Lymphocyte-rich HL has the characteristic of (HRS) cells in a lymphocyte-rich background. Although these histologies are associated with distinct architectural backgrounds, their prognosis and treatment strategies are very similar. It is thought that HRS cells are derived from preapoptotic germinal center B cells. They lack the typical B cell markers such as CD20, CD79b, or BCR [9–11]. However, detection of rearranged immunoglobulin heavy and light chains in HRS cells shows that they are derived from B cells.

Further, the identical *IgV* gene rearrangements in HRS cells of the same patient reveals their monoclonal nature [12,13]. Thus far, there is no pathognomonic genetic lesion representative of all HL cells; however, genetic lesions in BCL2, BCL6, MYC, MHC, TP53, TNFAIP3, JAK/STAT, and PD-L1 have all been found in HL cells [14–18]. Furthermore, HRS cells show constitutive activation of nuclear factor-kappa B (NF-KB) [18,20], Janus kinase (JAK)/signal transducers and activators of transcription (STAT) [21,22], and PI3K/AKT pathways [23].

LPHL is made up of lymphocyte-predominant cells, which carry one large multilobuted nucleus (popcorn cells). Their immunophenotype is very different from the HRS of cHL subtypes and resembles a B-cell lymphoma, with expression of CD20, CD79a, CD75, BOB1, and OCT-2 [8]. They are CD30- and CD15-negative. As such, they are treated similarly to other indolent B-cell lymphomas rather than HL [24].

Diagnosis and prognosis

Patients with HL typically present with painless and progressive lymphadenopathy. The most common sites are usually cervical and supra-clavicular, as they are the regions where disease is easily localized and detected. However, mediastinal lymphadenopathy is common as well and if bulky may cause chest pain, cough, and shortness of breath. Occasionally, patients present with superior vena cava syndrome. Although rare, HL can have extranodal involvement in organs such as the spleen, liver, lungs, and bone marrow. Patients with advanced HL typically also present with systemic symptoms such as fever, night sweats, weight loss, pruritus, and fatigue.

Although there is no diagnostic blood test for HL, often patients do present with laboratory abnormalities. Leukocytosis, leucopenia, neutro-philia, lymphopenia, eosinophilia, and anemia can all be observed, some of which are associated with a worse prognosis. An elevated erythrocyte sedimentation rate (ESR) and C-reactive protein are seen and have also been associated with a poor prognosis. The diagnosis of HL can only be made with an adequate tissue specimen using morphologic and immuno-histochemical criteria. Excisional, incisional, or core needle biopsies are accepted methods of obtaining tumor specimens. Fine-needle aspiration should never be used for diagnosing HL. The Ann Arbor Staging System is the same one used for lymphomas in general. Computed tomography (CT) and fluorine-18-dexoyglucose position emission tomography (FDG-PET-CT) are used for initial staging and for disease response assessment to treatment. The CT scan can give bidimensional measurements of lymph nodes, whereas the PET scan can measure the activity of the lymphoma. PET scans have been incorporated into several treatment clinical trials as predictive factors for prognosis based on early responses. For full workup please see Figure 12.1.

HL has been considered to be a curable lymphoma, as many patients can achieve durable remissions and have prolonged survival. In general, patients with stage I/II disease have a relatively high 5-year progression-free survival (PFS) and OS, and patients with stage III/IV disease have a relatively poor 5 year PFS and OS. However, there are other prognostic factors besides staging that are predictive of PFS and OS. The prognosis

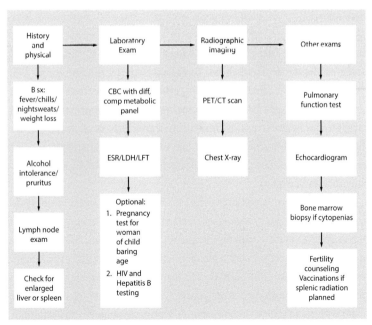

Figure 12.1 City of Hope treatment algorithm for working up a patient with Hodgkin lymphoma.
CBC, complete blood count; CT, computed tomography; ESR, erythrocyte sedimentation rate; LDH, lactate dehyrodgenase; LFT, liver function test; PET, position emission tomography.

for patients with early stage disease can be grouped into favorable or unfavorable depending on the risk factors involved, such as number of lymph node regions, bulky tumor mass, B symptoms, age, ESR, and early PET response [25,26]. Different study groups uses variations of these criteria to define risk (Table 12.1). For patients with advanced stage disease (III/IV), the Hasenclever score [25] is used to determine the rate of freedom from progression. Risk factors such as age ≥45 years, male sex, stage IV disease, hemoglobin ≤10.5 g/dl, serum albumin ≤4.0 g/dl, leukocytosis ≥15 x 10^9/l, and lymphopenia <0.6 x 10^9/l, are used to identify patients at high risk of progression after frontline therapy.

Early stage treatment (classical Hodgkin lymphoma)

Early stage disease is further subdivided into favorable and unfavorable. In the US, favorable is defined as stage I/II disease, no bulky mediastinal mass, age <40 years old, ESR <50 mm/h, and only ≤3 involved nodal regions. Other groups such as the European Organisation for Research and Treatment of Cancer (EORTC) Lymphoma Group, French Belgian Groupe d'Etude des Lymphomes de l'Adulte (GELA), and the German Hodgkin Study Group (GHSG) use variations of the same criteria to define favorable versus unfavorable [26,27]. Historically, patients with stage I/II favorable disease were treated with radiation alone, as HL tumors are very sensitive to radiation treatment. Initially, the radiation field was large and termed extended field radiotherapy (EFRT), and the approach later changed to involved-field radiotherapy (IFRT) and involved site radiotherapy (ISRT). This strategy has further evolved into combined modality therapy (CMT) and, finally, to limited chemotherapy only.

NCI-C/ECOG	GHSG	EORTC-GELA
Bulky mediastinal mass	Bulky mediastina mass	Bulky mediastinal mass
Age >40 years old	Extranodal disease	Age >50 years old
ESR >50 mm/h	Elevated ESR	Elevated ESR
Involved nodal regions >3	Involved nodal regions >2	Involved nodal regions >3
B symptoms		

Table 12.1 Unfavorable risk factors in limited stage Hodgkin lymphoma. EORTC-GELA, European organization for research and treatment of cancer/Groupe d'Etude des Lymphomes de l'Adulte; GHSG, German Hodgkin Study group; NCI-C/ECOG, National cancer institute/Eastern cooperative oncology group.

Stanford University pioneered the initial use of radiotherapy for HL using mantle field and subtotal nodal irradiation (STNI) techniques [28]. The total radiation dose was 40 Gy. Several studies done by the EORTC tested different radiation fields, the addition of chemotherapy, and the necessity of laparotomy for staging. STNI was considered the standard treatment for early favorable HL until the 1990s, but 25–30% of patients eventually relapsed. Additionally, late effects of radiation therapy, such as secondary malignancies, cardiovascular disease, pulmonary problems, and gonadal dysfunction, surfaced as many HL patients became long-term survivors [28]. The risk of cardiovascular disease and secondary malignancies was especially related to the radiation dose and field of radiation. A large Dutch study with a median follow up of 17 years showed that death from secondary cancer and cardiovascular disease was 22% and 9%, respectively [29].

Due to significant late-term toxicity and high relapse rate, many groups started investigating the addition of chemotherapy and reducing the radiation field and the dose termed CMT therapy. The German Hodgkin lymphoma study group (GHSG HD10) trial is the latest published analysis of the use of CMT. This study showed that two courses of adriamycin, bleomycin, vinblastine, and dacarbazine (ABVD) chemotherapy followed by 20 Gy of IFRT yields an OS of 97.5% and PFS of 93.2% [30] in patients with early-stage HL and a favorable prognosis. This study establishes the standard of CMT therapy in this population. However, investigators started to question whether or not radiotherapy is necessary given the long-term complications. The National Cancer Institute of Canada (NCIC) and Eastern Cooperative Oncology Group (ECOG) compared ABVD alone with ABVD plus STNI in early favorable and unfavorable patients. This study showed that CMT had a small PFS advantage, but there was no OS advantage after 12 years of follow-up [31]. Recently, investigators started using PET scans to determine the necessity of radiotherapy. Several studies in advanced HL showed that PET after two cycles is a predictive factor of long-term remission [32]. The UK National Cancer Research Institute (NCRI) Lymphoma Group RAPID trial performed in the UK removed radiation treatment for patients who achieved PET negative status after two cycles of ABVD. This study showed a minor 3.8% difference in 3-year PFS in favor of radiotherapy but no difference in OS [33]. The US Cancer and Leukemia Group B (CALGB) study had a similar design, but results are not yet available. However, the trend has been to avoid radiotherapy if patients are PET-negative at early assessment. A longer follow-up is needed in these trials to show conclusive evidence regarding whether radiotherapy can truly be avoided.

Patients with early stage unfavorable disease need either more cycles of chemotherapy or stronger doses of radiation. In the US, patients with adverse risk factors such as bulky disease or B symptoms are generally treated similarly to advanced stage disease (see below). Alternatively, they can also be treated with four cycles of ABVD followed by involved-field radiotherapy. The GHSG HD 11 study showed a 5-year OS of 95% and PFS of 88% based on this strategy [34].

Advanced stage treatment (classical Hodgkin lymphoma)

In the US and much of Europe, the standard of care for patients with advanced stage HL is ABVD chemotherapy for 6 cycles. The evolution of combination chemotherapy started with mechlorethamine, vincristine, procarbazine, and prednisone (MOPP) chemotherapy which showed a long-term remission of almost 50% [35]. A later study compared MOPP with a MOPP/ABVD hybrid regimen. Results show that MOPP/ABVD was superior to MOPP alone in terms of OS (83.9% versus 63.9%, $p<0.06$) and freedom from progression (64.6% versus 35.9%, $p<0.005$) [36]. The US intergroup then compared ABVD alone with MOPP or an ABVD/MOPP hybrid. The OS at 5 years was 73% for ABVD versus 66% for MOPP versus 75% for MOPP/ABVD. However, the hematologic toxicity is much higher for MOPP, and thus the standard of care has been ABVD alone [37]. Another regimen developed at Stanford University, called Stanford V, used a shorter course of chemotherapy followed by radiation to sites of initial disease [38]. This regimen was compared against ABVD (E2496) in a US cooperative group trial, and the results showed no difference in terms of 5-year PFS or OS [39]. As this method generally results in more myelosuppression and uses more radiation but has no confirmed survival advantage, it has generally gone out of favor in the US.

The patient in our case study was diagnosed with stage IVB HL. He was given six cycles of ABVD chemotherapy. He achieved complete remission documented by CT/PET scan, and has been in remission for 2 years.

While ABVD is the standard regimen for advanced HL in the US, the GHSG developed an increased dose density regimen called bleomycin, etoposide, doxorubicin, cyclophosphamide, vincristine, procarbazine, and prednisone (BEACOPP). This regimen has gone through many modifications, including escalation/deescalation and shortening the course to six cycles. The most recent standard is six cycles of escalated BEACOPP per the GHSG recommendations [40].

A variety of trials have taken place to compare BEACOPP with ABVD [41–43]. Most studies show improvements in response rate with the former regimen; however, there is no clear advantage in overall survival. BEACOPP is also associated with increased hematological toxicities, gonadal failures, and increased secondary malignancies and thus is not the standard of care in the US. The current research strategy involves using PET scans to determine which patients need more intense therapy. A US intergroup trial (NCT00822120) evaluated treatment intensification using six cycles of escalated BEACOPP if patients are PET-positive after two cycles of ABVD. The results are still pending. Figure 12.2 shows the City of Hope treatment pathway for patients with newly diagnosed HL.

Elderly patients

Although up to 70% of patients with advanced HL can be cured with ABVD, the elderly subset of patients typically have a worse outcome. About 20% of the total HL population fit into the elderly category (>60 years of age) [44]. The worse prognosis is in part due to the increased number of comorbidities and their impact on their ability to tolerate full doses of chemotherapy. Van Spronsen et al showed that elderly HL patients have cardiovascular disease (18%), chronic obstructive lung disease (13%), diabetes mellitus (10%), and hypertension (3%) [45]. Landgren et al showed that elderly HL patients who can tolerate >65% relative dose intensity (RDI)of chemotherapy had improved OS compared with patients who cannot tolerate 65% of RDI [46]. In addition, the North American E2496 trials showed increased hematologic toxicities, increased bleomycin lung toxicity (24%), increased treatment-related mortality (9%), and worse OS (48% versus 74% in young patients) with the use of ABVD [47]. It is clear that ABVD is not the optimal induction for elderly patients with comorbidities. Currently, a Phase II trial is underway evaluating the use of brentuximab vedotin either as a single agent or in combination with upfront treatment for elderly HL patients. Interim results show a high response rate, but more follow-up is needed to determine the true efficacy of such a strategy [48].

Relapsed/refractory disease

Although both advanced HL and early stage HL have efficacious upfront induction regimens, up to 30% of patients can still have relapsed/refractory disease. For these patients, high dose therapy followed by autologous stem cell transplantation (ASCT) is the standard treatment. This standard is based on two randomized studies showing improved event free survival in the ASCT group compared with the standard dose salvage

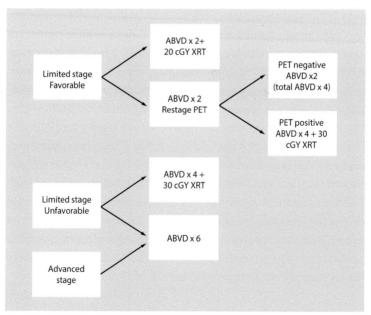

Figure 12.2 City of Hope treatment algorithm for patients with newly diagnosed Hodgkin lymphoma. ABVD, adriamycin, bleomycin, vinblastine, and dacarbazine; PET, positron emission tomography.

chemotherapy group [49,50]. A variety of salvage chemotherapy regimens are used in the US (ICE, DHAP, ESHAP, GVD, IGEV, GDP) [51–54], all with similar response rates (~70–80%). Similar to the salvage regimen, there are a variety of conditioning regimens used for ASCT with no clear benefit of one over the others. BCNU, etoposide, cytarabine, and melphalan (BEAM) [49,50] is the regimen of choice for most groups, and alternative regimens such as cyclophosphamide, carmustine, etoposide (CBV) [55] are a second choice for most centers. With regard to outcome post ASCT, several studies analyzed risk factors predictive of longer term remission rates. Primary refractory disease, early relapse post induction (<12 month), stage III/IV at relapse, extranodal disease at relapse, and B symptoms have all been identified as poor prognostic factors [56–58]. Perhaps the most important factor predictive of long-term remission outcome post-ASCT is the pre-ASCT PET status. Investigators at Memorial Sloan Kettering showed that patients with pre-ASCT PET-negative status had a 5-year EFS of 77% compared with 22% if patients were PET-positive at pre-ASCT [59].

Unfortunately for patients who fail ASCT, the treatment options are limited. For younger patients with an identified hematopoietic stem cell donor, good performance status, and adequate organ functions, reduced-intensity allogeneic stem cell transplantation is a viable option. There are several published regimens using either fludarabine plus melphalan, fludarabine plus low-dose total body irradiation (TBI), and alemtuzumab plus melphalan and fludarabine [60–62] as conditioning regimens. Although OS rates can be up to 50–60% at 3 years, relapses are common, and PFS rates are usually in the 20–30% range [60–62]. The most important predictive factor influencing outcome post allo-HCT is likely chemosensitive disease and comorbidity status prior to allo-HCT. Chen et al showed that, with the use of brentuximab vedotin, a novel antibody drug conjugate against CD30 in relapsed/refractory HL, PFS and OS can be improved post allo-HCT [63].

Novel targeted agents

A greater understanding of molecular and cell biology has allowed development of novel targeted therapies in treating HL. Brentuximab vedotin

(BV), an antibody drug conjugate, has changed the paradigm for relapsed/refractory HL. This drug has three components, an antibody targeted against CD30, the cytotoxic drug monomethyl auristatin E (MMAE), and a protease-cleavable linker. HL expresses CD30 on the surface of RS cells, and this drug is targeted to only deliver MMAE to CD30-expressing cells. In a pivotal Phase II trial, this drug showed a 73% ORR and 34% CR rate. It has received US Food and Drug Administration (FDA) approval for patients who failed ASCT or two lines of therapy prior to ASCT [64].

A separate Phase III randomized placebo-controlled trial using brentuximab vedotin as consolidation post-ASCT showed improved PFS in patients with high risk of relapse [65]. This drug has also been tested in the first salvage setting prior to ASCT and has shown a high response rate; it is therefore a suitable option for patients that want to avoid combination chemotherapy prior to ASCT [66,67]. Current trials incorporating brentuximab vedotin into induction regimens are ongoing and could change the standard regimen of ABVD and/or BEACOPP.

Besides BV, several other novel therapies are currently in development for relapsed/refractory (R/R) HL. Idelalisib, a phosphoinositide 3-kinase (PI3K) inhibitor approved for relapsed follicular lymphoma, has been tested in relapsed/refractory HL. Although the ORR is low (12%), several second-generation PI3K inhibitors are being used in clinical trials for R/R HL [68]. Histone deacetylase (HDAC) inhibitors such as vorinostat, panobinostat, etinostat, and mocetinostat have all been tested in R/R HL, with low ORR rates but relatively low toxicity profiles [69–71]. They are currently being used in the combination setting for R/R HL. Inhibitors of programmed cell death protein 1 (PD-1) and programmed death ligand 1 (PD-L1) are the most exciting novel agents for HL currently in development. PD-L1 is expressed on tumor cells, leading to immune escape through binding of PD-1 on T cells in the tumor microenvironment [72,73]. Nivolumab and pembrolizumab are both being tested, and preliminary results are very promising. Nivolumab was recently approved for the treatment of relapsed HL after failing stem cell transplant and BV [74].

Long-term complications

HL is a curative neoplasm and long-term survivors are common. The increasing length of time in which HL patients are surviving without a relapse has made the toxic effects of treatment more apparent adding to the burden of survivorship and quality of life. Upfront chemotherapy such as ABVD has two main acute toxicities: cardiotoxicities and pulmonary toxicities. Cardiotoxicites can present as arrhythmias or cardiomyopathy leading to congestive heart failure. They are usually caused by adriamycin, an anthracycline. Cardiotoxicites due to an anthracycline are dose-dependent and usually do not occur when cumulative doses are less than 300 mg/m^2, which is the standard dose given in six cycles of ABVD [75]. Another agent used in ABVD, bleomycin, can cause acute and late pulmonary toxicities. Patients may present with cough, dyspnea, and fever as well as the classic radiographic pattern of bibasilar reticular/nodular infiltrates [76]. The latter can be diagnosed with a FDG-PET scan or high resolution CT scan, and decreased diffusing capacity or transfer factor of the lung for carbon monoxide (DLCO) on pulmonary function test (PFT) exams. Treatment for these pulmonary toxicities includes cessation of bleomycin and steroid use, but these toxicities can be fatal, with one study reporting a 25% mortality rate [77]. Besides chemotherapy, radiation is also frequently used in upfront treatment and can also lead to cardiac and pulmonary toxicities. Radiation-associated heart disease can present as coronary artery disease, myocardial dysfunction, valvular heart disease, pericarditis, and arrhythmias [78–80]. Several studies have shown increased incidence of heart disease after radiation, even after a long-term follow up of 20 years [81–83]. Radiation therapy can also cause pneumonitis, resulting in dyspnea and cough and possibly leading to pulmonary fibrosis. The current treatment is use of high-dose steroids.

Gonadal dysfunction has been observed after induction chemotherapy, especially when high dose therapy such as BEACOPP or dose-escalated BEACOPP is given [84,85]. The risk of gonadal failure after ABVD is less common [86,87] and fertility preservation strategies may circumvent risk in these patients. Besides gonadal failures, secondary malignancies are unfortunately common after HL treatment because of the use of combination chemotherapy and radiation therapy. Leukemia is the most common secondary malignancy (22-fold risk), followed by non-Hodgkin lymphoma (6–14-fold), and connective tissue, bone, and thyroid cancer (4–11-fold) [88–92]. Solid tumors such as those in the lung, stomach, esophagus, colon, breast, and cervix may occur as well (two- to six-fold). Hence the goal remains to find strategies to minimize these long-term side effects of effective therapies. It is possible that the use of more targeted therapies like brentuximab vedotin in the upfront settings (currently in clinical trials) can circumvent these issues.

References

1 Ferlay J, Soerjomataram I, Ervik M, Dikshit R, Eser S, Mathers C et al. GLOBOCAN 2012 v1.0, Cancer Incidence and Mortality Worldwide: IARC CancerBase No. 11. Lyon, France: International Agency for Research on Cancer; 2013; http://globocan.iarc.fr. Accessed March 7, 2017.

2 Surveillance, Epidemiology, and End Results (SEER) Program. SEER*Stat Database: Incidence - SEER 18 Regs Research Data + Hurricane Katrina Impacted Louisiana Cases, Nov 2012 Sub (2000–2010) <Katrina/Rita Population Adjustment> - Linked To County Attributes - Total U.S., 1969–2011 Counties, National Cancer Institute, DCCPS, Surveillance Research Program, Surveillance Systems Branch, released April 2013, based on the November 2012 submission. www.seer.cancer.gov. Accessed March 7, 2017.

3 Mueller N, Grufferman S. *Cancer Epidemiology and Prevention, Hodgkin lymphoma*. 3rd edn. Oxford University Press: New York, 2006.

4 Evans AS, Gutensohn NM. A population-based case-control study of EBV and other viral antibodies among persons with Hodgkin's disease and their siblings. *Int J Cancer*. 1984;34: 149-157.

5 Weiss LM, Movahed LA, Warnke RA, Sklar J. Detection of Epstein-Barr viral genomes in Reed-Sternberg cells of Hodgkin's disease. *N Engl J Med*. 1989;320:502-506.

6 Frisch M, Biggar RJ, Engels EA, Goedert JJ. Association of cancer with AIDS-related immunosuppression in adults. *JAMA*. 2001;285:1736-1745.

7 Berenguer J, Miralles P, Ribera JM, et al. Characteristics and outcome of AIDS-related Hodgkin lymphoma before and after the introduction of highly active antiretroviral therapy. *J Acquir Immune Defic Syndr*. 2008;47:422-428.

8 Swerdlow SH, Campo E, Harris NL, et al. *WHO Classification of Tumours of Haematopoietic and Lymphoid Tissues*. Fourth edn, vol 2. Lyon: IARC 2008.

9 Kuzu I, Delsol G, Jones M, Gatter KC, Mason DY. Expression of the Ig-associated heterodimer (mb-1 and B29) in Hodgkin's disease. *Histopathology*. 1993;22:141-144.

10 Re D, Muschen M, Ahmadi T, et al. Oct-2 and Bob-1 deficiency in Hodgkin and Reed Sternberg cells. *Cancer Res*. 2001;61:2080-2084.

11 Watanabe K, Yamashita Y, Nakayama A, et al. Varied B-cell immunophenotypes of Hodgkin/Reed-Sternberg cells in classic Hodgkin's disease. *Histopathology*. 2000;36:353-361.

12 Kanzler H, Kuppers R, Hansmann ML, Rajewsky K. Hodgkin and Reed-Sternberg cells in Hodgkin's disease represent the outgrowth of a dominant tumor clone derived from (crippled) germinal center B cells. *J Exp Med*. 1996;184:1495-1505.

13 Kuppers R, Rajewsky K, Zhao M, et al. Hodgkin disease: Hodgkin and Reed-Sternberg cells picked from histological sections show clonal immunoglobulin gene rearrangements and appear to be derived from B cells at various stages of development. *Proc Natl Acad Sci USA*.1994;91:10962-10966.

14 Martin-Subero JI, Klapper W, Sotnikova A, et al. Chromosomal breakpoints affecting immunoglobulin loci are recurrent in Hodgkin and Reed-Sternberg cells of classical Hodgkin lymphoma. *Cancer Res*. 2006;66:10332-10338.

15 Gravel S, Delsol G, Al Saati T. Single-cell analysis of the t(14;18)(q32;q21) chromosomal translocation in Hodgkin's disease demonstrates the absence of this translocation in neoplastic Hodgkin and Reed-Sternberg cells. *Blood*. 1998;91:2866-2874.

16 Kato M, Sanada M, Kato I, et al. Frequent inactivation of A20 in B-cell lymphomas. *Nature*. 2009;459:712-716.

17 Mottok A, Renne C, Willenbrock K, Hansmann ML, Brauninger A. Somatic hypermutation of SOCS1 in lymphocyte-predominant Hodgkin lymphoma is accompanied by high JAK2 expression and activation of STAT6. *Blood*. 2007;110:3387-3390.

18 Green MR, Monti S, Rodig SJ, et al. Integrative analysis reveals selective 9p24.1 amplification, increased PD-1 ligand expression, and further induction via JAK2 in nodular sclerosing Hodgkin lymphoma and primary mediastinal large B-cell lymphoma. *Blood*. 2010;116: 3268-3277.

19 Cabannes E, Khan G, Aillet F, Jarrett RF, Hay RT. Mutations in the IkBa gene in Hodgkin's disease suggest a tumour suppressor role for IkappaBalpha. *Oncogene*. 1999;18:3063-3070.

20 Emmerich F, Meiser M, Hummel M, et al. Overexpression of I kappa B alpha without inhibition of NF-kappaB activity and mutations in the I kappa B alpha gene in Reed-Sternberg cells. *Blood*. 1999;94:3129-3134.

21 Kube D, Holtick U, Vockerodt M, et al. STAT3 is constitutively activated in Hodgkin cell lines. *Blood*. 2001;98:762-770.

22 Skinnider BF, Elia AJ, Gascoyne RD, et al. Signal transducer and activator of transcription 6 is frequently activated in Hodgkin and Reed-Sternberg cells of Hodgkin lymphoma. *Blood*. 2002;99:618-626.

23 Dutton A, Reynolds GM, Dawson CW, Young LS, Murray PG. Constitutive activation of phosphatidyl-inositide 3 kinase contributes to the survival of Hodgkin's lymphoma cells through a mechanism involving Akt kinase and mTOR. *J Pathol*. 2005;205:498-506.

24 Advani RH, Hoppe RT. XVIII. Management of nodular lymphocyte predominant Hodgkin lymphoma. *Hematol Oncol*. 2015;33 Suppl 1:90-95.

25 Hasenclever D, Diehl V. A prognostic score for advanced Hodgkin's disease. International Prognostic Factors Project on Advanced Hodgkin's Disease. *N Engl J Med*. 1998;339:1506-1514.

26 Ferme C, Eghbali H, Meerwaldt JH, et al. Chemotherapy plus involved-field radiation in early-stage Hodgkin's disease. *N Engl J Med*. 2007;357:1916-1927.

27 Engert A, Franklin J, Eich HT, et al. Two cycles of doxorubicin, bleomycin, vinblastine, and dacarbazine plus extended-field radiotherapy is superior to radiotherapy alone in early favorable Hodgkin's lymphoma: final results of the GHSG HD7 trial. *J Clin Oncol*. 2007;25: 3495-3502.

28 Hoppe RT, Coleman CN, Cox RS, Rosenberg SA, Kaplan HS. The management of stage I–II Hodgkin's disease with irradiation alone or combined modality therapy: the Stanford experience. *Blood*. 1982;59:455-465.

29 Aleman BM, van den Belt-Dusebout AW, Klokman WJ, Van't Veer MB, Bartelink H, van Leeuwen FE. Long-term cause-specific mortality of patients treated for Hodgkin's disease. *J Clin Oncol*. 2003;21:3431-3439.

30 Engert A, Plutschow A, Eich HT, et al. Reduced treatment intensity in patients with early-stage Hodgkin's lymphoma. *N Engl J Med*. 2010;363:640-652.

31 Meyer RM, Gospodarowicz MK, Connors JM, Pearcey RG, Wells WA, Winter JN et al. ABVD alone versus radiation-based therapy in limited-stage Hodgkin's lymphoma. *N Engl J Med*. 2012;366:399-408.

32 Hutchings M, Loft A, Hansen M, et al. FDG-PET after two cycles of chemotherapy predicts treatment failure and progression-free survival in Hodgkin lymphoma. *Blood*. 2006;107: 52-59.

33 Radford J, Illidge T, Counsell N, Hancock B, Pettengell R, Johnson P et al. Results of a trial of PET-directed therapy for early-stage Hodgkin's lymphoma. *N Engl J Med*. 2015;372:1598-1607.

34 Borchmann P, Diehl V, Goergen H, et al. Combined modality treatment with intensified chemotherapy and dose-reduced involved field radiotherapy in patients with early unfavourable Hodgkin lymphoma (HL): final analysis of the German Hodgkin Study Group (GHSG) HD11 trial. *Blood*. 2009;114:299-300.

35 Devita JVT, Simon RM, Hubbard SM, et al. Curability of Advanced Hodgkin's Disease with ChemotherapyLong-Term Follow-up of MOPP-Treated Patients at the National Cancer Institute. *Ann Intern Med*. 1980;92:587-595.

36 Bonadonna G, Valagussa P, Santoro A. Alternating non-cross-resistant combination chemotherapy or MOPP in stage IV Hodgkin's disease. A report of 8-year results. *Ann Intern Med*. 1986;104:739-746.

37 Canellos GP, Anderson JR, Propert KJ, Nissen N, Cooper MR, Henderson ES et al. Chemotherapy of advanced Hodgkin's disease with MOPP, ABVD, or MOPP alternating with ABVD. *N Engl J Med*. 1992;327:1478-1484.

38 Horning SJ, Hoppe RT, Breslin S, Bartlett NL, Brown BW, Rosenberg SA. Stanford V and radiotherapy for locally extensive and advanced Hodgkin's disease: mature results of a prospective clinical trial. *J Clin Oncol*. 2002;20:630-637.

39 Advani RH, Hong F, Fisher RI, et al. Randomized phase III trial comparing ABVD plus radiotherapy with the Stanford V regimen in patients with stages I or II locally extensive, bulky mediastinal Hodgkin lymphoma: a subset analysis of the North American intergroup E2496 trial. *J Clin Oncol*. 2015;33:1936-1942.

40 Engert A, Haverkamp H, Kobe C, et al. Reduced-intensity chemotherapy and PET-guided radiotherapy in patients with advanced stage Hodgkin's lymphoma (HD15 trial): a randomised, open-label, phase 3 non-inferiority trial. *Lancet*. 2012;379:1791-1799.

41 Federico M, Luminari S, Iannitto E, et al. ABVD compared with BEACOPP compared with CEC for the initial treatment of patients with advanced Hodgkin's lymphoma: results from the HD2000 Gruppo Italiano per lo Studio dei Linfomi Trial. *J Clin Oncol*. 2009;27:805-811.

42 Mounier N, Brice P, Bologna S, et al. ABVD (8 cycles) versus BEACOPP (4 escalated cycles >/=4 baseline): final results in stage III-IV low-risk Hodgkin lymphoma (IPS 0-2) of the LYSA H34 randomized trial. *Ann Oncol*. 2014;25:1622-1628.

43 Viviani S, Zinzani PL, Rambaldi A, Brusamolino E, Levis A, Bonfante V et al. ABVD versus BEACOPP for Hodgkin's lymphoma when high-dose salvage is planned. *N Engl J Med*. 2011;365:203-212.

44 Stark GL, Wood KM, Jack F, Angus B, Proctor SJ, Taylor PR. Hodgkin's disease in the elderly: a population-based study. *Br J Haematol*. 2002;119:432-440.

45 van Spronsen DJ, Janssen-Heijnen ML, Breed WP, Coebergh JW. Prevalence of co-morbidity and its relationship to treatment among unselected patients with Hodgkin's disease and non-Hodgkin's lymphoma, 1993-1996. *Ann Hematol*. 1999;78:315-319.

46 Landgren O, Algernon C, Axdorph U, et al. Hodgkin's lymphoma in the elderly with special reference to type and intensity of chemotherapy in relation to prognosis. *Haematologica*. 2003;88:438-444.

47 Evens AM, Hong F, Gordon LI, et al. The efficacy and tolerability of adriamycin, bleomycin, vinblastine, dacarbazine and Stanford V in older Hodgkin lymphoma patients: a comprehensive analysis from the North American intergroup trial E2496. *Br J Haematol*. 2013;161:76-86.

48 Forero-Torres A, Holkova B, Goldschmidt J, et al. Phase 2 study of frontline brentuximab vedotin monotherapy in Hodgkin lymphoma patients aged 60 years and older. *Blood*. 2015;126:2798-2804.

49 Linch DC, Winfield D, Goldstone AH, Moir D, Hancock B, McMillan A et al. Dose intensification with autologous bone-marrow transplantation in relapsed and resistant Hodgkin's disease: results of a BNLI randomised trial. *Lancet*.1993;341:1051-1054.

50 Schmitz N, Pfistner B, Sextro M, et al. Aggressive conventional chemotherapy compared with high-dose chemotherapy with autologous haemopoietic stem-cell transplantation for relapsed chemosensitive Hodgkin's disease: a randomised trial. *Lancet*. 2002;359:2065-2071.

51 Moskowitz CH, Nimer SD, Zelenetz AD, et al. A 2-step comprehensive high-dose chemoradiotherapy second-line program for relapsed and refractory Hodgkin disease: analysis by intent to treat and development of a prognostic model. *Blood*. 2001; 97:616-623.

52 Josting A, Rudolph C, Reiser M, et al. Time-intensified dexamethasone/cisplatin/cytarabine: an effective salvage therapy with low toxicity in patients with relapsed and refractory Hodgkin's disease. *Ann Oncol*. 2002;13:1628-1635.

53 Bartlett NL, Niedzwiecki D, Johnson JL, et al. Gemcitabine, vinorelbine, and pegylated liposomal doxorubicin (GVD), a salvage regimen in relapsed Hodgkin's lymphoma: CALGB 59804. *Ann Oncol*. 2007;18:1071-1079.

54 Magagnoli M, Spina M, Balzarotti M, et al. IGEV regimen and a fixed dose of lenograstim: an effective mobilization regimen in pretreated Hodgkin's lymphoma patients. *Bone Marrow Transplant*. 2007;40:1019-1025.

55 Morschhauser F, Brice P, Ferme C, et al. Risk-adapted salvage treatment with single or tandem autologous stem-cell transplantation for first relapse/refractory Hodgkin's lymphoma: results of the prospective multicenter H96 trial by the GELA/SFGM study group. *J Clin Oncol*. 2008;26:5980-5987.

56 Josting A, Franklin J, May M, Koch P, Beykirch MK, Heinz J, et al. New prognostic score based on treatment outcome of patients with relapsed Hodgkin's lymphoma registered in the database of the German Hodgkin's lymphoma study group. *J Clin Oncol*. 2002;20:221-230.

57 Sureda A, Constans M, Iriondo A, et al. Prognostic factors affecting long-term outcome after stem cell transplantation in Hodgkin's lymphoma autografted after a first relapse. *Ann Oncol*. 2005;16:625 633.

58 Moskowitz CH, Yahalom J, Zelenetz AD, et al. High-dose chemo-radiotherapy for relapsed or refractory Hodgkin lymphoma and the significance of pre-transplant functional imaging. *Br J Haematol*. 2010;148:890-897.

59 Moskowitz CH, Matasar MJ, Zelenetz AD, et al. Normalization of pre-ASCT, FDG-PET imaging with second-line, non-cross resistant, chemotherapy programs improves event-free survival in patients with Hodgkin lymphoma. *Blood*. 2012;119:1665-1670.

60 Chen R, Palmer JM, Thomas SH, et al. Brentuximab vedotin enables successful reduced-intensity allogeneic hematopoietic cell transplantation in patients with relapsed or refractory Hodgkin lymphoma. *Blood*. 2012;119:6379-6381.

61 Burroughs LM, O'Donnell PV, Sandmaier BM, et al. Comparison of outcomes of HLA-matched related, unrelated, or HLA-haploidentical related hematopoietic cell transplantation following nonmyeloablative conditioning for relapsed or refractory Hodgkin lymphoma. *Biol Blood Marrow Transplant*. 2008;14:1279-1287.

62 Sureda A, Canals C, Arranz R, et al. Allogeneic stem cell transplantation after reduced intensity conditioning in patients with relapsed or refractory Hodgkin's lymphoma. Results of the HDR-ALLO study - a prospective clinical trial by the Grupo Espanol de Linfomas/Trasplante de Medula Osea (GEL/TAMO) and the Lymphoma Working Party of the European Group for Blood and Marrow Transplantation. *Haematologica*. 2012;97:310-317.

63 Chen R, Palmer JM, Tsai NC, et al. Brentuximab vedotin is associated with improved progression-free survival after allogeneic transplantation for Hodgkin lymphoma. *Biol Blood Marrow Transplant*. 2014;20:1864-1868.

64 Younes A, Gopal AK, Smith SE, et al. Results of a pivotal phase II study of brentuximab vedotin for patients with relapsed or refractory Hodgkin's lymphoma. *J Clin Oncol*. 2012;30:2183-2189.

65 Moskowitz CH, Nademanee A, Masszi T, et al. Brentuximab vedotin as consolidation therapy after autologous stem-cell transplantation in patients with Hodgkin's lymphoma at risk of relapse or progression (AETHERA): a randomised, double-blind, placebo-controlled, phase 3 trial. *Lancet*. 2015;385:1853-1862.

66 Chen R, Palmer JM, Martin P, et al. Results of a multicenter phase II trial of brentuximab vedotin as second-line therapy before autologous transplantation in relapsed/refractory Hodgkin lymphoma. *Biol Blood Marrow Transplant*. 2015;21:2136-2140.

67 Moskowitz AJ, Schoder H, Yahalom J, et al. PET-adapted sequential salvage therapy with brentuximab vedotin followed by augmented ifosamide, carboplatin, and etoposide for patients with relapsed and refractory Hodgkin's lymphoma: a non-randomised, open-label, single-centre, phase 2 study. *Lancet Oncology*. 2015;16:284-292.

68 Meadows SA, Vega F, Kashishian A, et al. PI3Kdelta inhibitor, GS-1101 (CAL-101), attenuates pathway signaling, induces apoptosis, and overcomes signals from the microenvironment in cellular models of Hodgkin lymphoma. *Blood*. 2012;119:1897-1900.

69 Kirschbaum MH, Goldman BH, Zain JM, et al. A phase 2 study of vorinostat for treatment of relapsed or refractory Hodgkin lymphoma: Southwest Oncology Group study S0517. *Leuk Lymphoma*. 2011;53:259-292.

70 Younes A, Oki Y, Bociek RG, et al. Mocetinostat for relapsed classical Hodgkin's lymphoma: an open-label, single-arm, phase 2 trial. *Lancet Oncology*. 2011;12:1222-1228.

71 Younes A, Sureda A, Ben-Yehuda D, et al. Panobinostat in patients with relapsed/refractory Hodgkin's lymphoma after autologous stem-cell transplantation: results of a phase II study. *J Clin Oncol*. 2012;30:2197-2203.

72 Pardoll DM. The blockade of immune checkpoints in cancer immunotherapy. *Nat Rev Cancer*. 2012;12:252-264.

73 Keir ME, Butte MJ, Freeman GJ, Sharpe AH. PD-1 and its ligands in tolerance and immunity. *Annu Rev Immunol*. 2008;26:677-704.

74 Ansell SM, Lesokhin AM, Borello I, et al. PD-1 blockade with nivolumab in relapsed or refractory Hodgkin's lymphoma. *N Engl J Med*. 2015;372:311-319.

75 Swain SM, Whaley FS, Ewer MS. Congestive heart failure in patients treated with doxorubicin: a retrospective analysis of three trials. *Cancer*. 2003;97:2869-2879.

76 Buchler T, Bomanji J, Lee SM. FDG-PET in bleomycin-induced pneumonitis following ABVD chemotherapy for Hodgkin's disease--a useful tool for monitoring pulmonary toxicity and disease activity. *Haematologica*. 2007;92:e120-121.

77 Martin WG, Ristow KM, Habermann TM, Colgan JP, Witzig TE, Ansell SM. Bleomycin pulmonary toxicity has a negative impact on the outcome of patients with Hodgkin's lymphoma. *J Clin Oncol*. 2005;23:7614-7620.

78 Schultz-Hector S, Trott KR. Radiation-induced cardiovascular diseases: is the epidemiologic evidence compatible with the radiobiologic data? *Int J Radiat Oncol Biol Phys*. 2007;67:10-18.

79 Adams MJ, Lipshultz SE, Schwartz C, Fajardo LF, Coen V, Constine LS. Radiation-associated cardiovascular disease: manifestations and management. *Semin Radiat Oncol*. 2003;13: 346-356.

80 Ng AK. Review of the cardiac long-term effects of therapy for Hodgkin lymphoma. *Br J Haematol*. 2011;154:23-31.

81 Aleman BM, van den Belt-Dusebout AW, De Bruin ML, et al. Late cardiotoxicity after treatment for Hodgkin lymphoma. *Blood*. 2007;109:1878-1886.

82 Darby SC, Cutter DJ, Boerma M, et al. Radiation-related heart disease: current knowledge and future prospects. *Int J Radiat Oncol Biol Phys*. 2010;76:656-665.

83 Hull MC, Morris CG, Pepine CJ, Mendenhall NP. Valvular dysfunction and carotid, subclavian, and coronary artery disease in survivors of hodgkin lymphoma treated with radiation therapy. *JAMA*. 2003;290:2831-2837.

84 Sieniawski M, Reineke T, Josting A, Nogova L, Behringer K, Halbsguth T et al. Assessment of male fertility in patients with Hodgkin's lymphoma treated in the German Hodgkin Study Group (GHSG) clinical trials. *Ann Oncol*. 2008;19:1795-1801.

85 Behringer K, Mueller H, Goergen H, et al. Gonadal function and fertility in survivors after Hodgkin lymphoma treatment within the German Hodgkin Study Group HD13 to HD15 trials. *J Clin Oncol*. 2013;31:231-239.

86 Viviani S, Santoro A, Ragni G, Bonfante V, Bestetti O, Bonadonna G. Gonadal toxicity after combination chemotherapy for Hodgkin's disease. Comparative results of MOPP vs ABVD. *Eur J Cancer Clin Oncol*. 1985;21:601-605.

87 Bonadonna G, Santoro A, Viviani S, Lombardi C, Ragni G. Gonadal damage in Hodgkin's disease from cancer chemotherapeutic regimens. *Arch Toxicol Suppl.* 1984;7:140-145.

88 Hodgson DC, Gilbert ES, Dores GM, et al. Long-term solid cancer risk among 5-year survivors of Hodgkin's lymphoma. *J Clin Oncol.* 2007;25:1489-1497.

89 van Leeuwen FE, Klokman WJ, van't Veer MB, et al. Long-term risk of second malignancy in survivors of Hodgkin's disease treated during adolescence or young adulthood. *J Clin Oncol.* 2000;18:487-497.

90 Swerdlow AJ, Higgins CD, Smith P, Cunningham D, Hancock BW, Horwich A et al. Second cancer risk after chemotherapy for Hodgkin's lymphoma: a collaborative British cohort study. *J Clin Oncol.* 2011;29:4096-4104.

91 Dores GM, Metayer C, Curtis RE, Lynch CF, Clarke EA, Glimelius B et al. Second malignant neoplasms among long-term survivors of Hodgkin's disease: a population-based evaluation over 25 years. *J Clin Oncol.* 2002;20:3484-3494.

92 Swerdlow AJ, Barber JA, Hudson GV, et al. Risk of second malignancy after Hodgkin's disease in a collaborative British cohort: The relation to age at treatment. *J Clin Oncol.* 2000;18:498-509.

Lymphomas in special clinical situations

Acquired immunodeficiency syndrome-related lymphoma

Joseph Alvarnas

Case presentation

Patient X is a 50-year-old man who presented to his primary care physicians with rapidly progressing right cervical lymphadenopathy. The patient underwent an excisional biopsy, which was consistent with diffuse large B-cell lymphoma (DLBCL). A computed tomography (CT) positron emission tomography (PET) fusion study demonstrated evidence of fluorine-18-fluorodeoxy-D-glucose (FDG)-avid right cervical and mediastinal lymphadenopathy measuring up to 2 cm in maximum dimension. A bone aspirate and biopsy demonstrated no evidence of involvement by non-Hodgkin lymphoma (NHL). Screening for human immunodeficiency virus (HIV) infection and hepatitis B and C demonstrated that the patient was infected with HIV. His viral load was 500,000 copies/mL and the CD4+ T-cell count was 230/μL.

Lymphoma risk and human immunodeficiency virus infection

A syndrome of immunodeficiency was first identified in homosexual men in 1981 [1]. The acquired immunodeficiency syndrome (AIDS) was associated with both a significant risk of opportunistic infections and an increased risk of several malignancies, including NHL. By 1984 a lentivirus, known as HIV, was identified as the causative agent of AIDS.

© Springer International Publishing AG 2017

J. Zain and L.W. Kwak (eds.), *Management of Lymphomas: A Case-Based Approach*, DOI 10.1007/978-3-319-26827-9_13

In 1985, the first screening tests became available for detecting both HIV1 (the dominant form of HIV in the western world) and HIV2 [2]. As of 2014, 36.9 million people worldwide were living with HIV infection [3]. In the United States alone, the Centers for Disease Control and Prevention (CDC) organization estimates that there are 1,218,400 people infected with HIV; this includes 156,300 people who are unaware of their infection [4].

Incidence and spectrum of lymphomas in human immunodeficiency virus-infected patients

HIV infection is associated with a significantly increased risk for a number of cancers. The Swiss Cohort study observed 7304 HIV-infected individuals for a total of 28,836 people-years. The risk of NHL in this population increased 72-fold compared with that of the non-infected population [5]. Prior to the advent of combination antiretroviral therapy (cART), HIV-infected patients had an up to 200-fold increase in the risk of NHL. Following the widespread availability of cART, the risk of NHL has dropped but remains elevated compared with that of the non-infected population [5]. The current annual incidence of NHL among HIV-infected patients is 170 new cases per 100,000 [6]. The annual incidence of NHL in the general population is 19.7 new cases per 100,000 [7]. Between 1 and 6% of HIV-infected patients develop lymphoma annually [8]. NHL is an AIDS-defining diagnosis for HIV-infected patients [9].

HIV-infected patients are also at a greater risk for the development of Hodgkin lymphoma (HL). In the Swiss Cohort study, the incidence of HL increased 17.3-fold compared with the non-infected population [5]. The current estimate is that HIV infection increases the risk of HL between 5 and 25-fold compared with the general population [8]. Unlike NHL, the risk of HL has not decreased significantly following the availability of cART and may, in fact, be increasing in the post-cART era [5]. HL is not an AIDS-defining diagnosis for HIV-infected patients.

Lymphomas of B-cell origin account for approximately 95% of cases of NHL in HIV-infected patients. Peripheral T-cell lymphomas are rare in this population [10]. The spectrum of AIDS-related NHL includes DLBCL, Burkitt lymphoma (BL), primary central nervous system lymphoma

(PCNSL), plasmablastic lymphomas, and primary effusion lymphomas [11]. DLBCL (including both immunoblastic DLBCL and centroblastic DLBCL) and BL account for nearly 90% of AIDS-related NHL in the post-cART era [8]. Prior to the advent of effective anti-HIV therapy, PCNSL and plasmablastic lymphoma occurred more frequently, typically in severely immunocompromised patients such as those with a CD4 T-cell count <100/μL. HIV-infected patients with HL most commonly present with the lymphocyte-depleted or mixed cellularity histologies. The World Health Organization (WHO) Classification Scheme for lymphomas in HIV-infected patients is shown in Table 13.1 [11].

Oncogenic viruses play a significant role in the development of HIV-related lymphomas. More than 50% of patients with AIDS-related NHL have evidence of Epstein Barr virus (EBV) infection present in their lymphoma [8,12]. EBV infection of the NHL tumor clone plays an important role in the development of PCNSL, primary effusion lymphomas, and plasmablastic lymphoma of the oral cavity. Nearly 100% of patients with HL have evidence of EBV involvement [13,14]. In addition to EBV, human herpes virus 8 (HHV-8), also known as Kaposi sarcoma-associated virus (KSHV), infection plays a role in the development of primary effusion lymphomas and multicentric Castleman disease in HIV-infected patients [8,14].

Lymphoma category	Lymphoid malignancy
Lymphomas occurring in both HIV+ and immunocompetent patients	Burkitt and Burkitt-like lymphomas
	Diffuse large B-cell lymphomas:
	• Centroblastic
	• Immunoblastic
	Extranodal MALT lymphoma
	Peripheral T-cell lymphoma
	Classical Hodgkin lymphoma
Lymphomas occurring primarily in HIV-infected patients	Primary effusion lymphoma
	Plasmablastic lymphoma of the oral cavity
Lymphomas occurring in other immunodeficiency states	Polymorphic B-cell lymphoma (PTLD-like)

Table 13.1 World Health Organization classification of lymphoid malignancies occurring in human immunodeficiency virus-infected individuals. HIV, human immunodeficiency virus; MALT, mucosa-associated lymphoid tissue.

Clinical presentation

Patients with AIDS-related NHL frequently present with advanced stage disease with involvement at multiple extranodal sites, including the CNS (up to 20% of patients), bone marrow (30% of patients), and gastrointestinal tract (50% of patients). B symptoms are frequently present at the time of diagnosis [15–17]. At the time of diagnosis, patients should be evaluated carefully for the presence of extranodal disease; a lumbar puncture should be performed in all patients as part of initial staging. Patients with HIV-associated HL typically present with advanced stage disease [18]. In one trial, 67% of patients had stage IV disease [19]. Patients frequently have involvement at extranodal sites, including bone marrow involvement in up to 60% of patients at presentation. Peripheral blood cytopenias are common. Up to 75% of patients exhibit B symptoms at diagnosis [19–21].

Initial treatment of acquired immunodeficiency syndrome-related non-Hodgkin lymphoma

In the initial years of the AIDS pandemic, outcomes for patients with AIDS-related NHL were abysmal [22]. The ability to administer effective anti-lymphoma therapy was compromised by poor lymphoma response rate, patient intolerance of standard regimens, and an untenable risk of infectious complications [17]. Prior to the advent of cART, initial management of AIDS-related lymphoma often consisted of low-dose/dose-attenuated regimens, such as low-dose methotrexate, bleomycin, doxorubicin, cyclophosphamide, vincristine, and dexamethasone (m-BACOD).

In the National Institute of Allergy and Infectious Diseases AIDS Clinical Trials Group study comparing low-dose versus standard dose m-BACOD, 198 patients with untreated NHL were randomized to receive either low-dose (98) or standard dose (94) m-BACOD [23]. Forty-two of 81 evaluable patients who received the standard dose regimen and 39 of 94 patients who received the low-dose regimen achieved a complete response (CR). Overall and disease-free survival did not differ between the groups. Median survival for patients treated with standard-dose and low-dose regimens was only 35 weeks and 31 weeks, respectively [23].

Following the availability of effective anti-HIV therapy, the prognosis for patients with AIDS-related NHL has improved profoundly and now parallels that of non-infected patients. For patients with newly diagnosed AIDS-related NHL, the International Prognostic Index (IPI), has important prognostic utility [17,24,26]. In a series of 69 patients with AIDS-related NHL, the CR rates for patients with low, low-intermediate, intermediate, and high IPI risk were 100%, 88%, 50%, and 32%, respectively [25]. Of note, 52% of the patients presented with IPI high-risk disease. In addition to the IPI, the CD4 T-cell count at the time of diagnosis also has prognostic significance. In a multivariate risk analysis of 111 patients diagnosed with AIDS-related NHL, the IPI and a low CD4 T-cell count ($<100/\mu L$) at the time of diagnosis were the only two independent predictors for the risk of death [17,26].

The current standard of care for patients with AIDS-related NHL consists of treatment with combination chemotherapeutic regimens administered in standard dosing. For patients with DLBCL, regimens such as cyclophosphamide, doxorubicin, vincristine, prednisone (CHOP) and CHOP combined with rituximab (R-CHOP) can be administered successfully to patients with AIDS-related NHL. In a Phase II trial of 61 newly diagnosed patients, Boué et al evaluated the effectiveness of R-CHOP in this setting [27]. The median patient was 42 years of age, 42 patients had DLBCL, two had immunoblastic lymphoma, and 16 had BL. The median CD4 T-cell count at diagnosis was $172/\mu L$. Fifty-two patients were evaluable. CR was achieved in 42 of 52 evaluable patients. Estimated 2-year overall survival (OS) was 75% [27].

In the randomized Phase III trial AIDS Malignancy Consortium (AMC) 010 trial, 150 patients with AIDS-related NHL were randomized (2:1 randomization) to receive either R-CHOP (99 patients) or CHOP (50 patients) [28]. The overall response rate for the R-CHOP and CHOP groups was 57.6% and 47%, respectively. The was no statistically significant difference for the groups in their overall response rates (ORR), progression-free survival (PFS), and OS. Those patients with a CD4 T-cell count $<50/\mu L$ at the time of diagnosis who received rituximab appeared to have an increased risk of infection-related deaths [28].

Infusional chemotherapeutic regimens also appear to be quite effective in the treatment of AIDS-related DLBCL. In a 2003 National Cancer Institute (NCI) trial using EPOCH combined with rituximab (EPOCH-R) for 39 patients with AIDS-related NHL (31 with DLBCL), the CR rate was 74% and at a median follow-up of 53 months the OS was 60% [29].

In an AMC trial of dose-adjusted EPOCH, rituximab was given either concurrently prior to each cycle of chemotherapy or administered in six doses following completion of chemotherapy [30]. One hundred and six patients were treated on trial. In the concurrent treatment arm, 35 out of 48 evaluable patients achieved a CR/complete response unconfirmed (CRu) (73%) versus 29 out of 53 evaluable patients (55%) in the sequential treatment arm. Of note, patients with a CD4 T-cell count <50 at the time of diagnosis had a higher rate of infection-related deaths in the concurrent treatment arm [30].

More recently, NCI investigators have evaluated the role of an abbreviated course of EPOCH administered with dosing of rituximab on days 1 and 5 of each cycle (EPOCH-RR) for patients with AIDS-related DLBCL [31]. Patients underwent CT-PET imaging prior to treatment, following two cycles, and had repetition of the imaging study until they achieved a PET CR. Patients received one additional cycle of therapy past achieving a PET CR. The median number of chemotherapeutic cycles was three. The CR rate for the group was 91% and at a medial of five years, the PFS rate was 84% [31].

For patients with BL, CHOP, and CHOP-like regimens are inadequate. For this group of patients, treatment with a more intensive regimen is essential. Effective therapeutic regimens including cyclophosphamide, vincristine, doxorubicin, high-dose methotrexate alternating with ifosfamide, etoposides, and high-dose cytarabine (CODOX-M/IVAC) [32–34], cyclophosphamide, vincristine, doxorubicin, and dexamethasone alternating with high-dose methotrexate/cytarabine (hyper-CVAD) [35,36], or EPOCH-RR [36] represent the standard of care. In the AMC 048 trial, 34 patients with BL were treated with CODOX-M/IVAC-rituximab. For this group, the estimated one-year PFS and OS were 69% and 72%, respectively [32]. In 13 patients with AIDS-related BL or Burkitt leukemia who were treated with hyper-CVAD, Cortes et al found that 92%

achieved a CR and median survival was 12 months [34]. In a report on 11 patients with AIDS-related BL treated at the NCI using EPOCH-RR, OS and PFS were 100% and 90%, respectively, at a median follow-up of 73 months [37].

In a pooled analysis of 1546 patients treated on 19 prospective clinical trials for AIDS-related NHL, the investigators identified a number of factors that resulted in improved CR, PFS, and/or OS rates [38]. The investigators found that use of concomitant cART therapy during treatment was associated with an improved CR rate (odds ration 1.89). While the use of cART during chemotherapy did not achieve statistical significance in terms of improving OS, the investigators noted that there was a trend toward improved survival. The use of rituximab concomitantly with chemotherapy was associated with statistically significant improvements in the CR, PFS, and OS rates. The odds ratio for an improved CR rate was 2.89. Treatment with regimens more intensive than CHOP was also associated with improvements in CR rates, PFS, and OS. Finally, for patients with DLBCL, the use of infusional chemotherapeutic regimens was associated with improved OS rates. The investigators also confirmed the previous finding that patients with a pre-treatment CD4 T-cell count $<50/\mu L$ had an extremely poor prognosis [38].

The principles for the treatment of patients with AIDS-related NHL are to:

- include lumbar puncture and cerebrospinal fluid (CSF) evaluation as part of initial staging;
- consider initiation/continuation of cART throughout the treatment course;
- evaluate cART and chemotherapeutic regimens carefully to identify potential drug–drug interactions;
- consider the use of infusional chemotherapy regimens for patients with DLBCL;
- include rituximab for the treatment of CD20-expressing NHL; and
- use rituximab with caution in patients with CD4 T-cell counts $<50/\mu L$.

Patients with AIDS-related NHL should be evaluated carefully for extranodal involvement at the time of diagnosis, including lumbar puncture for assessment of possible CNS involvement. Patients with DLBCL should receive combination chemotherapy in standard dosing. Infusional chemo-therapy with a regimen, such as EPOCH, appears to produce superior outcomes. Patients should receive rituximab concomitantly with their chemotherapeutic regimen [39]. Rituximab should be used with caution in patients with CD4 T-cell count $<50/\mu L$. Patients with BL should not receive CHOP or CHOP-like regimens. They should be treated with more intensive regimens or treatment with infusion chemotherapy combined with rituximab should be considered.

Management of human immunodeficiency virus-related Hodgkin lymphoma

While HL is not an AIDS-defining diagnosis, the risk of HL is significantly increased among patients with HIV-infection. Unlike the risk of NHL, HL may occur in patients with higher CD4 T-cell counts at diagnosis and the risk has not decreased significantly following the availability of effective anti-HIV treatment [40]. Prior to the availability of cART, the outcomes for patients with HIV-related HL were poor with a high risk of infections and treatment-related mortality [19]. In a trial using doxorubicin, bleo-mycin, vinblastine, and dacarbazine (ABVD) in 21 HIV-infected patients with HL, the median survival was only 1.5 years. Only 42% of patients achieved a CR. Treatment was complicated by opportunistic infections in six patients [19].

Following the availability of cART, the prognosis for patients with HIV-related HL has improved dramatically. Xicoy et al reported the outcome for 62 patients with HIV infection who were treated using the ABVD regimen [41]. All of the patients had advanced stage disease at the time of diagnosis. At a median follow-up of 9 years, the estimated 14-year OS was 65% (95% confidence intervals: 47–83%) with an estimated event-free survival (EFS) of 59% (95% confidence intervals: 44–74%) [41].

In a prospective Phase II trial involving 59 patients with HIV-related HL, Spina et al used the Stanford V regimen (doxorubicin, vinblastine, mecloretamine, etoposide, vincristine, bleomycin, prednisone). The regimen was administered concomitantly with cART. The investigators noted that the regimen was well-tolerated and that 69% of patients did not require therapeutic interruption or dose-reductions. Spina et al also found that at a median follow-up of 17 months, the 3-year estimated OS and disease-free survival (DFS) were 51% and 68%, respectively [42].

Hartman et al treated 12 patients with HIV-related HD with the bleomycin, etoposide, doxorubicin, cyclophosphamide vincristine, procarbazine, and prednisone (BEACOPP) regimen. All of the patients achieved a CR. Nine of the patients remained in CR at the time of the publication of the report [43]. In a subsequent study from this group, 108 patients with HIV-related HL were treated with stage-adapted therapy. Patients with early stage/favorable HL received ABVD followed by involved-field radiotherapy. Patients with early stage/unfavorable disease were initially treated with BEACOPP but in light of the results of the German Hodgkin Study Group HD11 trials were subsequently treated with ABVD followed by involved-field radiotherapy. Patients with advanced stage disease received six to eight cycles of BEACOPP. Patients with advanced HIV infection received ABVD. The two-year estimated OS for the entire group was 90.7% with patients with advanced HL having an estimated survival of 86.8% [44].

The standard of care for the treatment of HIV-related HL is the use of standard, effective chemotherapeutic regimens for this group of patients. These include ABVD, Stanford V, and BEACOPP. Risk-adapted treatment strategies appear to be appropriate for this patient population.

Autologous transplant in patients with human immunodeficiency virus-related lymphomas

Autologous hematopoietic cell transplantation (AHCT) is the standard of care for patients with relapsed and persistent, chemotherapy-sensitive aggressive NHL and HL [45,46]. Initial attempts to use AHCT in patients with HIV-related lymphomas prior to the availability of cART were unsuccessful [47]. In 2000, following the availability of effective anti-HIV therapy, two groups published their initial experience using AHCT for patients with HIV-related lymphomas [48,49]. Gabarre et al published their experience using AHCT to treat eight patients with relapsed or persistent NHL [48]. This included one, previously reported, patient who had been unsuccessfully treated prior to the advent of cART [47]. All of the patients, except for the first, had an undetectable viral load at the time of AHCT. The patient group included four patients with HL, two with immunoblastic lymphoma, and two with BL. At the time of the report's publications, four patients were alive and in remission from their lymphoma.

Following an initial report in 2000, the City of Hope group published their outcomes for 20 patients using AHCT to treat patients with relapsed, persistent, and high-risk HIV-related lymphomas. The median CD4 T-cell count at AHCT was $174/\mu L$. Seventeen of the patients were prepared for transplant using a chemotherapy-only regimen (carmustine, etoposide, cyclophosphamide) and three received total body irradiation (TBI)-based preparative regimens. PFS and OS for the group were 85% at a median follow-up of 31.8 months [49].

A number of groups from both the United States and the European Union (EU) have published transplant trials using AHCT for patients with chemotherapy-sensitive relapsed and persistent lymphoma [50–56]. These groups have used a variety of preparative regimens (both chemotherapy only and total body irradiation [TBI]-based regimens). Overall, these studies demonstrate outcomes similar to those seen in non-HIV-infected patients. In a retrospective review of 68 patients treated at multiple centers in the EU who were followed for a median of 32 months post-transplant, the European Group for Blood and Marrow Transplantation (EBMT) reported an estimated three-year PFS of 56% and an OS of 61% [56].

The Bone Marrow Transplant Clinical Trials Network (BMT CTN 0803)/AMC 071 trial prospectively evaluated outcomes using a standardized preparative regimen and cART management strategy for patients with relapsed and persistent, chemotherapy-sensitive lymphoma [57]. A total of 40 patients underwent transplant; 15 had HL and 25 had NHL (including 16 with DLBCL and seven with BL or Burkitt-like lymphoma). Patients were prepared using the BEAM regimen (carmustine, etoposide, cytarabine, and melphalan). cART was interrupted at the time of initiation of the preparative regimen and resumed following recovery from peri-transplant gastrointestinal toxicities. At a median follow-up of 24 months, the estimated 1-year PFS was 82.3%. Outcomes were comparable for patients with HL and NHL. Transplant-related mortality at 1-year was 5.2% [57].

Three groups have performed case-control outcome comparisons for AHCT comparing HIV-infected and non-infected patients [57–59]. Outcomes between patient groups are comparable. Similarly, HIV-infected patients do not appear to have any unique difficulties in mobilizing an adequate cell dose of hematopoietic stem cells [60,61]. For those patients who fail to mobilize adequately using filgrastim with or without chemotherapy, the addition of plerixafor may allow for successful stem cell collection [61].

Based upon this information, AHCT should be considered the standard of care for treatment-responsive HIV-infected patients with relapsed/persistent chemotherapy-sensitive lymphoma provided that they meet standard transplant criteria.

Allogeneic transplant for human immunodeficiency virus-infected patients with non-Hodgkin lymphoma

Attempts to use allogeneic HCT for patients with HIV-infection prior to the availability of cART were unsuccessful [62–64]. There are limited data from the post-cART era that demonstrate that allogeneic transplantation may be feasible for patients with HIV infection and lymphoma [64,65]. The BMT CTN 0903/AMC 081 trial is a prospective, 15-patient trial and is assessing the toxicity and effectiveness of this approach. As of this time, allogeneic transplant for patients with HIV-related lymphomas has not been established as the standard of care.

Management of combination antiretroviral therapy in patients with human immunodeficiency virus-related lymphomas

A number of groups have interrupted cART during the treatment of patients with HIV-related lymphomas in order to reduce the risk of cytopenias and avoid significant drug–drug interactions that might be associated with these antiretroviral regimens. These interruptions do not appear to be associated with loss of virological control of the HIV infection [31,37]. Other groups, however, have successfully continued cART through the treatment course without evidence of significant related toxicities [16,27,42]. Based upon the multivariate analysis data from Barta et al, there may be advantages to continuing cART while patients undergo treatment. At this institution, patients with HIV-related lymphomas continue their cART regimens while receiving combination chemotherapy/chemoimmunotherapy [38].

The risk of significant drug–drug interactions may be significant when patients on cART receive standard chemotherapeutic regimens. The use of zidovudine (AZT) and ritonavir-boosted protease inhibitors may be problematic in the setting of chemotherapy. AZT may be associated with significant bone marrow toxicity and should be avoided in patients who are receiving chemotherapy [66]. Similarly the use of ritonavir-boosted protease inhibitors should be avoided in combination with chemotherapy [67,68]. Given their tissue penetration and limited drug interactions with chemotherapeutic agents, the integrase inhibitors may be excellent agents for consideration in the treatment of HIV-infected patients with lymphoma [68].

During and following completion of treatment for HIV-related lymphomas, patients may experience significant and protracted decreases in the CD4 T-cell count. Patients should remain on effective anti-viral, Pneumocytis jiroveci, and anti-fungal prophylaxis until their CD4 T cell count recovers to levels >300/μL.

Conclusions

The management of patients with HIV-related lymphomas has changed profoundly since the beginning of the HIV/AIDS pandemic. With the availability of effective cART, patients with HIV-related malignancies can be treated with the same therapeutic approaches that are applied to patients without HIV infection. Results for patients with HIV-related lymphomas are now comparable to patients without HIV infection. In treating patients with AIDS-related NHL, infusion chemotherapeutic regimens that include the use of rituximab produce particularly promising results. Those patients with relapsed and persistent HIV-related lymphoma who meet standard transplant criteria should be considered for AHCT.

In the case discussed above the patient was started on combination antiretroviral therapy (cART) with tenofovir/emtricitabine combined with raltegravir. The patient began treatment with short course double dose rituxi-mab, etoposide, vincristine, cyclophosphamide, and doxorubicin (EPOCH-RR). An initial lumbar puncture revealed no evidence of central nervous system (CNS) involvement by NHL. He received prophylactic intrathecal therapy with methotrexate through his course of EPOCH-RR. A restaging CT PET fusion study demonstrated a CR following two cycles of therapy. The patient received an additional cycle of therapy; a post-treatment CT PET study confirmed a continued CR. By 6 months post-completion of short course EPOCH-RR, the patient's HIV viral load was undetectable with a CD4+ T-cell count of 736/μL. Three years post-treatment, the patient remains clinically well in CR without evidence of opportunistic infection now.

References

1   Centers for Disease Control (CDC). Pneumocystis pneumonia–Los Angeles. *MMWR Morb Mortal Wkly Rep.* 1981;30:1-3.

2   Gallo RC, Salahuddin SZ, Popovic M, et al. Frequent detection and isolation of cytopathic retroviruses (HTLV-III) from patients with AIDS and at-risk for AIDS. *Science.* 1984;224:500-503.

3   World Health Organization. Global Health Observatory (GHO) data: HIV/AIDS. http://www.who.int/gho/hiv/en/. Accessed March 7, 2017.

4   Centers for Disease Control and Prevention. HIV/AIDS: HIV prevalence estimate. http://www.cdc.gov/hiv/statistics/overview/. Accessed March 7, 2017.

5   Clifford GM, Polesel J, Rickenbach M, et al. Cancer risk in the Swiss HIV cohort study: associations with immunodeficiency, smoking, and highly active antiretroviral therapy. *J Natl Cancer Inst.* 2005;97:425-432.

6   Achenbach CJ, Buchanan AL, Cole SR, Hou L, et al. HIV viremia and incidence of non-Hodgkin lymphoma in patients successfully treated with antiretroviral therapy. *Clin Infect Dis.* 2014;58:1599.

7   National Cancer Institute. SEER stat fact sheets: non-Hodgkin lymphoma. http://seer.cancer.gov/statfacts/html/nhl.html. Accessed March 7, 2017.

8   Bibas M and Antinori A. EBV and HIV-related lymphoma. *Mediterr J Hematol Infect Dis.* 2009;1:e2009032.

9   Centers for Disease Control. 1993 revised classification for HIV infection and expanded surveillance case definition for AIDS among adolescents and adults. *MMWR Recomm Rep.* 1992;41:961-962.

10 Gucalp A, Noy A. Spectrum of HIV lymphoma 2009. Curr Opin Hematol. 2010;17:362-367.

11 Swerdlow SH, Campo E, Harris NL, et al (eds). *World Health Organization Classification of Tumours of Haematopoietic and Lymphoid Tissues,* Vol 2. Lyon, France: IARC Press 2008.

12 Epeldegui M, Vendrame e, Martinez-Maza O. HIV-associated immune dysfunction and viral infection: role in the pathogenesis of AIDS-related lymphoma. *Immunol Res.* 2010;48:72-83.

13 Biggar RJ, Jaffe ES, Goedert JJ, Chaturvedi A, Pfeiffer R, Engels EA. Hodgkin lymphoma and immunodeficiency in persons with HIV/AIDS. *Blood.* 2006;108:3786.

14 Carbone J, Cesarman E, Spina, M, Gloghini A, Schulz TF. HIV-associated lymphomas and gamma-herpesviruses. *Blood.* 2009;113:1213-1224.

15 Levine AM. Acquired immunodeficiency syndrome-related lymphoma. *Blood.* 1992;80:8-20.

16 Vishnu P, Aboulafia DM. AIDS-related non-Hodgkin's lymphoma in the era of highly active antiretroviral therapy. *Adv Hematol.* 2012;2012:485943.

17 Vishnu P, Aboulafia DM. AIDS-related non-Hodgkin's lymphoma in the era of highly active antiretroviral therapy. *Adv Hematol*. 2012;2012:485943.

18 Thompson LD, Fisher SI, Chu WS, Nelson A, Abbondanzo SL. HIV-associated Hodgkin lymphoma: a clinicopathologic and immunophenotypic study of 45 cases. *Am J Clin Pathol*. 2004;121:727-738.

19 Levine AM, Li P, Cheung T, et al. Chemotherapy consisting of doxorubicin, bleomycin, vinblastine, and decarbazine with granulocyte-colony-stimulating factor in HIV-infected patients with newly diagnosed Hodgkin's disease: a prospective multi-institutional AIDS clinical trials group study (ACTG 149). *J Acquir Immune Defic Syndr*. 2000;24:444-450.

20 Martis N, Mounier N. Hodgkin lymphoma in patients with HIV infection. *Curr Hematol Malg Rep*. 2012;7:228-234.

21 Levine AM. Management of AIDS-related lymphoma. *Curr Opin Oncol*. 2008;20:522-528.

22 Hamilton-Dutoit SJ, Pallesen G, Franzmann MB, et al. AIDS-related lymphoma: histopathology, immunophenotype, and association with Epstein-Barr virus as demonstrated by in situ nucleic acid hybridization. *Am J Path*. 1991;138:149-163.

23 Kaplan LD, Straus DJ, Testa MA, et al. Low-dose compared with standard-dose m-BACOD chemotherapy for non-Hodgkin's lymphoma associated with human immunodeficiency virus infection. *New Engl J Med*. 1997;336:1641-1648.

24 Shipp MA, Harrington DP, Anderson JR, et al. A predictive model for aggressive non-Hodgkin's lymphoma. *New Engl J Med*. 1994;329:987-994.

25 Rossi G, Donisi A, Casari S, Re A, Cadeo G, Carosi G. The International Prognostic Index can be used as a guide to treatment decisions regarding patients with human immunodeficiency virus-related systemic non-Hodgkin lymphoma. *Cancer*. 1999;86:2391-2397.

26 Bower M, Bazzard B, Mandalia S, et al. A prognostic index for systemic AIDS-related non-Hodgkin lymphoma treated in the era of highly arctive antiretroviral therapy. *Ann Intern Med*. 2005;143:265-273.

27 Boué F, Gabarre J, Gisselbrecht C, et al. Phase II trials of CHOP plus rituximab in patients with HIV-associated non-Hodgkin's lymphoma. *J Clin Oncol*. 2006;24:4123-4128.

28 Kaplan LD, Lee JY, Ambinder RF, et al. Rituximab does not improve clinical outcome in a randomized phase 3 trial of CHOP with or without rituximab in patients with HIV-associated non-Hodgkin lymphoma: AIDS-Malignancies Consortium trial 010. *Blood*. 2005;106:1538-1543.

29 Little RF, Pittaluga S, Grant N, et al. Highly effective treatment of acquired immunodeficiency syndrome-related lymphoma with dose-adjusted EPOCH: impact of antiretroviral suspension and tumor biology. *Blood*. 2003;101:4653-4659.

30 Sparano JA, Lee JY, Kaplan, LD, et al. Rituximab plus concurrent infusional EPOCH chemotherapy is highly effective in HIV-associated B-cell non-Hodgkin lymphoma. *Blood*. 2010;115:3008-3016.

31 Dunleavy K, Little RF, Pittaluga S, et al. The role of tumor histogenesis, FDG-PET, and short-course EPOCH with dose-dense rituximab (SC-EPOCH-RR) in HIV-associated diffuse large B-cell lymphoma. *Blood*. 2010;115:3017-3024.

32 Noy A, Kaplan L, Lee JY. A modified dose-intensive CODOX-M/IVAC for HIV-associated Burkitt lymphoma and atypical Burkitt lymphoma (BL) demonstrates high cure rates and low toxicity: prospective multicenter trial of the AIDS Malignancy Consortium (AMC 048). *Blood*. 2013;122:639.

33 Rodrigo JA, Hicks LK, Cheung MC, et al. HIV-associated Burkitt lymphoma: Good efficacy and tolerance of intensive chemotherapy including CODOX-M/IVAC with or without rituximab in the HAART era. *Adv Hematol*. 2012;2012:735392.

34 Montoto S, Wilson J, Shaw K, et al. Excellent immunological recovery following CODOX-M/IVAC, an effective intensive chemotherapy for HIV-associated Burkitt's lymphoma. *AIDS*. 2010;24:851-856.

35 Cortes J, Thomas D, Rios A, et al. Hyperfractionated cyclophosphamide, vincristine, doxorubicin, and dexamethasone and highly active antiretroviral therapy for patients with acquired-immunodeficiency syndrome-related Burkitt lymphoma/leukemia. *Cancer*. 2002;94:1492-1499.

36 Kojima Y, Hagiwara S, Uehira T, et al. Clinical outcomes of AIDS-related Burkitt lymphoma: A multi-institution retrospective survey in Japan. *Jpn J Clin Oncol*. 2014;44:318-323.

37 Dunleavy K, Pittaluga S, Shovlin M, et al. Low-intensity therapy in adults with Burkitt's lymphoma. *New Engl J Med*. 2013;369:1915-1925.

38 Barta SK, Xue X, Wang D, et al. Treatment factors affecting outcomes in HIV-associate non-Hodgkin lymphomas: a pooled analysis of 1546 patients. *Blood*. 2013;122:3251-3262.

39 Dunleavy K, Wilson WH. The case for rituximab in AIDS-related lymphoma. *Blood*. 2006;107:3014-3015.

40 Kaplan LD. Management of HIV-associated Hodgkin lymphoma: How far we have come. *J Clin Oncol*. 2012;30:4056-4058.

41 Xicoy B, Miralles P, Morgades M, Rubio R, Valencia ME, Ribera JM. Long-term follow up of patients with human immunodeficiency virus infection and advanced stage Hodgkin's lymphoma treated with doxorubicin, bleomycin, vinblastine, dacarbazine. *Haematologica*. 2013;98:e85-e86.

42 Spina M, Gabarre J, Rossi G, et al. Stanford V regimen and concomitant HAART in 59 patients with Hodgkin disease and HIV infection. *Blood*. 2002;100:1984-1988.

43 Hartmann P, Rehwald U, Salzberger B, et al. BEACOPP therapeutic regimen for patients with Hodgkin's disease and HIV infection. *Ann Oncol*. 2003;14:1562-1569.

44 Hentrich M, Berger M, Wyen C, et al. Stage-adapted treatment of HIV-associated Hodgkin lymphoma: Results of a prospective multicenter study. *J Clin Oncol*. 2012;30:4117-4123.

45 Philip T, Guglielmi C, Hagenbeek A, et al. Autologous bone marrow transplantation as compared with salvage chemotherapy in relapses of chemotherapy-sensitive non-Hodgkin's lymphoma. *New Engl J Med*. 1995;333:1540-1545.

46 Nademanee A, O'Donnell MR, Snyder DS, et al. High-dose chemotherapy with or without total body irradiation followed by autologous bone marrow and/or peripheral blood stem cell transplantation for patients with relapsed and refractory Hodgkin's disease: results in 85 patients with analysis of prognostic factors. *Blood*. 1995;85:1381-1390.

47 Gabarre J, Leblond V, Sutton L, et al. Autologous bone marrow transplantation in relapsed HIV-related non-Hodgkin's lymphoma. *Bone Marrow Transplant*. 1996;18:1195-1197.

48 Gabarre J, Azar N, Autran B, Katlama C, Leblond V. High-dose therapy and autologous haematopoietic stem-cell transplantation for HIV-1-associated lymphoma. *The Lancet*. 2000;355:1071-1072.

49 Molina A, Krishnan AY, Nademanee A, et al. High dose therapy and autologous stem cell transplantation for human immunodeficiency virus-associated non-Hodgkin lymphoma in the era of highly active antiretroviral therapy. *Cancer*. 2000;89:680-689.

50 Krishnan A, Molina A, Zaia J, et al. Durable remissions with autologous stem cell transplantation for high-risk HIV-associated lymphomas. *Blood*. 2005;105:874-878.

51 Re A, Cattaneo C, Michieli M, et al. High-dose therapy and autologous peripheral-blood stem-cell transplantation as salvage treatment for HIV-associated lymphoma in patients receiving highly active antiretroviral therapy. *J Clin Oncol*. 2003;21:4423-4427.

52 Gabarre J, Marcelin AG, Azar N, et al. High-dose therapy plus autologous hematopoietic stem cell transplantation for human immunodeficiency virus (HIV)-related lymphoma: results and impact on HIV disease. *Haematologica*. 2004;89:1100-1108.

53 Serrano D, Carrión R, Balsalobre P, et al. HIV-associated lymphoma successfully treated with peripheral blood stem cell transplantation. *Exp Hematol*. 2005;33:487-494.

54 Spritzer TR, Ambinder RF, Lee JY, Ket al. Dose-reduced busulfan, cyclophosphamide, and autologous stem cell transplantation for human immunodeficiency virus-associated lymphoma: AIDS Malignancy Consortium study 020. *Biol Blood Marrow Transplant*. 2008;14:59-66.

55 Re A, Michieli M, Casari s, et al. High-dose therapy and autologous peripheral blood stem cell transplantation as salvage treatment for AIDS-related lymphoma: long-term results of the Italian Cooperative Group of AIDS and Tumors (GICAT) study with analysis of prognostic factors. *Blood*. 2009;114:1306-1313.

56 Balsalobre P, Díez-Martín JL, Re A, et al. Autologous stem-cell transplantation in patients with HIV-related lymphoma. *J Clin Oncol.* 2009;27:2192-2198.

57 Alvarnas J, Le Rademacher J, Wang Y, et al. Autologous hematopoietic stem cell transplantation (AHCT) in patients with chemotherapy-sensitive, relapsed/refractoary (CSRR) Human Immunodeficiency virus-related lymphoma (HAL): Results from the Blood and Marrow Transplant Clinical Trials Network (BMT CTN 0803)/AIDS Malignancy Consortium (AMC-071) trial. *Blood.* 2014; Abstract 674.

58 Krishnan A, Palmer JP, Zaia JA, Tsai NC, Alvarnas M, Forman SJ. HIV status does not affect the outcome of autologous stem cell transplantation (ASCT) for non-Hodgkin lymphoma (NHL). *Biol Blood Marrow Transplant.* 2010;16:1302-1308.

59 Díez-Martín JL, Balsalobre P, Re A, et al. Comparable survival between HIV+ and HIV- non-Hodgkin and Hodgkin lymphoma patients undergoing autologous peripheral blood stem cell transplantation. *Blood.* 2009;113:6011-6014.

60 Re A, Cattaneo C, Skert C, et al. Stem cell mobilization in HIV seropositive patients with lymphoma. *Haematologica.* 2013;98:1762-1768.

61 Attolico I, Pavone V, Ostuni An, et al. Plerixafor added to chemotherapy plus G-CSF is safe and allows adequate PBSC collection in predicted poor mobilizer patients with multiple myeloma or lymphoma. *Biol blood Marrow Transplant.* 2012;18:241-249.

62 Giri N, Vowels MR, Ziegler JB. Failure of allogeneic bone marrow transplantation to benefit HIV infection. *J Paediatr Child Health.* 1992;28:331-333.

63 Contu L, La Nasa G, Arras M, et al. Allogeneic bone marrow transplantation combined with multiple anti-HIV-1 treatment in a case of AIDS. *Bone Marrow Transplant.* 1993;12:669-671.

64 Gupta V, Tomblyn M, Pedersen TL, et al. Allogeneic hematopoietic cell transplantation in HIV-positive patients with hematological disorders: a report from the Center for International Blood and Marrow Transplant Research (CIBMTR). *Biol Blood Marrow Transplant.* 2009;15: 864-871.

65 Hütter G, Zaia JA. Allogeneic haematopoietic stem cell transplantation in patients with human immunodeficiency virus: the experiences of more than 25 years. *Clin Exp Immunol.* 2011;163:284-295.

66 Moh R, Danel C, Sorho S, et al. Haematological changes in adults receiving a zidovudine-containing HAART regimen in combination with cotrimoxazole in Cote d'Ivoire. *Antiviral Therapy.* 2004;10:615-624.

67 Cingolani A, Torti L, Pinnetti C, et al. Detrimental clinical interaction between ritonavir-boosted protease inhibitors and vinblastine in HIV-infected patients with Hodgkin's lymphoma. *AIDS.* 2010;24:2408-2412.

68 Torres HA, Rallapalli V, Saxena A, et al. Efficacy and safety of antiretrovirals in HIV-infected patients with cancer. *Clin Microbial Infect.* 2014;20:672-679.

Chapter 14

Central nervous system lymphoma
Matthew Mei

Case presentation

A 56-year-old woman began to experience vertigo, headaches, and frequent falls. A computed tomography (CT) scan of the brain revealed the presence of a 1.6 x 1.6 x 2.1 cm mass involving the fourth ventricle (Figure 14.1). A gadolinium-enhanced magnetic resonance imaging (MRI) scan confirmed the presence of the mass, and a stereotactic biopsy was performed that demonstrated a primary central nervous system lymphoma (PCNSL) with a diffuse large B-cell histology. Complete blood count (CBC), lactate dehydrogenase (LDH), and beta-2-microglobulin were normal. Systemic staging with a positron emission tomography (PET)/CT scan and bone marrow biopsy showed no evidence of lymphomatous involvement outside the CNS. An eye exam and lumbar puncture showed no evidence of either ocular or leptomeningeal involvement.

Epidemiology

PCNSL is relatively uncommon with an overall incidence of seven cases per million persons per year from 1998 to 2008 [1]. There is a strong association between immunodeficiency and PCNSL, as patients with human immunodeficiency virus (HIV)/acquired immune deficiency syndrome (AIDS) prior to the advent of highly active antiretroviral therapy (HAART) were more than 1000 times as likely to develop PCNSL compared with the general population with patients with lower CD4 counts being at

© Springer International Publishing AG 2017
J. Zain and L.W. Kwak (eds.), *Management of Lymphomas: A Case-Based Approach*, DOI 10.1007/978-3-319-26827-9_14

particularly high risk for developing PCNSL [2]. In the era of HAART, the overall incidence of PCNSL has declined although the incidence rate in older adults has risen. Other etiologies for immunodeficiency including iatrogenic immunosuppression in the setting of solid organ transplant also predispose to PCNSL [3].

Clinical presentation and pathology

The most common clinical presentation of PCNSL is in the form of one or more intracerebral masses, often located in the periventricular areas. However, leptomeningeal, intravitreal, and intradural involvement have all been described, and any given patient may have one or more of these sites of involvement [4]. Most patients come to clinical attention due to focal neurological deficits although other clinical manifestations include personality changes, seizures, and signs and symptoms related to elevated intracranial pressure [5]. Since none of the aforementioned sites of disease are specific to PCNSL and can be seen with a variety of malignancies and even infections, accurate pathologic diagnosis is needed, typically in the form of a stereotactic biopsy. The diagnosis can also be made less invasively through cerebrospinal fluid (CSF) sampling, but the

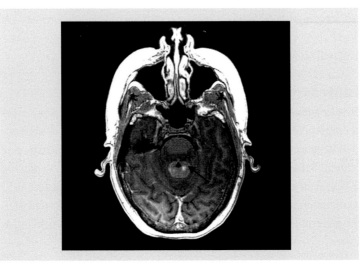

Figure 14.1 Primary central nervous system lymphoma located around the fourth ventricle (see arrow).

sensitivity is limited, and any diagnostic uncertainty essentially mandates a surgical biopsy. Histologically, most PCNSL cases are classified as high grade B-cell lymphomas and are usually indistinguishable from diffuse large B-cell lymphoma (DLBCL) although other morphologies including low-grade lymphoma and T-cell lymphomas have been reported as well [6,7]. Aside from CD20 positivity, PCNSL is typically positive for BCL-2 and BCL-6, and gene expression profiling has suggested that the cell of origin is a late germinal B-cell [8].

Workup and staging

Although involvement outside of the CNS is uncommon, complete systemic staging with either a contrast-enhanced CT scan of the chest, abdomen, and pelvis or PET/CT scan as well as a bone marrow biopsy are important to rule out systemic disease, which is present in a small percentage of patients [9]. A CBC with differential, chemistry panel, LDH, serologic testing for HIV, and hepatitis serologies should all be performed as well prior to treatment. Evaluation of cognition and performance status is also very important. Testicular imaging should be performed in all elderly males as well as in any younger male with an abnormal clinical testicular exam given the high propensity for testicular lymphoma to present with CNS involvement as well.

Initial treatment

Owing to its rarity, treatment of PCNSL has not been completely standardized, and many of the available treatment options have not undergone prospective comparison against each other. Nonetheless, the following principles of treatment are supported by the current data:

- The most active agent in PCNSL is high-dose methotrexate (MTX), which should be given at a dose of at least 3 gm/m^2.
- Combination therapy including high-dose MTX is probably better than single-agent MTX.
- Whole-brain radiotherapy (WBRT) appears to add significant neurotoxicity when used in conjunction with chemotherapy. Given the high response rates with high-dose MTX-based treatment, it is not recommended as part of upfront therapy.

- Most patients who achieve a response, even a complete response (CR), will relapse, and consolidation therapy should be considered. However, the optimal consolidation regimen is not known, and autologous stem-cell transplantation (ASCT), non-myeloablative chemotherapy, and radiation therapy are all reasonable options.

There are three upfront combination regimens with reasonably robust clinical data, and any of the three are reasonable choices for the fit patient. MTX 3.5 gm/m^2 and high-dose cytarabine (ara-C) dosed at 2 gm/m^2 for four doses was tested against MTX 3.5 gm/m^2 alone in a Phase II trial, with systemic therapy administered every 3 weeks. CR rates were 46% and 18%, respectively with 3-year failure-free survival (FFS) of 38% versus 21%. Overall survival at 3 years was 46% in the combination arm compared with 32% with MTX alone although the difference did not achieve statistical significance. Toxicity was significantly increased in the combination arm with severe hematological toxicity noted due to the addition of ara-C [10]. Induction therapy with rituximab, MTX, procarbazine, and vincristine (R-MPV) followed by consolidation ASCT conditioned with thiotepa, cyclophosphamide, and busulfan resulted in a 2-year progression-free survival (PFS) of 79% and 2-year overall survival (OS) of 81%; no events were observed beyond 2 years [11]. Finally, CALGB 50202 tested the regimen of MTX given every 2 weeks, rituximab given weekly for six doses, and temozolomide given over 5 days every 4 weeks followed by non-myeloablative consolidation with high-dose ara-C and etoposide. The CR rate after induction was 66%, and 2-year PFS was 57%; median OS was not reached. Toxicities were overall mild during induction although hematological toxicity during consolidation was significant as expected [12].

Finally, our institution participated in CALGB 51101, which was a prospective Phase II trial for newly diagnosed PCNSL using a modified version of the rituximab, MTX, and temozolomide mentioned above given every 2 weeks as induction followed by one cycle of high-dose ara-C (Figure 14.2). There is no head-to-head comparison between any of the aforementioned trials, so the specific choice of therapy should be made with consideration of the patient's comorbidities. The administration of multiple cycles of high-dose ara-C is associated with significant hematological toxicities and often requires inpatient monitoring whereas procarbazine is rarely used in oncology, and many practitioners may not have much experience with this medication. As such, the preferred City of Hope induction regimen for newly diagnosed PCNSL is the regimen from CALGB 51101, which is outlined in Figure 14.3.

The choice of consolidation therapy is also similarly fraught due to a lack of data. The first three regimens above each were followed up by a separate mode of consolidation (ASCT, WBRT, and non-myeloablative chemotherapy). These have not been compared head to head. Due to the long-term cognitive sequelae of WBRT and the highly morbid nature of recurrent disease, we favor consolidation with ASCT using a thiotepa-based conditioning regimen, preferably thiotepa, busulfan, and cyclophosphamide [13,14] for patients with adequate organ function and performance status. Thiotepa and carmustine (BCNU) is an alternative ASCT conditioning regimen, which may be easier to tolerate for patients who may not be adequately fit for thiotepa, busulfan, and cyclophosphamide [14]. A City of Hope algorithm for primary treatment of PCNSL is given in Figure 14.3.

Case presentation continued

She was treated with five cycles of rituximab, methotrexate, procarbazine, and vincristine and achieved complete remission (CR) with complete resolution of the enhancing lesion. She then proceeded to autologous stem cell transplantation conditioned with thiotepa, busulfan, and cyclophosphamide. She remains in remission 2 years later.

Cycles 1–4 (28 day cycle)

Methotrexate 8 gm/m^2 IV days 1, 15

Temozolomide 200 mg/m^2 PO days 7-11 (150 mg/m^2 for cycle 1 only)

Rituximab 375 mg/m^2 IV on days 3, 10, 17, and 24 of cycle 1 and days 3, 10 of cycle 2 (6 weekly doses)

Cycle 5

Cytarabine 2 gm/m^2 IV every 12 hours x 4 dose

Figure 14.2 Recommended induction therapy for primary central nervous system lymphoma.

Patients with comorbidities

Given that the average age of PCNSL has been increasing over time, many patients with PCNSL have other medical comorbidities, which may influence their eligibility for intensive induction treatment. That notwithstanding, poor performance status alone should not be a contraindication for therapy as the response rate tends to be high and neurologic

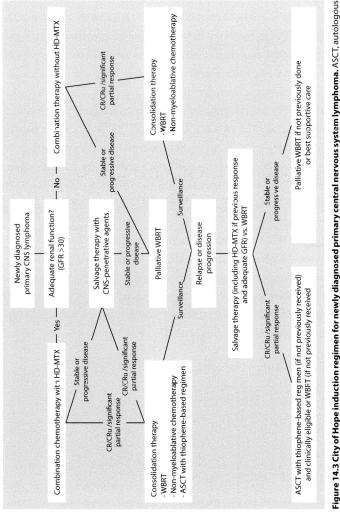

Figure 14.3 City of Hope induction regimen for newly diagnosed primary central nervous system lymphoma. ASCT, autologous stem cell transplantation; CNS, central nervous system; CR, complete response; CRU, unconfirmed complete response; GFR, glomerular filtration rate; HD-MTX, high-dose methotrexate; WBRT, whole barin radiotherapy.

improvements are often seen quickly. The single most important agent is high-dose MTX which, although cleared by the kidney, can be safely given with a CrCl down to 30 mL/min. Patients who are unable to receive high-dose methotrexate can be treated with other CNS-penetrating chemotherapeutic agents such as high-dose cytarabine, etoposide, and temozolomide. WBRT is reasonable as well for palliation.

Response evaluation and surveillance

The International Primary CNS Lymphoma Collaborative Group has outlined response criteria [9]:

- CR requires resolution of contrast-enhancing lesions without the need for corticosteroids. Any abnormalities in the CSF or ophthalmic exam should be resolved as well.
- An unconfirmed complete response (CRu) is as per CR but with the need for ongoing corticosteroids or with an ongoing minor abnormality in imaging.
- A partial response (PR) requires a 50% decrease in the enhancing lesion or a decrease in the lymphoma burden in the CSF.
- Progressive disease (PD) requires a 25% increase in the size of the enhancing lesion.

Response assessment should be performed within 2 months of the completion of all planned therapy. While there is no specific recommended schedule for surveillance, most relapses are limited to the CNS alone and occur within 5 years. Therefore, in the absence of symptoms concerning for recurrent disease, we typically perform an MRI every 3–4 months for the first two years and every 6 months afterwards for the next 3 years.

Treatment of relapsed or refractory primary central nervous system lymphoma

Unfortunately, the prognosis of patients with relapsed or refractory disease is poor. If high-dose MTX was previously administered with a good response, repeat administration can be considered. Use of other chemotherapeutic agents with CNS penetration such as high-dose cytarabine, etoposide, and/or temozolomide, if not administered previously, can be considered. If not previously performed in the front-line setting,

ASCT can be considered in select patients with a response to salvage chemotherapy with an appropriate performance status in which case a thiotepa-based conditioning regimen is recommended. WBRT can also be given in the salvage setting.

References

1   O'Neill BP, Decker PA, Tieu C, Cerhan JR. The changing incidence of primary central nervous system lymphoma is driven primarily by the changing incidence in young and middle-aged men and differs from time trends in systemic diffuse large B-cell non-Hodgkin's lymphoma. *Am J Hematol*. 2013;88:997-1000.

2   Haldorsen IS, Krakenes J, Goplen AK, Dunlop O, Mella O, Espeland A. AIDS-related primary central nervous system lymphoma: a Norwegian national survey 1989-2003. *BMC Cancer*. 2008;8:225.

3   Schabet M. Epidemiology of primary CNS lymphoma. J Neurooncol. 1999;43:199-201.

4   Hochberg FH, Miller DC. Primary central nervous system lymphoma. *J Neurosurg*. 1988;68: 835-853.

5   Bataille B, Delwail V, Menet E, Vandermarcq P, Ingrand P, Wager M et al. Primary intracerebral malignant lymphoma: report of 248 cases. *J Neurosurg*. 2000;92:261-266.

6   Krogh-Jensen M, D'Amore F, Jensen MK, et al. Clinicopathological features, survival and prognostic factors of primary central nervous system lymphomas: trends in incidence of primary central nervous system lymphomas and primary malignant brain tumors in a well-defined geographical area. Population-based data from the Danish Lymphoma Registry, LYFO, and the Danish Cancer Registry. *Leuk Lymphoma*. 1995;19:223-233.

7   Gijtenbeek JM, Rosenblum MK, DeAngelis LM. Primary central nervous system T-cell lymphoma. *Neurology*. 2001;57:716-718.

8   Montesinos-Rongen M, Brunn A, Bentink S, et al. Gene expression profiling suggests primary central nervous system lymphomas to be derived from a late germinal center B cell. *Leukemia*. 2008;22:400-405.

9   Abrey LE, Batchelor TT, Ferreri AJ, et al. Report of an international workshop to standardize baseline evaluation and response criteria for primary CNS lymphoma. *J Clin Oncol*. 2005;23:5034-5043.

10   Ferreri AJ, Reni M, Foppoli M, et al. High-dose cytarabine plus high-dose methotrexate versus high-dose methotrexate alone in patients with primary CNS lymphoma: a randomised phase 2 trial. *Lancet*. 2009;374:1512-1520.

11   Omuro A, Correa DD, DeAngelis LM, et al. R-MPV followed by high-dose chemotherapy with TBC and autologous stem-cell transplant for newly diagnosed primary CNS lymphoma. *Blood*. 2015;125:1403-1410.

12   Rubenstein JL, Hsi ED, Johnson JL, et al. Intensive chemotherapy and immunotherapy in patients with newly diagnosed primary CNS lymphoma: CALGB 50202 (Alliance 50202). *J Clin Oncol*. 2013;31:3061-3068.

13   Cote GM, Hochberg EP, Muzikansky A, et al. Autologous stem cell transplantation with thiotepa, busulfan, and cyclophosphamide (TBC) conditioning in patients with CNS involvement by non-Hodgkin lymphoma. *Biol Blood Marrow Transplant*. 2012;18:76-83.

14   Cheng T, Forsyth P, Chaudhry A, et al. High-dose thiotepa, busulfan, cyclophosphamide and ASCT without whole-brain radiotherapy for poor prognosis primary CNS lymphoma. *Bone Marrow Transplant*. 2003;31:679-685.

Chapter 15

Conclusion

Jasmine Zain and Larry W Kwak

In this book, we have made an attempt to present a concise description of the major subtypes of both non-Hodgkin and Hodgkin lymphoma and the current treatment guidelines as practiced by experts at City of Hope National Medical Center, California, USA. At City of Hope we see over 2000 patients with lymphoma per year and our hematopathology department consults on over 1500 cases a year. It remains one of the lead institutions for developing National Comprehensive Cancer Network guidelines that serve as the standard of care and most of our experts serve on panels that define these treatment guidelines. We have an active clinical trials program backed by fundamental and translational research at the Beckman Research Institute and California Institute of Technology. There is a strong culture of collaboration between clinicians and scientists at the institution and worldwide. Hence, we feel strongly in endorsing the treatment guidelines that have been recommended in the chapters and hope that they will lead to successful treatment of patients all over.

© Springer International Publishing AG 2017
J. Zain and L.W. Kwak (eds.), *Management of Lymphomas:
A Case-Based Approach*, DOI 10.1007/978-3-319-26827-9_15

Printed in the United States
By Bookmasters